Network-Informed Complex Evaluation

Lixin Zhang

Network-Informed Complex Evaluation

Evaluating Complex Health Programs Using Social Network Analysis

Springer

Lixin Zhang
School of Medicine
Case Western Reserve University
Cleveland, OH, USA

ISBN 978-3-032-27494-6 ISBN 978-3-032-27495-3 (eBook)
https://doi.org/10.1007/978-3-032-27495-3

This Springer imprint is published by the registered company Springer Nature Switzerland AG
The registered company address is: Gewerbestrasse 11, 6330 Cham, Switzerland

The Beauty of Evaluation

Evaluation, at its core, is a disciplined
practice of truth-telling.
It seeks to understand programs as they are
implemented in real-world contexts,
asking not only whether they work,
but how,
for whom,
under what circumstances,
and why.

Personally, I find its beauty in this
commitment,
to evidence grounded in context,
to judgment informed by understanding,
to serving those whom programs are meant to
benefit,
and to the learning that emerges through
evaluative inquiry.

This commitment deepens through
network-informed approaches to complex
evaluation.
Here, attention shifts from isolated program
components
to relationships, interactions, and patterns of
influence.

What was once treated as background
becomes central.
What was once assumed becomes examined.

Social network analysis reveals dimensions
often hidden from view:
the structures that connect actors,
the relationships through which
collaboration unfolds,
the flows of resources, ideas, and information,
the pathways through which influence travels,
and the dynamics through which outcomes
emerge
over time and across social–ecological
systems.

In this book, evaluation does not attempt to
simplify complexity.
It learns to see it.
It reveals the stories embedded within systems
by tracing the relationships, structures, and
patterns
through which change unfolds.

And in doing so, evaluation becomes not only
a method of inquiry,
but a way of seeing the systems we seek to
change.

Preface

A set of persistent questions has guided my scholarly and professional journey: What forces shape program outcomes, and how can evaluation methods capture these forces within the complexity of real-world systems? These questions first arose during my early career as a Registered Nurse, when I observed that patients' health outcomes were influenced not only by clinical care, but also by the complex interplay of social, institutional, and environmental determinants. This experience demonstrated that many factors affecting well-being extend beyond clinical practice boundaries, emerging from dynamic interactions among individuals, organizations, communities, and policy environments. My interest in these dynamics deepened after I transitioned to a training and development role within local government, where I frequently encountered questions central to evaluation practice: Which theoretical frameworks inform program and intervention design? How can stakeholders develop a meaningful understanding of a program's theory of change? How can evaluation methods remain both rigorous and responsive to the contextual complexity in which programs operate? My subsequent work as an evaluator in university extension programs further clarified the interconnected nature of social drivers and their impact on program outcomes across individual, organizational, community, and policy levels.

Through my experiences in clinical, governmental, and institutional settings, I have observed various factors that influence outcomes. From these observations, I have identified three adaptable principles that provide practical guidance for evaluators in different contexts:

- *Boundary Scanning.* Evaluators who intentionally integrate insights from multiple disciplines and sectors are able to identify connections and influences that are often overlooked within narrowly defined boundaries. This approach encourages moving beyond disciplinary silos to uncover hidden factors shaping program outcomes.
- *Relational Mapping.* Systematic mapping and tracing of relational frameworks allows evaluators to clarify complex networks within program implementation.

This principle uncovers patterns of collaboration, influence, and resource flows that shape outcomes in multifaceted environments.
- *Methodological Reflexivity.* Evaluators who systematically review and refine their methodologies ensure that evaluations remain both relevant and meaningful. This process demands continuous critical reflection and adaptation to evolving program contexts and stakeholder priorities.

Recognizing the value of systems thinking and relational dynamics steadily transformed my methodological viewpoint. Early in my career, I utilized foundational network theories, which examine how patterns of relationships among actors structure system behavior, to enhance my understanding of complex systems. However, while these frameworks offer key insights, they often emphasize static structures rather than context-specific adaptation and change. Additionally, evaluators often apply network analysis in isolation rather than integrating it into evaluation practice. This is where Network-Informed Complex Evaluation (NCE) meaningfully departs from standalone network science: NCE treats networks as evolving hypotheses to be explored and re-examined as programs unfold, rather than static maps to be measured once and archived. Recognizing this gap led me to develop NCE, an approach that combines social network analysis (SNA), systems thinking, and a focus on relational context. Through NCE, I examine not only structural patterns but also the evolving interplay and adaptation among actors, organizations, and institutions over time.

At its best, evaluation allows practitioners to move beyond surface measures and reveal the deeper dynamics that drive change in complex systems. This book is fueled by scholarship and extensive experience evaluating a range of programs, including public health initiatives to improve community health and well-being, training and education programs that strengthen organizations, leadership programs that promote culturally responsive schools, and family violence prevention efforts that seek better institutional responses. Despite their diverse goals and structures, each setting shares a consistent pattern: all are shaped by complex networks of interdependence. Outcomes depend on relationship networks, mutual influences, and adaptive interactions among people, organizations, and environments. By naming this recurring theme—interconnectedness—the book offers a framework for recognizing similar patterns in other contexts. This core idea shows that NCE's challenges and opportunities extend far beyond any single sector and reflect the foundation of all social programs.

Addressing such complexity demands evaluation approaches that examine relationships and structures across multiple levels of social organization, which traditional methods often overlook. Yet, established methods still hold value. For instance, logic models clarify program resources, actions, and expected results, enabling evaluators and stakeholders to align efforts around common goals. These frameworks help communicate program logic, build stakeholder consensus, and support accountability in straightforward settings. Building on these strengths, NCE advances evaluation by broadening the scope of conventional methods. Instead of viewing programs as machines designed for predictable outcomes, NCE frames them as interconnected webs of individuals, actions, and influences. Programs are dynamic and adaptive, shaped by patterns of interaction among all participants and stakeholders. This framework helps evaluators see how relationships drive collaboration, information flow, resource sharing, and outcomes. By combining traditional and network-informed methods, NCE enhances evaluators' capacity to tackle complexity while retaining the advantages of established tools.

This book invites evaluators to expand their conceptualization and examination of social programs embedded in complex systems. Before exploring detailed theoretical frameworks, consider whether any of the following challenges resonate with your evaluation work:

- Do unpredictable outcomes often arise despite careful planning?
- Do the relationships and influences among stakeholders exceed the explanatory power of existing evaluation models?
- Do classic evaluation tools fall short in capturing the real complexity of program settings?

If these challenges sound familiar, you are not alone. Many evaluation practitioners face such complexities without clear direction. This book draws on knowledge from complex adaptive systems, network theory, and evaluation theory to address these issues. The NCE approach equips evaluators to examine how relationships, structures, and context shape processes and outcomes. Rather than treating complexity as a barrier, this approach places it at the center of real-world evaluation. The book blends theory with practical guidance, encouraging evaluators, researchers, and practitioners to focus on relational and systemic drivers of change. For example, early chapters introduce the "Network-Informed Approach to Stakeholder Identification in Evaluation" and the "Network-Informed Context Assessment Checklist." This work extends beyond outcome measurement by uncovering structures and interactions that facilitate social change through network-informed context assessment, program theory development, and evaluation design.

How the Book Is Organized

This book facilitates a shift in evaluation mindsets, promotes the application of practical network-informed methods, and aims to enhance system impact in complex programs. Evaluators of contemporary social interventions frequently encounter challenges in assessing the intricate relationships and networks that influence program outcomes. The book presents a conceptual and methodological framework for the systematic analysis of these dynamics. To address this complexity, it first establishes foundational assumptions about complexity, relational systems, and knowledge construction, explaining the limitations of traditional models and the necessity of new evaluation perspectives. Subsequently, the book outlines iterative steps for network-informed evaluations to guide practical implementation. Finally, it explores the broader theoretical and practical implications of this approach. Fig. 1 illustrates

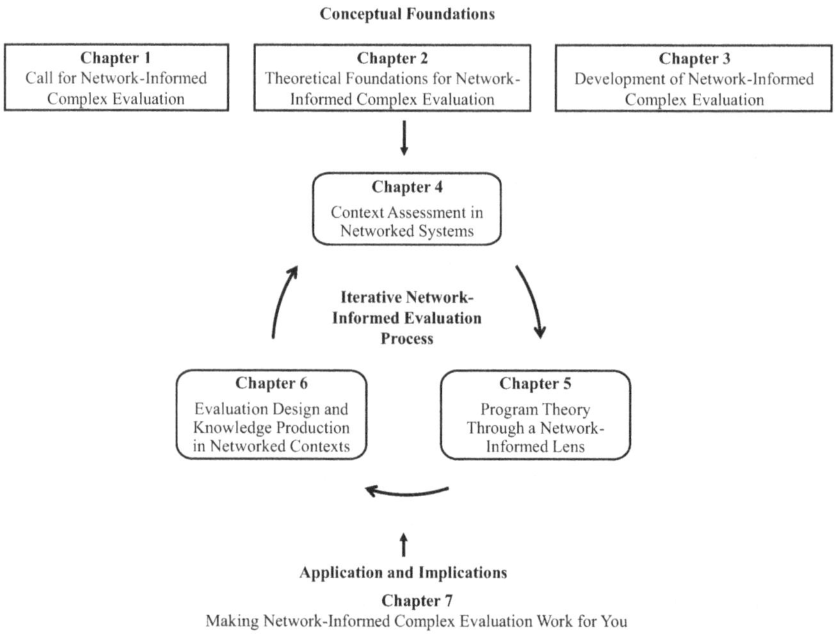

Fig. 1 Organizational framework of the book

the book's structure, showing the connections among its conceptual foundations, methods, and applications.

The first three chapters establish the conceptual foundation for NCE. Chapter 1 situates this approach within the broader challenges of evaluating complex programs, especially those targeting health equity. It examines the limitations of conventional evaluation models and demonstrates how network-based perspectives provide novel insights into program dynamics. After completing Chapter 1, readers should be able to identify common barriers to evaluating complex programs and explain how network perspectives address these limitations. The following questions are proposed for reflection: Where do evaluation efforts most often encounter persistent blind spots? Which stakeholder voices remain unheard in current approaches? What assumptions about causality or context might limit current evaluation practices? How might evaluation practice change if these challenges were reframed through a network-informed lens?

Chapter 2 examines theoretical foundations by integrating complex adaptive systems, social–ecological theory, and network analysis across multiple social–ecological levels. These theories converge within the NCE framework to establish a cohesive approach: complexity science provides the overarching logic of emergence and adaptation; social–ecological theory situates actors and processes within layered contexts; and social network analysis connects these dimensions by revealing relational pathways through which interactions occur and influence outcomes (see

Fig. 2.1 and Table 2.1 for illustration). The chapter also presents selected theories that support the development of NCE across social–ecological levels. After completing Chapter 2, readers will be able to articulate key theories underpinning network-informed complex evaluation and understand their influence on evaluation strategies across diverse contexts.

Chapter 3 applies these theoretical insights to develop a practical framework that outlines guiding principles, essential network concepts, and specific step-by-step procedures for conducting network-informed complex evaluations. Upon completing Chapter 3, readers will understand foundational network concepts and concrete methods required to design and implement network-informed evaluations in practice.

Chapters 4–6 form the book's analytical core by demonstrating the practical application of the NCE framework. Chapter 4 reconceptualizes context assessment as the analysis of relational networks consisting of actors, institutions, and governance arrangements. To facilitate immediate practitioner use, it translates criteria for evaluating program readiness for network-informed evaluation into a practical checklist. This chapter provides a ready-to-use checklist (e.g., Table 4.1) to determine whether a program is prepared to benefit from a network-informed approach. After completing Chapter 4, readers will be able to map relational networks within their program settings and apply this checklist to assess both program and stakeholder readiness for network-informed evaluation.

Chapter 5 reconceptualizes the input stage of program theory from a network perspective, framing programs as relational systems where actors, resources, and actions interact within complex environments. It presents conceptual and analytical tools for developing program theories that incorporate governance dynamics, contextual constraints, influence flows, and the inclusion or exclusion of actors within collaborative networks. Appendix A: Network-Informed Complex Evaluation Program Theory Template offers a practical resource for constructing network-informed program theories.

Chapter 6 addresses evaluation design and knowledge production, highlighting the interaction between methodological decisions and network structures. These decisions affect the generation and utilization of evaluative knowledge, support stakeholder engagement, and improve the practical application of findings. The chapter further explores how design choices can alter power dynamics within program environments. Upon completing Chapter 6, readers will be equipped to design evaluations that leverage network structures to foster comprehensive knowledge creation, stakeholder involvement, and effective use of findings. Appendix B: Network-Informed Complex Evaluation Design and Planning Template offers tools for evaluation planning, design, and reporting to facilitate practical implementation.

The concluding chapter synthesizes the book's conceptual and methodological contributions and examines their implications for evaluation theory and practice. Chapter 7 situates the NCE framework within the broader evaluation scholarship and explores how network-informed perspectives can transform evaluation practices in complex, networked environments. Upon completing Chapter 7, readers will understand the broader implications of adopting a network-informed evaluation approach and gain practical resources to apply it across diverse contexts.

What This Book Is For

This book advocates a paradigm shift: from viewing programs as linear cause-and-effect chains to understanding them as dynamic networks of connection and influence. Traditional logic models represent a direct sequence: "if activity A occurs, then outcome B follows." In contrast, a network-informed approach examines "who interacts with whom, and how these relationships drive change." The objective is to establish network-informed evaluation as a foundational perspective within complexity-oriented research. Rather than viewing networks as supplementary tools, this perspective asserts that network approaches transform all aspects of evaluation, including conceptualization, context analysis, causal theory, design, and knowledge utilization. NCE reframes evaluation as the study of relationships that generate outcomes. In complex systems, relationships themselves constitute the intervention.

Central to the book is the articulation of the NCE framework. NCE reconceptualizes networks as ontological and epistemological foundations for evaluation practice rather than as mere measurement tools. Through systematic analysis and critical comparison of established evaluation theories, this framework extends causal theorization beyond organizational boundaries to encompass policy networks, cross-sector partnerships, and multilevel social–ecological systems from a network-informed perspective. In policy evaluation, network-informed complex evaluation supports decision-making by demonstrating how policy networks influence outcomes, identifying key actors and their relationships, and mapping the flow of resources and information. Consequently, NCE clarifies how policies affect stakeholders and outcomes. This book advances theoretical and methodological discourse in evaluation by emphasizing the complexities of social programs operating within or across social–ecological levels.

Who Will Benefit and How

Interpreting unpredictable results and complex relationships in multifaceted programs presents considerable challenges. NCE offers a network-informed approach to address these complexities and generate more robust and insightful evaluations within dynamic environments. This volume examines the challenges posed by the scale and unpredictability of complex programs, where outcomes emerge from interactions among actors, relationships, and contexts that linear models fail to explain adequately. To demonstrate the book's relevance, the following subsections outline specific benefits for key audiences involved in complexity-focused evaluation contexts.

The primary audience consists of evaluation scholars and researchers dedicated to developing theoretical frameworks for complexity-oriented evaluation. Chapters 1–3 establish the conceptual and analytical foundations essential for rigorous scholarly inquiry. These chapters introduce models and arguments that critically engage with and advance current debates concerning causality, context, and complexity in evaluation research. By framing evaluation through a network-informed perspective, these chapters offer theoretical bases for interrogating and enriching theoretical discourse. Each chapter concludes with curated reflection questions intended to foster sustained, critical engagement with foundational issues in evaluation theory.

Graduate students in evaluation, public health, education, organizational studies, and related disciplines will find this book valuable as they explore emerging approaches to evaluating complex programs. The book provides a comprehensive framework that supports advanced coursework in evaluation theory, public health program evaluation, and network analysis, including detailed evaluation procedures and templates to enhance learning and practical application.

Another key audience includes evaluation practitioners working in complex program environments, such as public health systems, educational institutions, nonprofit organizations, and government agencies. These practitioners frequently encounter programs characterized by multiple stakeholders, adaptive implementation processes, and unpredictable outcomes. This book provides conceptual frameworks and practical tools to address these complexities while enhancing the rigor and utility of evaluation. Furthermore, Chapters 1 through 6 conclude with applied activities and reflection questions to facilitate the immediate application of the NCE concepts introduced in each chapter.

I hope that, regardless of your role or discipline, this book provides both theoretical insights and practical guidance for navigating the complexities of contemporary evaluation. As you engage with the content, I encourage you to look beyond surface-level indicators and examine the structural relationships that shape your program outcomes. Exploring these relational dynamics will reveal the networks through which information, influence, and resources circulate, offering new ways to understand how program outcomes emerge and how evaluation findings can inform action. Rather than merely reflecting on your evaluation practice, I invite you to experiment with re-envisioning your current evaluation approach through a network-informed perspective. Consider how this perspective might reveal connections, patterns of influence, or opportunities for change that remain hidden within conventional frameworks. Ultimately, I hope this book motivates you to explore the relational dimensions of programs more deeply and inspires you to illuminate the complex systems through which social change unfolds.

Cleveland, OH, USA Lixin Zhang
March 2026

Acknowledgments This book is founded on a core belief: the true responsibility of evaluation lies in our relationships with others. Every insight presented here emerges from the generous guidance, thoughtful collaboration, and steadfast support I have received throughout my evaluation journey. Because evaluation is fundamentally relational, it is fitting that this book expresses my deep gratitude to the many individuals who shaped its ideas and enabled its creation.

I begin by honoring my Ph.D. advisor and academic mentor, the late Dr. David R. Johnson, whose guidance profoundly shaped my academic trajectory and understanding of evaluation. From him, I learned that evaluation extends beyond methods or models; it embodies responsibility: asking difficult questions with humility, engaging complexity without reductionism, and remaining accountable to communities affected by programs and policies. Dr. Johnson often emphasized that true evaluation thrives on "rigor with humility," a principle balancing methodological precision with deep respect for the people and contexts studied. His commitment to ethical grounding and clarity of thought continues to influence my work. Although he is no longer present to see this book, his mentorship has had a lasting impact on my evaluation practice. I carry his example forward with gratitude and aspire to offer my students the same generosity of mentorship he extended to me.

I am deeply grateful to Dr. Emily Becher, whose evaluation practice grounded my academic training in lived complexity. Collaborating with her during my early professional years to evaluate programs aimed at promoting community health and well-being demonstrated that theory must remain accountable to practice. She integrated rigorous evaluation design with respect for communities, treating both as essential commitments. She approached evidence with discipline, listened attentively to stakeholder voices, and maintained a clear focus on purpose. Her example deeply influenced my perspective on evaluation, demonstrating that it is not only a matter of technical skill and careful practice, but also a meaningful professional commitment.

I acknowledge the anonymous reviewers who evaluated the original book proposal. Their thoughtful critiques and encouragement during the formative stage refined the project's conceptual boundaries and clarified its intended contribution. Their insights facilitated a clearer distinction between network-informed approaches and traditional evaluation models. Their feedback ensured that the theory addressed both systemic connections and practical challenges faced by evaluators. Although their names remain unknown, their intellectual generosity strengthened the foundation of this work.

I extend my gratitude to the manuscript reviewers, whose rigorous and collegial engagement strengthened this book. Dr. Axel Kaehne provided clear connective logic and incisive guidance on the conceptual framing and structure of the Network-Informed Complex Evaluation framework. His capacity to clarify and link the framework's argument enhanced its coherence and intellectual positioning. His affirmation of the framework's originality and relevance to evaluation science and practice was especially encouraging.

Dr. Muhammad Khalifa offered thoughtful reflections on narrative flow, accessibility, and scholarly positioning. His encouragement to articulate the intellectual journey behind the framework more explicitly and to clarify transitions across chapters improved readability and resonance, ensuring that readers can follow the framework's evolution with ease. I am especially grateful for his recognition of the book's potential to serve scholars and practitioners committed to equity-focused, community-engaged evaluation across diverse contexts.

I am grateful to Dr. Yue Zhang for her detailed and constructive review. Her careful analysis of theoretical integration (how the ideas fit together) and methodological articulation (how the methods are described and connected), as well as the framework's practical implications, enhanced its coherence as an evaluative perspective. Her recommendations on case illustrations, implementation boundaries, and practical guidance strengthened the balance between conceptual depth and applied relevance.

I gratefully acknowledge the editorial and production team at Springer Nature for their essential contributions to this book's development. I especially thank Janet Kim, whose guidance during the initial book proposal, contract negotiations, and ongoing oversight shaped the project's direction and established a strong foundation. Dhivya Savariraj provided expert supervision throughout the production process, ensuring clear and timely communication that facilitated the manuscript's smooth transition from draft to publication. Sophie Li offered thoughtful coordination and attentive support, enabling efficient and careful management of all details. Brian Halm and his production team managed the logistics and final preparations that brought the book to market. Their professionalism, attention to detail, and commitment to scholarly excellence, often behind the scenes, were instrumental in bringing this book to fruition. I sincerely appreciate the expertise and dedication that guided this project to completion.

Finally, I express my deepest gratitude to my family. Writing a book requires time, solitude, and sustained focus, which are never granted lightly. The care they provide daily exemplifies the evaluative relationships advocated in this book, grounded in mutual support, attentiveness, and generosity. They continually remind me that relationships are not peripheral to meaningful work but form its foundation. This book embodies not only years of scholarship and practice but also the love, support, and trust that enabled such sustained effort, all united by the evaluative care that initiated this endeavor.

Competing Interests The author has no competing interests to declare that are relevant to the content of this manuscript.

Contents

1 Call for Network-Informed Complex Evaluation 1
Introduction 1
Addressing Evaluation Challenges with Network-Informed Approaches 2
Technical–Rational Model 3
Myth of Neutrality 6
Donor-Centric Accountability 6
Technocratic Reductionism 7
Toward a Network-Informed Lens 8
Navigating Complexity Challenges with Network-Informed Complex Evaluation 8
Expanding the Case for Network Lenses in Health Equity 8
Mapping Social Determinants of Health to the Social–Ecological Model 10
Complex Adaptive Systems as a Framework for Evaluating Health Equity Initiatives 13
Network Theory as a Foundation for Network-Informed Complex Evaluation 14
How Network-Informed Complex Evaluation Meets Challenges of Complexity 15
What Is Network-Informed Complex Evaluation? 19
Positioning the Evaluator in Network-Informed Complex Evaluation 20
Situating Network-Informed Complex Evaluation within Established Evaluation Theories 21
Chapter Summary 25
Reflection Questions 26
Applied Activities 26
References 27

2 Theoretical Foundations of Network-Informed Complex Evaluation 31
Introduction 31
Conceptual Foundations 32
Network-Informed Complex Evaluation at the Individual Level 36
Individual Level as a Complex Adaptive System 36
Linking Network-Informed Complex Evaluation to Individual-Level Theories 36
Network-Informed Complex Evaluation at the Organizational Level 40
Organizational Level as a Complex Adaptive System 40
Linking Network-Informed Complex Evaluation to Organizational-Level Theories 41
Network-Informed Complex Evaluation at the Community Level 44
Community Level as a Complex Adaptive System 45
Linking Network-Informed Complex Evaluation to Community-Level Theories 45
Network-Informed Complex Evaluation at the Policy Level 49
Policy Level as a Complex Adaptive System 49
Linking Network-Informed Complex Evaluation to Policy-Level Theories 50
Example: Reconceptualizing the BeSD Framework from a Network Perspective 53
Chapter Summary 57
Reflection Questions 58
Applied Activities 58
References 60

3 Development of Network-Informed Complex Evaluation 65
Introduction 65
Principles of Network-Informed Complex Evaluation 65
Systems and Complexity Orientation 67
Social–Ecological Orientation 67
Network Orientation 68
Standards 69
Adaptive and Participatory Learning 71
Sustainability and Capacity-Building 72
Cultural and Contextual Responsiveness 72
Network Terminology in Complex Evaluation 73
Network Concepts in Network-Informed Complex Evaluation 73
Network Variables in Network-Informed Complex Evaluation 75
Network Measures in Network-Informed Complex Evaluation 78
Approaches to Conducting Network-Informed Complex Evaluation 87
Context Stage 93
Input Stage 94
Process Stage 94

Product Stage 95
Chapter Summary 95
Reflection Questions 96
Applied Activities 97
References 98

4 Context Assessment in Networked Systems 101
The Critical Role of Context Assessment in Network-Informed Complex Evaluation 101
Conducting Network-Informed Context Assessment 104
Section A: Needs and Opportunity Analysis 104
Section B: Intended Users and Uses 112
Section C: Stakeholder Landscape and Engagement 113
Section D: Network Boundaries and Data Availability 114
Section E: Organizational and Technical Readiness 117
Section F: Ethical Considerations 118
Network-Informed Complex Evaluation Readiness 119
Identifying Stakeholders in a Network-Informed Approach 119
Network-Informed Stakeholder Identification Criteria 120
Network-Informed Stakeholder Identification Steps 121
Network-Informed Stakeholder Identification Example 123
Utilizing Context Assessment Findings 123
Implications for the Input Stage 123
Implications for the Process Stage 126
Implications for the Product Stage 126
Chapter Summary 127
Reflection Questions 128
Applied Activities 128
References 129

5 Program Theory Through a Network-Informed Lens 131
Network-Informed Complex Evaluation: Why Input Stage Matters 131
Supporting Stakeholders in Clarifying Their Program Theory 132
Defining Program Scope in Networked Systems 134
Defining Action Plan in Networked Systems 138
Defining Program Effects in Networked Systems 145
Addressing Contextual Factors in Network-Informed Complex Evaluation 148
Why Contextual Factors Matter in Network-Informed Complex Evaluation 148
Conceptualizing Contextual Dimensions Through a Network Lens 149
Addressing Assumptions in Network-Informed Complex Evaluation 154
Why Assumptions Matter in Network-Informed Complex Evaluation 155

Conceptualizing Assumptions Through a Network Lens 155
Chapter Summary 158
Reflection Questions 159
Applied Activities 159
References 159

6 **Evaluation Design and Knowledge Production in Networked Contexts** 161
Introduction 161
Formulating Network-Informed Evaluation Objectives and Questions 163
How Program Theory Shapes Evaluation Objectives and Questions 163
Developing Network-Informed Objectives and Questions 164
Defining Network Scope and Boundaries 165
Boundary Specification Strategies 165
Network Boundaries at Social-Ecological Levels 170
Aligning Evaluation Methods with Questions and Network Boundaries 172
Developing Data Collection and Analysis Plans 173
Network Data-Collection Procedures in Evaluation 174
Analytic Strategies in Network-Informed Complex Evaluation 180
Data Collection and Analysis Planning in Network-Informed Complex Evaluation 184
Designing Reporting and Knowledge-Use Strategies 185
Developing Effective Evaluation Reports 186
Facilitating Sense-Making and Action Translation 187
Integrating Feedback and Adaptive Learning Loops 192
Prioritizing Equity-Centered Communication and Use 193
Network-Informed Complex Evaluation Design and Reporting Checklist 193
Chapter Summary 201
Reflection Questions 202
Applied Activities 202
References 203

7 **Making Network-Informed Complex Evaluation Work for You** 207
What Network-Informed Complex Evaluation Offers 207
Accountability and Control 207
Social Inquiry 208
Method 208
Value 209
Use 209
Foundational Questions in Network-Informed Complex Evaluation 210
Is Network-Informed Complex Evaluation a Theoretically Coherent Framework? 210

Is Network-Informed Complex Evaluation a Good Evaluation Theory? 211
How Does Network-Informed Complex Evaluation Advance and Operationalize Complexity-Oriented Evaluation Frameworks? 214
How Can Network-Informed Complex Evaluation Be Operationalized in Real-World Evaluation Settings? 215
Does Network-Informed Complex Evaluation Provide Sufficient Methodological Rigor to Ensure Credible and Valid Evaluation? 219
How Does Network-Informed Complex Evaluation Ensure that Network Mapping and Analysis Do not Perpetuate Inequity? 220
How Can Evaluators Build Capacity for Network-Informed Complex Evaluation? 220
What Are Other Common Applications of Network-Informed Complex Evaluation? 222
Can Network-Informed Complex Evaluation Be Applied in Other Contexts? 223
Conclusion 225
A Call to Action for Evaluation Scholars and Practitioners 226
Final Reflection 227
References 229

Appendix A: Network-Informed Complex Evaluation Program Theory Template 233

Appendix B Network-Informed Complex Evaluation Design and Planning Template 239

Index 249

About the Author

Lixin Zhang, Ph.D., is the Assistant Director of Research Evaluation at Case Western Reserve University and an alumna of the University of Minnesota in the United States. Her research integrates social network analysis, complexity theory, and systems thinking to advance the conceptual foundations and practical applications of program evaluation. She earned her Ph.D. in Evaluation Studies from the University of Minnesota, where she developed the SNA–Evaluation Conceptual Framework, a theory-driven approach that integrates social network analysis into evaluation design, implementation, and interpretation. This framework advances evaluation methodology in complex, multi-stakeholder environments by repositioning social network analysis as a conceptual lens for examining relational structures, collaborative infrastructures, and system-level change.

Dr. Zhang has designed and implemented mixed-method and network-informed approaches for federally and state-funded initiatives in public health, violence prevention, nutrition education, rural development, and translational science. Her work has been presented at international and national forums, including the United Nations Development Programme National Evaluation Capacities (NEC) Conference and the American Evaluation Association Conference, and has been published in peer-reviewed journals such as *Frontiers in Public Health.* With interdisciplinary training in nursing, human resource development, and evaluation science, she brings a complexity-oriented and human-centered perspective to her work. Through her publications, development of evaluation systems, and professional service, she remains committed to advancing evaluation methodology to address complex social and health challenges.

List of Figures

Fig. 2.1	Network-informed complex evaluation (NCE) framework	33
Fig. 3.1	Core principles for network-informed complex evaluation (NCE)	66
Fig. 3.2	Network-informed complex evaluation (NCE) approach	93
Fig. 4.1	Network-informed approach to stakeholder identification in evaluation	121
Fig. 5.1	Network-informed program theory: Scope, action plans, and effects	134
Fig. 7.1	Network-informed complex evaluation of health equity programs	212
Fig. 7.2	Criteria framework for determining when network-informed complex evaluation is methodologically warranted	218

List of Tables

Table 1.1 Limitations of conventional evaluation and corresponding network-informed evaluation approaches for advancing health equity ... 4
Table 1.2 Alignment of social determinants of health (SDOH) with the social–ecological model (SEM) and social network analysis (SNA) ... 11
Table 1.3 Analytical challenges in complex adaptive systems (CAS) and corresponding network-informed evaluation responses ... 16
Table 1.4 Positioning network-informed complex evaluation (NCE) in relation to established evaluation approaches ... 23
Table 2.1 Conceptual alignment of complex adaptive systems (CAS) principles across socio–ecological levels and implications for network-informed evaluation ... 34
Table 2.2 Individual-level theories interpreted through network analysis ... 37
Table 2.3 Organizational-level theories interpreted through network analysis ... 42
Table 2.4 Community-level theories interpreted through network analysis ... 46
Table 2.5 Policy-level theories interpreted through network analysis ... 51
Table 2.6 Network- and complexity-informed mapping of the WHO BeSD framework ... 54
Table 3.1 Core relational and positional concepts of network structure across levels of analysis ... 76
Table 3.2 Network measures for network-informed complex evaluation across levels ... 88
Table 4.1 Network-informed context assessment checklist ... 105
Table 4.2 Stakeholder landscape for network-informed complex evaluation ... 115
Table 4.3 Example of network-informed stakeholder identification results ... 124

Table 5.1 Network-informed interpretation of program scope 135
Table 5.2 Network-informed interpretation of action plan components 140
Table 5.3 Network-informed interpretation of program effects 146
Table 5.4 Network-informed conceptualization of contextual factors 150
Table 5.5 Network-informed conceptualization of assumptions 156
Table 6.1 Boundary specification strategies in network-informed complex evaluation across social-ecological levels 166
Table 6.2 Common network data-collection methods by social-ecological level 177
Table 6.3 Network analytic approaches in network-informed complex evaluation (NCE) 181
Table 6.4 Network-informed complex evaluation reporting products by audience, purpose, timing, and format 188
Table 6.5 Network-informed complex evaluation design and reporting checklist 194
Table 7.1 Comparison of network-informed complex evaluation (NCE), developmental evaluation, realist evaluation, and systems thinking in evaluation 216
Table A.1 Network-informed program scope with examples 234
Table A.2 Network-informed program action plan with examples 236
Table A.3 Network-informed program effects with examples 238

Chapter 1
Call for Network-Informed Complex Evaluation

Introduction

Health equity, broadly understood as the absence of avoidable, unfair, and unjust health differences among social groups, remains a central objective in global public health and a top priority for governments, non-governmental organizations, and international agencies (Braveman et al., 2018; Whitehead, 1992). Advancing health equity requires sustained attention to the social, economic, political, and environmental determinants that shape health outcomes across populations. These determinants—including access to resources such as wealth, power, and prestige—are distributed through policy decisions and institutional arrangements that operate within complex, multilevel systems. Such systems are characterized by feedback loops, nonlinear dynamics, and historically embedded patterns of inequality that influence the distribution of health opportunities.

Despite the need to evaluate programs operating within these complex environments, evaluation practice often relies on models originally designed for more stable, predictable contexts. These models typically assume fixed interventions, clear causal pathways, and linear progressions of change. Such assumptions risk obscuring the interconnected and dynamic conditions that shape outcomes in real-world settings. Complex social programs frequently involve multiple interacting components, evolving relationships among actors, and emergent effects that cannot be fully anticipated (Renger, 2022; Rogers, 2008). Nevertheless, many evaluations continue to use structured approaches that specify program theories or logic models, indicators, and intended outcomes in advance and employ systematic designs to assess program implementation and effects (Rossi et al., 2003; Weiss, 1998). While these approaches provide valuable tools for assessing program performance, they may overlook the relational networks, power dynamics, and contextual conditions through which complex social interventions actually produce—or fail to produce—equitable outcomes.

L. Zhang, *Network-Informed Complex Evaluation*,
https://doi.org/10.1007/978-3-032-27495-3_1

Network-Informed Complex Evaluation (NCE) addresses these limitations by revealing hidden relational structures and power dynamics. For instance, in a rural maternal health initiative, traditional evaluation methods may quantify prenatal visits but overlook transportation barriers faced by disadvantaged women, resulting in resource misallocation. A network perspective can identify leverage points, such as key community connectors who influence and mobilize resources. Engaging these connectors can improve access to healthcare services. Another leverage point involves streamlining bureaucratic procedures that impede service delivery, and network analysis can help identify them. Network-informed evaluation clarifies the interactions among relationships, structures, and systems that shape health outcomes, enabling evaluators to address the root causes of health inequities. This approach advances evaluation beyond surface-level analysis by identifying leverage points, exposing hidden structural barriers, and promoting equity-focused change. The rationale for network-informed complex evaluation is summarized in the central question: *How can a network-informed evaluation approach enhance health equity by addressing the limitations of current program evaluation methods?*

Addressing Evaluation Challenges with Network-Informed Approaches

The increasing complexity and interconnectedness of contemporary systems reveal important limitations in conventional linear accountability models used in evaluation practice. These models assume stable program environments, predictable cause-and-effect relationships, and relatively bounded interventions. In practice, however, evaluators frequently encounter settings characterized by evolving stakeholder relationships, shifting priorities, and nonlinear dynamics. For example, in one multisector opioid prevention initiative I evaluated, changes in policy priorities and community advocacy rapidly altered partnerships and resource flows, making program pathways far from linear. Such experiences illustrate how conventional logic models can become unstable as leadership structures, partnerships, and institutional contexts evolve.

Much of evaluation practice has historically been shaped by technical–rational traditions emphasizing causal attribution, standardized measurement, and procedural rigor (Chelimsky & Shadish, 1997; Rossi et al., 2003). While these approaches contribute valuable methodological tools for assessing program effectiveness and accountability, they often prove insufficient when applied to complex social systems characterized by uncertainty, contested values, and dynamic local contexts (Schwandt, 2015; Weiss, 1998). Scholars of complexity and systems evaluation likewise argue that linear models struggle to capture emergent change processes and adaptive responses within complex environments (Patton, 2011; Preskill et al., 2014). As a result, evaluators increasingly seek approaches that can examine the relationships, feedback loops, and contextual influences that shape program outcomes.

NCE responds to these challenges by emphasizing shared sense-making with diverse stakeholders and by employing network mapping techniques to visualize relationships among actors. These strategies help surface marginalized voices and reveal patterns of interaction that influence program implementation and outcomes. By examining how relationships shape the flow of information, resources, and influence, NCE enables evaluators to identify structural and relational dynamics that affect equity outcomes. The following section, supported by Table 1.1, outlines several limitations of traditional evaluation models, their implications for health outcomes, and opportunities to strengthen evaluation practice through a network-informed perspective.

Technical–Rational Model

The technical–rational model conceptualizes programs as bounded interventions governed by predictable cause-and-effect relationships and clear causal attribution (Chelimsky & Shadish, 1997, Chap. 3; Rossi et al., 2003). This approach often produces evaluation designs centered on linear logic models and predefined indicators for measuring program outputs and outcomes. While these tools provide useful structure for monitoring program implementation, they may also risk oversimplifying the complex and evolving conditions that define many health and social interventions. Critics have argued that technical–rational approaches privilege linear evidence-to-decision models, despite the reality that implementation is shaped by complex social, political, and organizational processes that cannot be fully understood through predefined causal pathways alone (Schwandt, 1997).

These limitations are particularly evident in evaluations of healthcare access initiatives. For example, a public health initiative aimed at improving healthcare access in underserved communities may overlook critical questions such as "Which patients are missing care, and why?" Focusing exclusively on increases in average clinic visit numbers oversimplifies the dynamic, relational, and nonlinear conditions inherent in many health and social interventions. More broadly, a narrow focus on whether a program achieved its planned outcomes, such as increased clinic visits, limits the scope of evaluation inquiry and overlooks critical questions about who benefited, under what conditions, and why. Weiss (1998) emphasizes that this limitation is especially problematic for equity-oriented initiatives, where understanding differential effects and local contexts is essential.

NCE offers an alternative perspective that emphasizes relationships, interdependencies, and emergent outcomes within collaborative systems. In the healthcare access example, network-informed evaluation moves beyond counting clinic visits to examine how interactions among clinics, community organizations, policymakers, and local leaders shape program outcomes. Rather than attributing change solely to individual program components, NCE conceptualizes outcomes as products

Table 1.1 Limitations of conventional evaluation and corresponding network-informed evaluation approaches for advancing health equity

Limitation	Conventional assumption	Implications for health outcomes	NCE response
Technical rational model	Programs are conceptualized as linear, bounded, and controllable systems in which cause-and-effect relationships are assumed to be predictable and measurable.	Oversimplifies the dynamic, relational, and nonlinear realities of health systems, which can constrain organizational learning and limit adaptive responses to complex and evolving conditions.	• Emphasizes relational dynamics, complexity, and emergent outcomes. • Understands outcomes as coproduced within interconnected networks of actors. • Values adaptive learning and participation over rigid technical precision.
Myth of neutrality	Evaluation is assumed to be objective, value-free, and politically neutral.	Obscures the value-laden and political dimensions of evaluation practice, often reinforcing dominant priorities and existing power relations within health systems.	• Positions evaluators as embedded actors within systems rather than detached observers. • Encourages reflexivity, transparency, and co-creation with diverse stakeholders. • Replaces neutrality with transparency and negotiated meaning-making.

(continued)

Table 1.1 (continued)

Limitation	Conventional assumption	Implications for health outcomes	NCE response
Donor-centric accountability	Program success is primarily defined by upward accountability to donors and external authorities.	Marginalizes local knowledge, community priorities, and lived experiences, thereby limiting the evaluation's capacity to support equity-oriented learning, accountability, and system transformation.	• Promotes multidirectional accountability to donors, communities, and implementing partners. • Frames evaluation as a shared learning process across networks. • Reorients accountability toward strengthening collective capacity, trust, and systems resilience.
Technocratic reductionism	Program performance and impact can be adequately captured through standardized, predominantly quantitative indicators.	Neglects structural conditions, social context, and systemic drivers of inequity, resulting in partial or misleading interpretations of impact.	• Applies systems thinking and complexity-oriented evaluation approaches. • Expands analytic scope to include relationships, interdependencies, and adaptive change processes. • Values local knowledge, qualitative insight, and diverse epistemic perspectives with quantitative data.

Source Author synthesis from the evaluation and development literature on technical–rational models, values and power in evaluation, accountability systems, and complexity-informed approaches (e.g., Chambers, 1997; Chelimsky & Shadish, 1997; Edwards & Hulme, 1996; House & Howe, 1999; Merry, 2011; Mertens, 2008; Patton, 2011; Preskill et al., 2014; Rossi et al., 2003; Weiss, 1998) of collaborative interactions among stakeholders operating within broader institutional and social contexts. This perspective highlights adaptive learning, stakeholder participation, and the role of relational dynamics in shaping program trajectories.

Myth of Neutrality

A second challenge concerns the assumption that evaluation can be conducted as a purely value-neutral activity. Extensive scholarship demonstrates that evaluative practice inevitably involves value commitments, as reflected in decisions about problem framing, evidence standards, indicator selection, and the prioritization of particular stakeholder perspectives (House & Howe, 1999; Mertens, 2008). These choices influence which outcomes are considered important and whose experiences are recognized in evaluation findings.

Historically, metrics defined by donors, international funders, and governmental agencies have dominated evaluation, shaping definitions of success that may overlook the realities of marginalized groups (Chambers, 1997; Edwards & Hulme, 1996). Although such indicators facilitate comparability and accountability, they may also obscure local realities and marginalize qualitative knowledge from communities most affected by interventions. For instance, in public health initiatives, evaluators often prioritize quantitative clinic-visit data over qualitative insights from marginalized community members, especially when funders require measurable outputs, such as visit counts. Although quantitative indicators provide statistical rigor, they may inadvertently marginalize qualitative insights essential for understanding context-specific dynamics. This situation raises a critical question for evaluators: Which outcomes remain invisible when only clinic visit numbers are considered?

NCE addresses this issue by positioning evaluators as participants embedded within program systems rather than detached observers. This perspective encourages reflexivity about the assumptions and priorities that shape evaluation decisions. Through collaborative interpretation and dialogue with stakeholders, NCE promotes transparency in evaluative judgments and enables diverse perspectives to inform evaluation processes and findings.

Donor-Centric Accountability

A third limitation concerns the frequent dominance of upward accountability, where evaluation questions and success criteria are set primarily by funders or external authorities (Bakewell & Garbutt, 2005; Edwards & Hulme, 1996). Information about programs and their outcomes is typically collected from local communities and conveyed to donors or funding agencies through implementing partners. Throughout this process, community perspectives and priorities are often diminished or lost before reaching final decision-makers. Accountability structures that prioritize efficiency, cost-effectiveness, and compliance reduce community decision-making power, marginalizing local priorities and knowledge in program design and interpretation. Chambers (1997) argues that such patterns can contribute to epistemic injustice by privileging external expertise over local knowledge.

NCE responds directly to this limitation by transforming accountability from a traditional, upward-facing structure to a multidirectional, dynamic system grounded in relationships among donors, communities, and implementing partners. Instead of relying on linear information flows and top-down decisions, NCE leverages distributed knowledge and influence within stakeholder networks, establishing mechanisms like community advisory teams where all parties regularly convene to discuss clinic access, health priorities, and emerging challenges. This approach incorporates diverse perspectives, especially those of community members, into evaluation and program adaptation. For instance, when quantitative data indicate increased clinic visits but network members identify persistent barriers for specific groups, the advisory team collaboratively analyzes these patterns and adjusts resources or interventions to address inequities. Embedding evaluation within these network-based processes enhances transparency, inclusivity, and adaptability, enabling communities to influence evaluation criteria and outcomes while promoting equity and responsiveness to local contexts.

Technocratic Reductionism

Conventional evaluation often demonstrates technocratic reductionism by prioritizing standardized, predominantly quantitative indicators as sufficient measures of impact (Merry, 2011). While measurement and quantification are essential, reliance on a limited set of indicators can underrepresent structural conditions, social context, and systemic drivers of inequity, leading to partial or misleading interpretations of program outcomes. For example, in a public health initiative, exclusive dependence on average clinic visit numbers concealed persistent barriers faced by marginalized groups. This limitation obscured significant disparities among populations and highlighted the need to re-examine the evaluation framework.

NCE expands its analytical framework by applying systems thinking and complexity approaches that emphasize relationships, interdependencies, and adaptive change mechanisms. In practice, this approach combines quantitative indicators, qualitative insights, and network analysis to capture a more comprehensive picture of program dynamics. For instance, network measures such as betweenness centrality may identify key community actors who facilitate access to healthcare resources. At the same time, qualitative interviews reveal how trust and local knowledge influence participation in the program. By integrating multiple forms of evidence, NCE produces contextually grounded interpretations better suited to understanding complex social systems.

Toward a Network-Informed Lens

Table 1.1 synthesizes key limitations of conventional evaluation approaches discussed in the literature and contrasts them with network-informed evaluation perspectives. The limitations presented in Table 1.1 should not be interpreted as a rejection of conventional evaluation methods, but rather as evidence that accountability-oriented assumptions may be insufficient for assessing interventions within the complex, interconnected networks that influence health inequities. NCE offers a network-informed perspective by emphasizing relational dynamics, power structures, and contextual conditions, thereby ensuring that evaluation practices capture the adaptive and interdependent nature of real-world social systems. Advancing evaluation through this framework requires moving beyond linear, technical-rational models to adopt approaches that recognize outcomes as emergent properties of evolving networks, promote reflexivity and transparency regarding normative commitments, expand accountability to operate in multidirectional ways among all network actors, and integrate qualitative insights and diverse knowledge forms alongside quantitative indicators. By centering the network perspective, NCE positions evaluation as a catalyst for organizational learning and enhances understanding of the structural and relational determinants affecting health outcomes.

Navigating Complexity Challenges with Network-Informed Complex Evaluation

Addressing persistent health disparities requires acknowledging that traditional evaluation frameworks that focus on individual outcomes or isolated interventions can be limiting. At the core of NCE is a network lens that emphasizes examining structural relations and their impacts on health equity. This perspective enables the identification of hidden connections, resource flows, and power dynamics that perpetuate inequities. Complexity theory highlights the adaptive and emergent behavior of complex systems, whereas network theory underscores the importance of relational structures in shaping access to resources, opportunities, and power. By identifying critical leverage points, evaluators can facilitate meaningful change. This section explores how established theories can be integrated through a network lens to address the complex, interconnected mechanisms underlying health outcomes.

Expanding the Case for Network Lenses in Health Equity

The persistence of health inequities underscores the need for evaluation frameworks that extend beyond individual outcomes and isolated interventions. Although traditional methods are valuable for assessing program effectiveness, they often overlook the relational contexts that generate and sustain health outcomes. A network perspective addresses this limitation by analyzing patterns of relationships among individuals, organizations, and institutions that collectively influence health equity. This approach is particularly relevant in policy and system change contexts, where complex public health challenges often exceed the capacity of any single organization, requiring coordinated action among multiple agencies, community organizations, and sectors.

Research on public sector organizational networks demonstrates that collaborative arrangements enable organizations to pool resources, share information, and coordinate strategies to address challenges beyond the capacity of individual institutions (Provan & Lemaire, 2012). Common strategies in policy and systems change, such as coalition building, policy advocacy, and cross-sector partnerships, fundamentally operate through relational processes. These processes depend on connections among diverse stakeholders to mobilize resources, build consensus, and align actions across institutional boundaries. At the community and systems levels, multisector partnerships and public health coalitions function as networks that coordinate actions among governmental, nonprofit, and community actors to address population health challenges and equity objectives (Woulfe et al., 2010). Because these initiatives rely on patterns of collaboration among organizations and stakeholders, evaluating their effectiveness requires approaches that consider network structure, governance, and the relational processes through which information, resources, and influence circulate.

Extensive research demonstrates that social and organizational networks influence the dissemination of health outcomes and innovations within populations and institutions. In social epidemiology, Berkman and Glass (2000) propose a multilevel framework wherein broader social conditions affect health partly through their impact on social network structures. These networks influence health via mechanisms such as social support, social influence, social engagement, and access to informational and material resources. Evidence from this and related epidemiological studies indicates that individuals with greater social integration often exhibit lower mortality risk, even after controlling for socioeconomic status and health behaviors. Network structures also affect the diffusion of health innovations and interventions. Greenhalgh et al. (2004), in their systematic review of innovation diffusion in health service organizations, demonstrate that adoption patterns are shaped by communication channels, opinion leaders, and the configuration of professional and organizational networks. Similarly, research on social networks and health behavior reveals that patterns of interpersonal and organizational ties influence the diffusion of health information, behavioral norms, and interventions within communities (Valente, 2010). Collectively, this literature underscores the critical role of relational structures in shaping both health outcomes and the dissemination of health interventions.

This body of evidence indicates that evaluations that exclude relational mechanisms risk underestimating the barriers and facilitators that influence progress toward health equity. The rationale for adopting a network perspective rests on three interconnected arguments. First, health inequities arise and persist through relational mechanisms, such as segregation, exclusion, and unequal access to social and institutional resources, which shape opportunities and constraints across populations. Second, many interventions aimed at advancing equity rely on relational strategies, including coalition building, peer support, cross-sector collaboration, and the diffusion of innovations through social and organizational networks. Third, evaluating these interventions requires methodological approaches capable of capturing and analyzing the relational structures and dynamics through which influence, resources, and information circulate. Integrating network analysis within broader structural and relational systems can enhance evaluation practices beyond isolated outcome measurement. NCE conceptualizes networks both as mechanisms of change and as objects of systematic evaluation, facilitating the examination of relational processes across multiple levels, including individuals, organizations, communities, and policy systems, and providing a framework to assess how patterns of connection influence the coordination of collective action and the advancement of health equity.

Mapping Social Determinants of Health to the Social–Ecological Model

Advancing health equity requires integrating SDOH, SEM, and SNA. This approach highlights that health outcomes emerge from complex, multilayered systems and are shaped by relationships at multiple ecological levels (Bronfenbrenner, 1979; McLeroy et al., 1988). SEM demonstrates how social determinants interact at individual, interpersonal, organizational, community, and policy levels to produce and sustain inequities. SNA reveals how social ties, organizational collaborations, and policy coalitions influence access to resources, the diffusion of innovation, and participation in decision-making.

Integrating these frameworks enables evaluators to understand not only where inequities emerge within the ecological system but also how relational mechanisms may reinforce or mitigate those disparities. Table 1.2 illustrates how SDOH manifests across SEM levels and highlights the unique contributions of a network lens for evaluation. For example, evaluators can use SNA to identify referral bottlenecks, structural holes, and weak partnerships that undermine system effectiveness, revealing opportunities to strengthen coordination and advance equity. By moving beyond traditional metrics, a network-informed, multilayered approach enables evaluators to engage more deeply with the underlying patterns that drive health inequities.

Table 1.2 Alignment of social determinants of health (SDOH) with the social–ecological model (SEM) and social network analysis (SNA)

SDOH	Individual	Organizational	Community	Policy	SNA Application
Economic stability	Employment status, income security, financial literacy, and the ability to meet basic needs are strong predictors of health outcomes.	Workplace wages, benefits, and job security influence opportunities for economic stability and well-being.	Access to stable employment, affordable housing, childcare, and food security strengthens community resilience.	Minimum wage policies, food assistance programs, and housing subsidies help reduce poverty and health inequities.	SNA can identify gaps in referral pathways among job training, housing, and food assistance services, revealing how weak or fragmented ties limit access to economic opportunities.
Education access and quality	Educational attainment is associated with life expectancy, health literacy, and healthier behaviors.	Educational institutions influence health through curricula, teacher capacity, institutional resources, and supportive learning environments.	Community-based literacy programs, after-school support, and early childhood education initiatives help reduce educational disparities.	Policies mandating equitable funding and access to early education reduce systemic disparities.	SNA can assess partnerships among schools, community organizations, and families to identify structural holes and strengthen coordination in educational support systems.

(continued)

Table 1.2 (continued)

SDOH	Individual	Organizational	Community	Policy	SNA Application
Health care access and quality	Preventive service use, health literacy, and chronic disease self-management are critical to health.	Workplace health screenings and school-based health services increase accessibility to preventive care.	Community clinics, mobile health units, and culturally competent providers expand care in underserved areas.	Policies that improve affordability, insurance coverage, and access to care shape equity in access to health services.	Mapping patient–provider and interorganizational ties can reveal referral bottlenecks, trust gaps, and opportunities to strengthen care coordination in underserved populations.
Neighborhood and built environment	Exposure to unsafe housing, traffic risks, or toxins increases the risk of disease.	Safe school and workplace facilities reduce exposure to environmental and occupational hazards.	Neighborhood walkability, parks, and access to healthy food retailers shape community health.	Urban planning, zoning regulations, transportation policies, and environmental protections influence neighborhood health conditions and disparities.	SNA can map connections among residents, organizations, and planning bodies to assess how information and resources related to safety and environmental risks circulate.
Social and community context	Discrimination, resilience, and supportive relationships shape stress and health outcomes.	Inclusive organizational cultures and health-focused institutional policies can mitigate discrimination and promote health and well-being.	Social cohesion, peer-mentoring, and civic engagement foster resilience.	Civil rights protections, anti-discrimination policies, and investments in community development promote social equity.	SNA can examine social support networks, identify socially isolated groups, and highlight bridging connections that strengthen cohesion and inclusion.

Source Author synthesis based on Bronfenbrenner, 1979; CDC, 2024; Hahn, 2021; Healthy People 2030; Low & Low, 2006; Marmot et al., 2008; Marmot & Wilkinson, 2005; McLeroy et al., 1988; Whitman et al., 2022; WHO, 2008

Complex Adaptive Systems as a Framework for Evaluating Health Equity Initiatives

Traditional evaluation approaches rely on linear theories of causality, presuming stable contexts and predictable relationships among inputs, activities, and outcomes. While effective for bounded interventions, these models are inadequate for health equity initiatives operating in dynamic social, political, and economic environments shaped by intersecting systems of power and disadvantage (Walton, 2014). Health equity initiatives often evolve through feedback, adaptation, and multilevel interactions. Complex adaptive systems (CAS) theory, initially proposed by Holland (1992) and further developed in subsequent works (Holland, 1995, 2012), conceptualizes systems as networks of interacting agents, adaptive processes, and evolving boundaries. This theory provides a comprehensive framework for evaluating health equity initiatives within complex social systems. A CAS consists of multiple interacting agents whose collective behavior cannot be fully understood by analyzing components in isolation. CAS theory highlights five characteristics especially relevant for evaluating health equity initiatives: dynamic behavior, massive entanglement, scale independence, transformative change, and emergence (Eoyang & Berkas, 1998).

- *Dynamic Systems.* A CAS is inherently dynamic, operating under conditions of continuous change "driven by the number of agents, their association with their own rules of behavior and the interdependence between the agents and their environments" (Eoyang & Berkas, 1998, p. 4). In health equity initiatives, this dynamism manifests through policy shifts, funding changes, community mobilization, and evolving institutional practices. As a result, evaluators cannot assume that causal pathways remain constant over time. Accordingly, evaluation designs should be adaptive and iterative, supporting ongoing sense-making rather than relying solely on retrospective assessment (Patton, 2011; Preskill et al., 2014). From a network-informed perspective, longitudinal network analysis enables monitoring of changes in relationships and influence patterns, revealing whether interventions enhance adaptive capacity or reinforce existing exclusions.
- *Massively Entangled Systems.* Complex systems are described as "massively entangled," with outcomes resulting from dense interdependencies among actors, variables, and subsystems (Eoyang & Berkas, 1998). Factors such as economic insecurity, housing instability, and access to care (Krieger, 2024; Link & Phelan, 1995) reinforce one another through interconnected pathways. Traditional evaluation methods that isolate variables may overlook these complexities. Embracing network-informed evaluation enables evaluators to examine relationships, resource flows, and coordination patterns across organizations and sectors, further empowering stakeholders to understand and address these entanglements.
- *Scale Independence.* A CAS exhibits scale independence, indicating that similar patterns of interaction and influence occur across multiple levels (Eoyang & Berkas, 1998; Holland, 1992). In health equity contexts, dynamics such as exclusion, trust, and power concentration may operate concurrently at neighborhood, organizational, and system-wide levels. Evaluations limited to a single level risk

misrepresenting mechanisms of change. Complexity-informed evaluation emphasizes cross-scale interactions, acknowledging that changes at one level can amplify or suppress dynamics at another (Rogers, 2008; Westhorp, 2012). Network-informed evaluation facilitates this multilevel analysis by examining relational structures both within and across scales.

- *Transformative Potential.* A CAS has the capacity for transformation because "the interdependent agents of a CAS are transformed and transforming in their interactions" (Eoyang & Berkas, 1998, p. 6). Under specific conditions, systems may reorganize around new norms, roles, or resource flows, resulting in distinct behavioral patterns (Eoyang & Berkas, 1998). In health equity initiatives, transformative change may involve shifts in governance structures, redistribution of decision-making authority, or redefinition of valued knowledge. These changes are often initiated at leverage points, which are strategic locations within a system where small interventions can yield significant effects (Meadows, 1997). Evaluations focused on transformation prioritize identifying and testing leverage points rather than strict adherence to predetermined activities. Network-informed evaluation identifies leverage points by locating actors whose structural positions enable them to influence coordination, information flows, or collective action.
- *Emergent Outcomes.* A CAS is characterized by emergence, in which system-level outcomes arise from interactions among agents and cannot be fully anticipated (Eoyang & Berkas, 1998). Health equity or inequity emerges not from a single policy or program but from patterned interactions embedded within historical and structural contexts (WHO, 2008). This complexity challenges evaluation models that depend on predefined indicators and outcomes. Evaluators must remain attentive to unintended consequences, novel forms of collaboration, and evolving power relations as they emerge (Rogers, 2008). Network-informed evaluation facilitates the study of emergence by revealing relational configurations, such as the formation of new alliances or the increasing centrality of previously marginalized actors, that indicate changes in system behavior.

Network Theory as a Foundation for Network-Informed Complex Evaluation

While complexity theory provides a macro-level framework for understanding dynamic interactions, network theory offers a complementary lens for examining the relational structures that shape outcomes across SEM levels. Network theory emphasizes that an actor's position within a network and the structure of ties among actors determine access to resources, opportunities, and power (Scott & Carrington, 2011). SNA operationalizes network theory by providing rigorous methodological tools for mapping, measuring, and interpreting relational patterns (Borgatti et al., 2024; Wasserman & Faust, 1994). For NCE, this capacity is transformative because SNA makes relational inequities visible, quantifiable, and actionable. By uncovering structural barriers embedded in social and organizational systems, network-informed evaluation provides the evidence needed to design interventions that address inequitable relational patterns.

SNA provides an analytical toolkit for conceptualizing inequity as a relational phenomenon that can be observed, measured, and transformed. By embedding network theory within its framework, NCE positions itself to intervene at the relational level, both within and across social–ecological levels. Key concepts that inform this approach are examined in detail in Chap. 3.

How Network-Informed Complex Evaluation Meets Challenges of Complexity

SDOH emerge from interactions among individuals, organizations, communities, and policy systems, all of which operate at interdependent, multilevel social–ecological levels (McLeroy et al., 1988; WHO, 2008). These systems exhibit CAS characteristics, including distributed agency, nonlinearity, feedback, adaptation, and the emergence of system-level patterns that cannot be understood by examining isolated components (Holland, 1992; Plsek & Greenhalgh, 2001). NCE addresses these challenges by structuring evaluative inquiries around the structural, relational, adaptive, and dynamic properties of social systems. Table 1.3 and the subsequent section present common analytical challenges in CAS: sense-making in dynamic systems, managing interdependence, identifying leverage points in scale-independent systems, interpreting emergence, and facilitating transformation. Each challenge is contextualized within CAS theory, the social–ecological model (SEM), and SDOH, with corresponding implications for network-informed evaluation.

Challenge 1: Sense-Making in Dynamic and Uncertain Systems

CASs evolve continuously as agents respond to internal feedback mechanisms and external social drivers (Eoyang & Berkas, 1998; Holland, 1992). In systems addressing SDOH, these drivers include policy reforms, economic conditions, labor and housing markets, and institutional priorities, all of which shape the ongoing evolution of system behavior (WHO, 2008). These factors reshape relationships, incentives, and resource distributions, making program contexts inherently dynamic. Consequently, evaluation practitioners and decision-makers encounter persistent sense-making challenges: they must interpret emerging patterns, understand the persistence of specific outcomes, and make decisions while navigating interactions between local actions and broader structural forces (Snowden & Boone, 2007). This makes it difficult to see what is changing, why it matters, and how to respond in practice.

Table 1.3 Analytical challenges in complex adaptive systems (CAS) and corresponding network-informed evaluation responses

Analytical Challenge	CAS Principle	Implications for SEM–SDOH Analysis	Network-Informed Evaluation Response
Sense-making under uncertainty	Dynamism and adaptation	Continually shifting social, institutional, and policy environments complicate causal inference and limit the usefulness of linear attribution models.	Supports collective sense-making through iterative relational analysis, tracking evolving patterns of coordination, collaboration, and information exchange across time.
Managing interdependence	Dense interconnection	Actions across individual, organizational, community, and policy domains generate indirect and often unintended system effects.	Maps relational structures to identify structural holes, coordination bottlenecks, and governance misalignments, and assesses network governance configurations.
Identifying leverage points	Scale independence	Structural inequities and coordination dynamics recur across micro-, meso-, and macro-levels of the system.	Identifies high-leverage network positions, brokerage roles, and connectivity patterns that may support strategic intervention across levels.
Interpreting emergence	Emergent patterning	System outcomes arise from distributed interactions rather than centralized control or planned program design.	Detects emergent subgroups, brokerage dynamics, and shifts in network centralization, conceptualizing interventions as events within evolving systems.
Supporting and evidencing transformation	Transformability	Structural change involves shifts in institutional rules, governance arrangements, norms, and power relations shaping social conditions.	Documents network reconfiguration, evolving authority structures, and changes in governance arrangements through longitudinal social network analysis.

Source Author's original synthesis informed by CAS theory and the network evaluation literature (e.g., Holland, 1992; Patton, 2011; Plsek & Greenhalgh, 2001; WHO, 2008)

NCE addresses these challenges by systematically examining the evolution of relationships and interaction patterns over time. By mapping relational structures and tracking network indicators such as connectivity, coordination patterns, influence pathways, and information flows, NCE enables evaluators to observe system dynamics across changing contexts. Longitudinal network analysis reveals shifts in collaboration, leadership, and resource exchange that reflect the system's adaptive responses to internal feedback and external pressures. Through this iterative relational analysis, NCE provides evaluators and decision-makers with a structured approach for interpreting evolving system behavior, supporting ongoing sense-making, and facilitating more adaptive responses to change. In practice, this helps identify where to focus attention and where to adjust responses.

Challenge 2: Managing Interdependence in Massively Entangled Systems

In CASs, agents are interconnected through multiple, interdependent relationships, causing actions in one part of the system to propagate indirect effects throughout the system (Eoyang & Berkas, 1998; Holland, 1992; Plsek & Greenhalgh, 2001). In systems that address SDOH, health outcomes are co-produced by interconnected sectors such as education, housing, employment, transportation, and governance. Although these systems operate with distinct mandates, their interactions generate shared consequences that shape population health and equity (Marmot et al., 2008). This interdependence poses a challenge for evaluation because outcomes cannot be attributed to isolated programs or sectors; instead, they emerge from dynamic interactions among actors and institutions, which evaluators must capture.

NCE addresses this challenge by conceptualizing relationships as mechanisms that shape system behavior and outcomes. Through network analysis, evaluators map collaboration patterns, governance arrangements, power distributions, and resource flows among actors and organizations. This analysis enables the identification of structural holes, coordination bottlenecks, and governance misalignments that influence how actors interact within the system. By examining these relational structures over time, NCE helps evaluators understand how interdependencies facilitate coordination, enable resource exchange, or constrain collective action across sectors.

Challenge 3: Identifying Leverage in Scale-Independent Systems

Scale-independent, or scale-free, patterns refer to the tendency of complex systems to exhibit similar structural features across multiple levels (Barabási, 2002; Eoyang & Berkas, 1998). In systems addressing SDOH, inequitable distributions of power, resources, and opportunities often occur at individual, organizational, community, and policy levels (Krieger, 2012). Because these patterns operate across scales, evaluating change at only one level may overlook how dynamics at other levels reinforce or constrain system behavior.

NCE addresses this challenge by examining relational structures across social–ecological levels. Using network analysis, evaluators identify structural features such as centrality, brokerage, marginalization, and bottlenecks that shape the flow of information, influence, and resources. By mapping relationships among individuals, organizations, coalitions, and institutions, NCE reveals how similar structural dynamics reproduce coordination challenges or inequities across scales. This multi-level perspective allows evaluators to identify leverage points where strategic changes in relationships or connectivity can generate disproportionate system-wide effects.

Challenge 4: Interpreting Emergence in Complex Systems

Emergence refers to system-level patterns or behaviors that arise from the cumulative effects of local interactions among agents and cannot be fully explained by the intentions or actions of individual actors or programs (Eoyang & Berkas, 1998; Holland, 1992). Within initiatives addressing the SDOH, emergent phenomena may include the spontaneous formation of informal referral networks, the development of shared norms within cross-sector coalitions, or the creation of adaptive service pathways that were not explicitly planned during program design. These outcomes result from ongoing interactions among organizations, community members, and institutions in dynamic environments.

Because emergent outcomes result from distributed interactions rather than discrete interventions, they challenge traditional evaluation approaches that emphasize attribution to individual programs or actors. Instead, evaluators must attend to how system responses evolve through patterns of interaction and adaptation. Recognizing and interpreting emergence, therefore, shifts the focus of evaluation from attributing outcomes to isolated interventions to understanding the adaptive responses of complex systems and the generative mechanisms through which change unfolds (Hawe et al., 2009; Patton, 2011, pp. 126–131).

NCE addresses this challenge by examining patterns of relationships and interactions within the system. Through network analysis and systematic observation of relational structures over time, NCE enables evaluators to identify emerging configurations of collaboration, information exchange, and resource flows. Changes in network structure, such as the formation of new clusters, bridging relationships, or informal coordination pathways, may indicate the development of new system-level behaviors. By documenting the evolution of these relational dynamics, NCE facilitates the interpretation of emergence as an inherent system property, offering insights into adaptive responses and the generative mechanisms that drive change.

Challenge 5: Enabling Transformation in Complex Adaptive Systems

Transformation constitutes a qualitatively distinct process within complex systems, distinct from both emergence and routine adaptation. Walker et al. (2004) define transformability as "the capacity to create a fundamentally new system when ecological, economic, or social (including political) conditions make the existing system untenable" (p. 8). Chaffin et al. (2016) further emphasize that transformation involves establishing new feedback mechanisms, governing rules, and institutional arrangements that reconfigure system structure and function.

NCE enables evaluators to document such transformation by directly linking longitudinal network change to structural reorganization and institutional change over time. Longitudinal network analysis allows evaluators to map evolving relationships among actors, resources, and institutions and to identify shifts in network structure, including the emergence of new actors, the formation of new connections, and the reconfiguration of governance arrangements and authority structures. These changes signal the development of new pathways for coordination, resource exchange, and decision-making. By tracking how incremental relational changes accumulate into broader structural reorganization, NCE provides empirical evidence of transformability within complex systems.

What Is Network-Informed Complex Evaluation?

In this book, Network-Informed Complex Evaluation is defined as follows:

> Network-Informed Complex Evaluation (NCE) is a systematic evaluation method that integrates network analysis and complexity theory to assess how relational structures, interactions, and system dynamics influence program implementation and outcomes in complex systems. NCE conceptualizes change as emerging through networks of actors operating across multiple social-ecological levels and employs network-informed methods to assess program readiness, refine program theory, and analyze relational mechanisms of change. By illuminating how context, power, and interdependence influence program processes and outcomes, NCE enables evaluators to identify structural relationships that sustain inequities and generate evidence to inform adaptive decision-making and system transformation.

NCE advances program evaluation by integrating insights from CAS, SNA, and SEM into a coherent evaluative framework. Each of these perspectives contributes a distinct analytical lens for understanding programs operating in complex environments. CAS emphasizes the adaptive, nonlinear, and emergent characteristics of complex systems. SNA provides conceptual and methodological tools to examine relational structures and interaction patterns among actors. SEM situates these dynamics within interconnected social–ecological levels that influence individual, organizational, community, and policy processes. For instance, in a youth program, informal peer hubs within schools (SNA) can reorganize and adjust their influence as new challenges arise (CAS), with these adaptations occurring across the school environment, family engagement, and evolving policy expectations (SEM). Collectively, these perspectives demonstrate that program outcomes emerge not solely from discrete activities but through interaction patterns among actors embedded within broader social systems.

Within this framework, evaluation extends beyond measuring program outputs and outcomes to analyzing the relational and structural conditions through which change occurs. Applying NCE involves examining how actors, organizations, and institutions connect within networks and how these relationships influence collaboration, information exchange, and resource flows across systems. Evaluators map relational networks across social–ecological levels, analyze structural configurations shaping system behavior, and identify leverage points for systemic change. This approach facilitates assessment of how relational and structural forces enable or constrain opportunities, affect the distribution of power and resources, and influence program implementation and impacts.

By situating program evaluation within the broader networked systems in which interventions operate, NCE provides a framework for generating evidence that informs contextually responsive and adaptive interventions. Consequently, NCE reframes program evaluation from assessing isolated interventions to understanding how relational dynamics and system structures shape the emergence of program outcomes within complex social systems. This perspective enhances evaluators' capacity to support learning, guide adaptive decision-making, and contribute to systemic efforts promoting equity and sustainable social change.

Positioning the Evaluator in Network-Informed Complex Evaluation

NCE requires a redefinition of the evaluator's role. Within CASs, evaluators serve as interpreters of system patterns and engage with evolving networks of actors whose interactions generate system-level outcomes across individual, organizational, community, and policy levels. Rather than acting as designers of change or system managers, evaluators are positioned as methodologically disciplined interpreters of system behavior. Their primary responsibility is to produce credible, theory-informed explanations of how relational dynamics influence outcomes over time. The evaluator's role encompasses three interrelated functions: interpreting system dynamics, analyzing interdependence and governance, and identifying strategic leverage and system constraints.

- *Evaluators as Interpreters of System Dynamics.* Dynamic systems challenge the assumption that causal mechanisms and contextual conditions remain sufficiently stable to support linear inference (Plsek & Greenhalgh, 2001). Among SDOH systems, ongoing policy changes, funding instability, institutional turnover, and social inequities continually reshape the context for interventions (WHO, 2008). In such environments, evaluators facilitate collective sense-making by enabling system actors to interpret emerging behavioral patterns and changes. Rather than treating emergence as unexpected variation, NCE evaluators examine how adaptive interactions and evolving relationships generate system-level change over time. System actors engage in a learning process by drawing on insights from sense-making to adjust strategies and refine intervention approaches. NCE evaluators design inquiries that emphasize relational dynamics and temporal change rather than static indicators. They maintain analytic independence by treating sense-making as evidence-informed interpretation, not consensus-building or facilitation.

- *Evaluators as Analysts of Interdependence and System Governance.* NCE evaluators play a critical role in revealing interdependence within systems. By treating relationships as analytic units, evaluators can examine patterns of collaboration, governance structures, power distributions, and resource flows that shape system performance. This approach shifts the evaluative focus from organizational outputs to the analysis of how collective arrangements enable or constrain action. This role is consistent with realist and system-oriented evaluation traditions that emphasize mechanisms embedded in social relationships rather than focusing solely on program activities (Pawson & Tilley, 1997; Williams & Hummelbrunner, 2010). Instead of prescribing governance solutions, evaluators generate evidence about the functioning of existing governance and network configurations, thereby enabling system actors to make informed decisions regarding coordination and alignment.
- *Evaluators as Identifiers of Leverage Points and System Constraints.* NCE evaluators enhance strategic focus by identifying leverage points and structural constraints within relational structures. By analyzing factors such as centrality (how connected an actor is within the network), brokerage (the ability of an actor to connect otherwise disconnected parts), marginalization (actors who are on the periphery and may have less influence), and bottlenecks (points where flow is restricted within the system), evaluators determine where minor changes in relationships or governance arrangements may produce significant system-level effects and where structural barriers may limit collaboration or system performance. In this context, the evaluator's role remains analytic rather than prescriptive. Leverage is conceptualized as a hypothesis supported by network evidence and theory, not as a guaranteed outcome. This approach keeps the evaluation focused on where change may matter most and increases the strategic utility of findings.

Situating Network-Informed Complex Evaluation within Established Evaluation Theories

Evaluation is a dynamic field shaped by ongoing methodological debates and evolving theoretical perspectives that respond to increasing demands for scientific rigor, inclusivity, and contextual relevance. Early traditions emphasized experimental and quasi-experimental designs to establish credibility and causal validity. Later developments introduced participatory and empowerment-oriented approaches to enhance stakeholder engagement and promote equity. Within this context, NCE builds on foundational evaluation principles and introduces a relational perspective as its core contribution. Table 1.4 summarizes the conceptual relationships and shows how NCE interacts with established evaluation traditions. The following discussion elaborates on these relationships by examining how NCE aligns with and extends several influential evaluation approaches.

- *NCE and Theory-Driven Evaluation.* Chen (1990, 2005, 2014) argued that evaluation should be grounded in theories of change that clarify how interventions are expected to achieve outcomes. Building on this perspective, NCE situates interventions within dynamic networks. Programs are not viewed as isolated inputs that produce predictable outputs but as embedded within relational environments that shape outcomes over time. This approach expands theories of change by emphasizing how interactions at the individual, organizational, community, and policy levels influence program results.
- *NCE and Utilization-Focused Evaluation.* Patton (2008) argued that evaluation should be assessed by the usefulness of its findings to intended users. NCE aligns with this principle and extends it by incorporating network perspectives. This approach provides stakeholders with insights into partnership functioning, communication breakdowns, and exclusion from decision-making or resource allocation. These relational diagnostics are both informative and actionable, enabling coalitions to restructure their collaboration. NCE expands utilization-focused evaluation by redefining 'use' to include the transformation of network structures.
- *NCE and Equity-Focused Evaluation.* Equity-focused evaluation has highlighted systemic inequities and sought to reveal them through disaggregated outcome data (Thomas & Madison, 2010). NCE complements this approach by shifting attention from outcomes alone to the relational structures that perpetuate inequity: *Who influences decision-making? Which organizations hold disproportionate power? How are resources and information distributed in ways that reinforce or challenge exclusion?* From a relational perspective, NCE positions equity as both a diagnostic focus and a transformative opportunity.
- *NCE and Complexity-Oriented Approaches.* NCE is closely aligned with complexity-oriented evaluation approaches. System-informed evaluation emphasizes feedback loops and nonlinear dynamics (Gates et al., 2021); in contrast, NCE addresses these elements through relational analysis. Developmental evaluation prioritizes adaptability (Patton, 2011), whereas NCE identifies relational mechanisms that either facilitate or impede adaptation. Realist evaluation aims to determine what works, for whom, under which conditions, and why (Pawson & Tilley, 1997). NCE shares this explanatory objective but focuses its analysis on relational mechanisms.

Table 1.4 situates NCE within the broader evaluation landscape by comparing it with several influential evaluation approaches. NCE advances these approaches by introducing a relational perspective that highlights patterns of interaction, influence, and exclusion as central to evaluative inquiry. From this perspective, programs and policies are not isolated interventions producing outcomes independently; instead, they are activities embedded within networks of relationships that shape the circulation of resources, information, authority, and opportunities over time. Analyzing these relational structures enables evaluators to move beyond assessing intervention success toward understanding how collaboration, coordination, and power dynamics influence both effectiveness and equity.

Table 1.4 Positioning network-informed complex evaluation (NCE) in relation to established evaluation approaches

Evaluation Approach	Core Emphasis	Strengths	Limitations for Addressing Complexity and Health Equity	How NCE Extends the Approach
Theory-driven evaluation	Development and testing of explicit theories of change linking interventions to outcomes (Chen, 1990, 2005, 2014).	Strengthens explanatory power by clarifying causal pathways and mechanisms.	Often privileges linear and individual-level mechanisms, potentially oversimplifying complex relational contexts.	Embeds theories of change within dynamic, multilevel relational networks, highlighting relational mechanisms of connection, exclusion, and influence shaping outcomes.
Utilization-focused evaluation	Designing evaluations to maximize use by intended users (Patton, 2008).	Ensures stakeholder relevance and adaptability across diverse contexts and decision-making needs.	May underspecify relational and structural barriers that shape whether use actually occurs.	Enhances utility by making otherwise invisible relational dynamics visible (e.g., influence patterns, gaps, and exclusion), enabling stakeholders to act collectively and strategically.
Equity-focused evaluation	Intentionally foregrounding inequities and justice in the design and interpretation of evaluations (Mertens, 2008; Thomas & Madison, 2010).	Aligns evaluation practice with ethical and justice commitments while making disparities visible.	Often emphasizes outcome disparities without systematically diagnosing the relational processes that reproduce inequities.	Introduces a network perspective revealing how inequities are generated and sustained through organizational and social structures, highlighting pathways for systemic change.
Systems- and complexity-informed evaluation	Drawing on systems thinking and complexity science to guide evaluation as adaptive, relational, and emergent rather than linear (Gates et al., 2021; Renger, 2022).	Elevates systems and complexity perspectives in evaluation and encourages shifts toward learning and adaptive judgment.	Applications vary widely; evaluators may struggle to operationalize complex concepts, set system boundaries, or link equity to relational mechanisms.	Operationalizes systemic perspectives by mapping network structures and interactions, making interdependencies empirically observable and actionable.

(continued)

Table 1.4 (continued)

Evaluation Approach	Core Emphasis	Strengths	Limitations for Addressing Complexity and Health Equity	How NCE Extends the Approach
Developmental evaluation	Supporting innovation and adaptation in emergent and rapidly changing contexts (Patton, 2011).	Provides real-time, iterative feedback that facilitates learning and responsiveness.	Strong in supporting adaptive learning but less diagnostic in explaining why particular adaptations succeed or fail.	Adds network-based relational diagnostics that clarify the structural conditions enabling or constraining adaptation within evolving networks.
Realist evaluation	Identifying context–mechanism–outcome configurations to explain what works, for whom, and under what conditions (Pawson & Tilley, 1997).	Provides strong explanatory depth by integrating contextual sensitivity with causal reasoning.	Mechanisms are often conceptualized as individual causal processes rather than relational or structural dynamics.	Illuminates relational mechanisms and network configurations (e.g., bridging actors, exclusionary clusters, network position) that shape outcomes.

Source Author

By emphasizing relational dynamics as the primary unit of analysis, NCE integrates methodological rigor, practical utility, and explicit value commitments into a coherent framework for evaluating complex systems. Network analysis and relational methods make systemic interdependencies empirically observable while also addressing the ethical and political dimensions of evaluation practice. In doing so, NCE complements existing approaches by enhancing their capacity to diagnose structural barriers, identify leverage points for change, and facilitate collective learning within multilevel systems. More broadly, advancing evaluation practice in contexts characterized by complexity and persistent inequities requires not only methodological innovation but also a reconceptualization of causality, collaboration, and system change.

Chapter Summary

This chapter established the normative and conceptual foundation of NCE by demonstrating how dominant evaluation paradigms often fall short in advancing health equity within complex social systems. Drawing on evaluation scholarship, the chapter examined the widespread reliance on linear logic models, technocratic measurement traditions, and donor-driven accountability frameworks. While these approaches support methodological standardization and performance monitoring, their assumptions of causal linearity, contextual stability, and evaluator neutrality constrain inquiry and obscure the dynamic interactions, feedback processes, and power relations that shape health outcomes.

In response to these limitations, the chapter introduced NCE as a complexity-responsive alternative grounded in CAS theory. CAS concepts, including emergence, nonlinearity, and adaptation, were integrated with complementary frameworks to capture the multidimensional nature of health inequities. The SDOH framework was used to situate inequities within broader political and material contexts, while the SEM provided a structure for analyzing interactions across individual, organizational, community, and policy levels. SNA was incorporated to examine relational structures, influence pathways, and resource flows within these interconnected systems. Through this synthesis, inequity was reconceptualized as an emergent property arising from interactions among actors and institutions embedded in complex systems.

A central contribution of the chapter is the reframing of relationships as the primary unit of analysis. Networks are conceptualized as structural configurations that shape access to resources, information, and decision-making power, revealing mechanisms of inclusion and exclusion that affect health outcomes. The chapter further explores the epistemological and ethical implications of complexity-informed evaluation, positioning evaluators as embedded actors whose positionality influences inquiry, interpretation, and application of findings. This raises a reflective question about the evaluator's position within a network and its impact on the interpretation of results and stakeholder engagement. Reflexivity, transparency, and sustained stakeholder engagement are identified as essential conditions for methodological rigor in complex evaluation contexts. By emphasizing complexity, relationality, and structural context as core analytic commitments, This chapter establishes the intellectual foundation for the NCE framework. Chapter 2 builds on this foundation by elaborating the integrated theoretical framework underpinning NCE and extending it across social–ecological levels.

Reflection Questions

1. How have your beliefs about rigor, validity, evidence, and evaluator neutrality shaped your approach to establishing evaluation criteria? When applying these criteria, which perspectives have been prioritized, marginalized, or excluded from the definition of knowledge?
2. How has the distribution of power among funders, implementers, policymakers, and community members shaped your evaluation questions? How has this dynamic affected your selection of methods and criteria for credible evidence?
3. In what ways have standardized or quantitative metrics limited your methodological ability to recognize the influence of relationships on marginalized groups or to identify the structural factors and patterns of exclusion affecting them?

Applied Activities

Scenario: A multisector community health initiative aims to improve food security and access to preventive care in a large metropolitan area. This initiative integrates community-based organizations, public health agencies, clinical providers, and local food distributors. Given the fluid policy and economic environment, the initiative was designed to support continuous learning and adaptation rather than a fixed implementation. Midway through implementation, several contextual disruptions occurred:

- A major federal funding stream was reduced.
- Local housing policy reforms modified eligibility criteria for supportive services.
- A newly elected municipal administration shifted budget priorities toward public safety.
- Economic instability increased community demand for services.

Service delivery continued; however, outcome indicators, such as food access rates, preventive visit completion, and referral follow-through, fluctuated unpredictably. Stakeholders disagreed over interpretation: some argued that the initiative was losing effectiveness, while others maintained that the volatility in outcomes reflected contextual turbulence rather than program decline. The primary users of this evaluation (e.g., initiative leadership, funding agencies, and local policymakers) must decide whether to scale, pivot, or suspend specific components. The evaluator is responsible for measuring performance and interpreting system behavior under stress.

Activity: This case raises a central evaluative question: when outcomes fluctuate in unstable environments, how can evaluators distinguish failure from adaptation? As you develop an evaluation strategy to interpret evolving system dynamics, consider the following:

- Which relationships and coordination patterns warrant examination? Consider connections that influence resource flow, decision authority, and access, especially those that may reinforce or disrupt structural privilege affecting historically excluded groups.
- Which relational or governance indicators might signal adaptive reconfiguration, such as redistribution of coordination roles, increased cross-sector reciprocity, emergence of new problem-solving routines, or other specific signs of adaptation?
- How can evaluators differentiate temporary disruption from meaningful system adjustment? When formulating criteria, explicitly define equity thresholds and decision rules. For example:
  - Do fluctuations widen or narrow racialized disparities in access?
  - Are historically marginalized groups disproportionately affected during periods of volatility? If so, does that indicate failure or a need to adapt the intervention?
  - Do adaptive responses redistribute burdens or benefits within the system?
- Which forms of repeated measurement, event logging, and structured reflection would enable interpretation over time rather than reliance on single-point performance assessments, and which adaptive signals should these methods track?

References

Alkin, M. C. (2004). *Evaluation roots: Tracing theorists' views and influences* (1st ed.). Sage Publications.

Bakewell, O., & Garbutt, A. (2005). *The use and abuse of the logical framework approach: A review of international development NGOs' experiences*. Swedish International Development Cooperation Agency.

Barabási, A. L. (2002). *The new science of networks*. Perseus.

Berkman, L. F., & Glass, T. (2000). Social integration, social networks, social support, and health. In L. F. Berkman & I. Kawachi (Eds.), *Social Epidemiology*. Oxford University Press. https://doi.org/10.1093/oso/9780195083316.003.0007

Borgatti, S. P., Everett, M. G., Johnson, J. C., & Agneessens, F. (2024). Analyzing social networks (3rd ed.). Sage Publications Ltd.

Braveman, P., Arkin, E., Orleans, T., Proctor, D., Acker, J., & Plough, A. (2018). What is health equity? *Behavioral Science & Policy, 4*(1), 1–14. https://doi.org/10.1177/237946151800400102

Bronfenbrenner, U. (1979). *Ecology of human development: Experiments by nature and design* (1st ed.). Harvard University Press.

Centers for Disease Control and Prevention. (2024, May 15). *Social determinants of health*. U.S.. https://www.cdc.gov/about/priorities/why-is-addressing-sdoh-important.html.
Chaffin, B. C., Garmestani, A. S., Gunderson, L. H., Benson, M. H., Angeler, D. G., Arnold, C. A., & Cosens, B., Craig, R. K., Ruhl, J. B., & Allen, C. R. (2016). Transformative environmental governance. *Annual Review of Environment and Resources, 41*(1), 399–423. https://doi.org/10.1146/annurev-environ-110615-085817
Chambers, R. (1997). *Whose reality counts?* Intermediate Technology Publications.
Chelimsky, E., & Shadish, W. R. (Eds.). (1997). *Evaluation for the 21st century: A handbook*. Sage.
Chen, H. (1990). Theory-driven evaluations. *Sage*. Publications.
Chen, H. T. (2005). *Practical program evaluation: Assessing and improving planning, implementation, and effectiveness*. Sage.
Chen, H. T. (2014). *Practical program evaluation: Theory-driven evaluation and the integrated evaluation perspective*. Sage Publications.
Edwards, M., & Hulme, D. (1996). Too close for comfort? The impact of official aid on nongovernmental organizations. *World Development, 24*(6), 961–973. https://doi.org/10.1016/0305-750X(96)00019-8
Eoyang, G., & Berkas, T. (1998). Evaluation in Complex adaptive system. In M. Lissack & H. Gunz (Eds.), *Managing complexity in organizations*. Quorum Books.
Gates, E. F., Walton, M., Vidueira, P., & McNall, M. (2021). Introducing systems- and complexity-informed evaluation. *New Directions for Evaluation, 2021*(170), 13–25. https://doi.org/10.1002/ev.20466
Greenhalgh, T., Robert, G., Macfarlane, F., Bate, P., & Kyriakidou, O. (2004). Diffusion of innovations in service organizations: Systematic review and recommendations. *The Milbank Quarterly, 82*(4), 581–629. https://doi.org/10.1111/j.0887-378X.2004.00325.x
Hawe, P., Shiell, A., & Riley, T. (2009). Theorising interventions as events in systems. *American Journal of Community Psychology, 43*(3–4), 267–276. https://doi.org/10.1007/s10464-009-9229-9
Hahn, R. A. (2021). What is a social determinant of health? Back to basics. *Journal of Public Health Research, 10*(4). https://doi.org/10.4081/jphr.2021.2324
Healthy People 2030. (n.d.). *Social determinants of health*. Office of Disease Prevention and Health Promotion. https://health.gov/healthypeople/objectives-and-data/social-determinants-health
Holland, J. H. (1992). Complex adaptive systems. *Daedalus, 121*(1), 17–30. http://www.jstor.org/stable/20025416
Holland, J. H. (1995). *Hidden order: How adaptation builds complexity*. Addison-Wesley.
Holland, J. H. (2012). *Signals and boundaries: Building blocks for complex adaptive systems* (1st ed.). MIT Press. https://doi.org/10.7551/mitpress/9412.001.0001
House, E. R., & Howe, K. R. (1999). *Values in evaluation and social research* (1st ed.).
Krieger, N. (2012). Methods for the scientific study of discrimination and health: An Ecosocial approach. *American Journal of Public Health (1971), 102*(5), 936–944. https://doi.org/10.2105/AJPH.2011.300544
Krieger, N. (2024). *Epidemiology and the People's health: Theory and context* (2nd ed.). Oxford University Press. https://doi.org/10.1093/oso/9780197695555.001.0001
Link, B. G., & Phelan, J. (1995). Social conditions as fundamental causes of disease. *Journal of Health and Social Behavior, 35*, 80–94. https://doi.org/10.2307/2626958
Low, B. J., & Low, M. D. (2006). Education and education policy as social determinants of health. *AMA Journal of Ethics, 8*(11), 756–761. https://doi.org/10.1001/virtualmentor.2006.8.11.pfor1-0611
Marmot, M., Friel, S., Bell, R., Houweling, T. A. J., & Taylor, S. (2008). Closing the gap in a generation: Health equity through action on the social determinants of health. *The Lancet, 372*(9650), 1661–1669.
Marmot, M., & Wilkinson, R. (Eds.). (2005). *Social determinants of health*. Oup Oxford.

McLeroy, K. R., Bibeau, D., Steckler, A., & Glanz, K. (1988). An ecological perspective on health promotion programs. *Health Education Quarterly, 15*(4), 351–377. https://doi.org/10.1177/109019818801500401

Meadows, D. (1997). Places to intervene in a system. *Whole Earth, 91*(1), 78–84.

Merry, S. E. (2011). Measuring the world: Indicators, human rights, and global governance. *Current Anthropology, 52*(S3), S83–S95. https://doi.org/10.1086/657241

Mertens, D. M. (2008). *Transformative research and evaluation.* Guilford Press.

Patton, M. Q. (2008). Utilization-focused evaluation. *Sage.* publications.

Patton, M. Q. (2011). *Developmental evaluation: Applying complexity concepts to enhance innovation and use.* Guilford Press.

Pawson, R., & Tilley, N. (1997). *Realistic evaluation.* Sage.

Plsek, P. E., & Greenhalgh, T. (2001). Complexity science: The challenge of complexity in health care. *BMJ, 323*(7313), 625–628. https://doi.org/10.1136/bmj.323.7313.625

Preskill, H., Cook, J., Mack, K., & Gopal, S. (2014). Evaluating complexity: Propositions for improving practice.

Provan, K. G., & Lemaire, R. H. (2012). Core concepts and key ideas for understanding public sector organizational networks: Using research to inform scholarship and practice. *Public Administration Review, 72*(5), 638–648. https://doi.org/10.1111/j.1540-6210.2012.02595.x

Renger, R. (2022). *System evaluation theory: A blueprint for practitioners evaluating complex interventions operating and functioning as systems.* IAP.

Rogers, P. J. (2008). Using programme theory to evaluate complicated and complex aspects of interventions. *Evaluation, 14*(1), 29–48. https://doi.org/10.1177/1356389007084674

Rossi, P. H., Lipsey, M. W., & Freeman, H. E. (2003). *Evaluation: A systematic approach.* Sage publications.

Schwandt, T. A. (1997). Evaluation as practical hermeneutics. *Evaluation, 3*(1), 69–83. https://doi.org/10.1177/135638909700300105

Schwandt, T. A. (2015). *Evaluation foundations revisited: Cultivating a life of the mind for practice* (1st ed.). Stanford Business Books, an imprint of Stanford University Press. https://doi.org/10.1515/9780804795722

Scott, J., & Carrington, P. J. (2011). The SAGE handbook of social network analysis. *SAGE.* publications.

Snowden, D. J., & Boone, M. E. (2007). A leader's framework for decision making. A leader's framework for decision making. *Harvard Business Review, 85*(11), 68.

Thomas, V. G., & Madison, A. (2010). Integration of social justice into the teaching of evaluation. *American Journal of Evaluation, 31*(4), 570–583. https://doi.org/10.1177/1098214010368426

Valente, T. W. (2010). *Social networks and health: Models, methods, and applications* (1st ed.). Oxford University Press. https://doi.org/10.1093/acprof:oso/9780195301014.001.0001

Walker, B., Holling, C. S., Carpenter, S. R., & Kinzig, A. (2004). Resilience, adaptability and transformability in social–ecological systems. *Ecology and Society, 9(2), Article art5.* https://doi.org/10.5751/ES-00650-090205

Walton, M. (2014). Applying complexity theory: A review to inform evaluation design. *Evaluation and Program Planning, 45*, 119–126. https://doi.org/10.1016/j.evalprogplan.2014.04.002

Wasserman, S., & Faust, K. (1994). *Social network analysis: Methods and applications.* Cambridge University Press.

Weiss, C. H. (1998). *Methods for studying programs and policies.* Wiki-Devel. Sugarlabs.

Westhorp, G. (2012). Using complexity-consistent theory for evaluating complex systems. *Evaluation, 18*(4), 405–420. https://doi.org/10.1177/1356389012460963

Whitehead, M. (1992). The concepts and principles of equity and health. *International Journal of Health Services, 22*(3), 429–445. https://doi.org/10.2190/986L-LHQ6-2VTE-YRRN

Whitman, A., De Lew, N., Chappel, A., Aysola, V., Zuckerman, R., & Sommers, B. D. (2022). Addressing social determinants of health: Examples of successful evidence-based strategies and current federal efforts. *Off Heal Policy, 1*, 1–30.

WHO Commission on Social Determinants of Health, & World Health Organization. (2008). *Closing the gap in a generation: Health equity through action on the social determinants of health: Commission on social determinants of health final report*. World Health Organization.
Williams, B., & Hummelbrunner, R. (2010). *Systems concepts in action: A practitioner's toolkit* (1st ed.). Stanford University Press. https://doi.org/10.1515/9780804776554
Woulfe, J., Oliver, T. R., Zahner, S. J., & Siemering, K. Q. (2010). Multisector partnerships in population health improvement. *Preventing Chronic Disease, 7*(6), A119.

Chapter 2
Theoretical Foundations of Network-Informed Complex Evaluation

Introduction

Health outcomes are determined by structural differences in resources, exposures, and opportunities, rather than by individual choices alone. These systemic factors prompt critical evaluative questions: *Who benefits from existing arrangements? Who controls resource allocation? Who bears the disadvantages?* Addressing these questions requires a framework that clarifies how structural inequities are produced and maintained. The social-ecological model (SEM) provides such a lens by organizing social determinants of health (SDOH) across nested levels: individual, organizational, community, and policy (Bronfenbrenner, 1979). Although SEM is effective for mapping determinants, it does not capture the dynamic processes and interdependencies among them. Consequently, an analytical approach is needed to reveal the flows of resources, opportunities, and power, and to identify opportunities to reconfigure these flows to advance health equity. Social network analysis (SNA) fulfills this need by making visible the relational structures—such as trust, collaboration, referrals, and influence—through which resources and norms circulate (Borgatti et al., 2024; Wasserman & Faust, 1994). By quantifying both network structures (e.g., density, modularity, centralization) and positions (e.g., centrality, brokerage, structural holes), SNA enables evaluators to understand how relationships shape opportunities and outcomes.

However, networks are embedded within broader systems that exhibit nonlinear, often unpredictable behavior. Health systems and communities can be conceptualized as complex adaptive systems (CAS), in which diverse actors interact, adapt, and generate emergent outcomes (Greenhalgh & Papoutsi, 2018; Mitchell, 2009; Plsek & Greenhalgh, 2001). Unlike traditional linear models, which assume a cause-and-effect relationship, CAS theory accounts for the complexity of real-world interactions in which outcomes are not simply the sum of their parts, highlighting the significance of historical context, path dependence, and local dynamics. This complexity calls for adaptive rather than prescriptive interventions. Integrating network theory and CAS

L. Zhang, *Network-Informed Complex Evaluation*,
https://doi.org/10.1007/978-3-032-27495-3_2

within SEM enables evaluators to move beyond mechanistic or reductionist models toward more context-sensitive approaches.

To facilitate this integration, the Network-informed Complex Evaluation (NCE) is introduced. Recognizing the static limitations of SEM, NCE intentionally integrates SEM with network and CAS theories to address these constraints. This synthesis supports a dynamic and adaptive approach to health equity. The NCE framework bridges theoretical gaps by introducing network-informed measures to advance equity in health outcomes. At each SEM level, NCE (1) justifies the classification of the level as a CAS, (2) identifies the most applicable SDOH, and (3) links relevant theories to network measures. As networks adapt and evolve, NCE connects dynamic network interactions with adaptive systems, demonstrating how emerging patterns can reveal hidden equity challenges. Evaluators using NCE are encouraged to identify key network actors, foster adaptive relationships, and continuously measure network dynamics to inform social programs.

Conceptual Foundations

The NCE framework employs a network-informed approach by integrating SEM, CAS theory, and SNA to evaluate health programs. This integration allows evaluators to examine how dynamic, nonlinear, and adaptive interactions among individuals, organizations, communities, and policy actors shape emergent outcomes and influence health equity.

While SEM provides a well-established multilevel framework for understanding how health outcomes emerge from interactions across levels, traditional approaches often lack analytical tools to operationalize these cross-level dynamics. NCE addresses this limitation by applying SNA to map and assess interdependencies across SEM levels. This operationalization of SEM provides evaluators with diagnostic and explanatory tools to capture the inherent multilevel complexity of social systems, ultimately helping address cross-level misalignments and reduce health disparities. Incorporating CAS theory, the NCE framework further advances evaluation by operationalizing principles such as emergence, feedback, and adaptation. Integrating network analysis within this context enables evaluators to observe the evolution of interaction patterns, the formation of coalitions and norms, and the influence of feedback loops on system adaptation. This multilevel, system-oriented approach is essential for understanding and mitigating structural inequities in complex social systems.

Figure 2.1 and Table 2.1 present the integration of key theoretical and methodological components within the NCE framework. Figure 2.1 conceptualizes health equity as an emergent property resulting from interconnected relational systems that operate as complex adaptive systems. Individual, organizational, community, and policy networks represent distinct yet interdependent domains through which health-related behaviors, practices, norms, and policies arise from ongoing social interactions. Feedback loops reinforce structural patterns across these domains, while adaptive learning processes allow the system to evolve in response to changing conditions. Within the context of SDOH, these interacting networks shape dynamic pathways that either sustain health inequities or promote equity. Table 2.1 integrates complexity theory, social–ecological perspectives, and SNA to align CAS principles across individual, organizational, community, and policy levels. Instead of viewing these levels as discrete or hierarchical, the table conceptualizes them as dynamically interconnected domains where relational processes influence patterns of behavior, coordination, and governance.

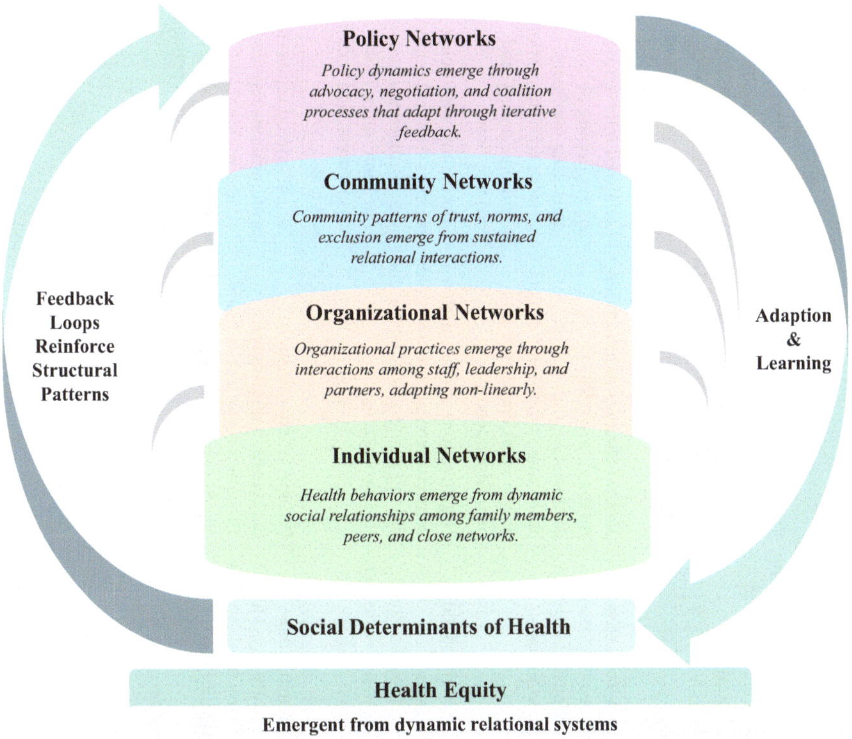

Fig. 2.1 Network-informed complex evaluation (NCE) framework. The figure presents author's conceptual framework showing how health equity emerges from interactions across individual, organizational, community, and policy networks

Table 2.1 Conceptual alignment of complex adaptive systems (CAS) principles across socio–ecological levels and implications for network-informed evaluation

CAS principles	Individual	Organizational	Community	Policy
Emergence	Health behaviors emerge from patterned interaction within ego-centered networks (family, peers, caregiving ties)	Organizational routines, norms, and cultures self-organize through repeated interaction among staff, leadership, clients, and partners	Collective phenomena such as trust, solidarity, stigma, and exclusion emerge from self-organizing patterns of community interaction	Policy agendas and outcomes emerge through iterative negotiation and coalition formation among political actors and institutions
Dynamics (nonlinearity and adaptation)	Minor shifts in trust, stigma, or peer reinforcement may generate nonlinear changes in behavioral trajectories	Modest changes in leadership, funding, or workforce composition may trigger cascading institutional effects due to interdependence and path dependency	Localized interventions may trigger tipping points, generating nonlinear network reconfiguration of coalitions, norms, and resource flows	Incremental policy adjustments may generate disproportionate and unintended system-wide consequences through feedback amplification
Embeddedness (cross-level interdependence)	Individuals are embedded within overlapping interpersonal, organizational, and institutional networks that shape constraints and opportunities	Organizations operate within dense interorganizational fields linking funders, regulators, and service systems	Community well-being emerges from entangled systems that span housing, education, safety, the environment, and social services	Policy processes are embedded in multilevel governance networks spanning local, national, and transnational domains
Scale-independent patterning	Micro-level interactional norms recursively reproduce macro-level structural patterns such as inequality and exclusion	Patterns of coordination, brokerage, and resource allocation recur across teams, organizations, and sectors	Neighborhood relational configurations replicate broader regional and structural inequalities and exhibit scale-independent properties	Governance dynamics exhibit recurring configurations of influence, brokerage, and coalition alignment across institutional scales

(continued)

Table 2.1 (continued)

CAS principles	Individual	Organizational	Community	Policy
Transformative feedback	Individuals adapt relational strategies in response to social feedback, reinforcing or disrupting prevailing behavioral norms	Organizational policies and practices evolve in response to feedback from clients, partners, and regulatory environments	Crises, mobilization, or investment generate feedback loops that reshape the structures of inclusion, resilience, and opportunity	Policies evolve through feedback from implementation, public response, and political cycles
Network-informed evaluation implications	Map ego networks of support, influence, and stigma; assess homophily, social reinforcement, opinion leadership, and behavioral diffusion	Identify boundary spanners, brokers, structural holes, redundancy, resilience, and practice diffusion	Map bonding and bridging ties, coalition structures, hidden brokers, structural holes, fragmentation, and network resilience	Analyze influence networks, advocacy coalitions, gatekeepers, agenda-setting dynamics, and structurally absent actors

Note This table reflects the author's conceptual synthesis informed by established literature on complex adaptive systems, social–ecological models, and social network analysis.
Source Author

Network-Informed Complex Evaluation at the Individual Level

Addressing health equity at the individual level requires integrating theoretical perspectives with the principles of the CAS and SDOH. This section synthesizes how key theories, such as social support, social positioning, and the diffusion of innovations, intersect with CAS principles to shape health outcomes through dynamic network processes. The overview below clarifies these conceptual linkages and provides a practical foundation for translating theory into measurable network constructs at the individual level.

Individual Level as a Complex Adaptive System

Figure 2.1 and Table 2.1 illustrate that programs at the individual-level function as CASs. Health behaviors emerge from continuous, dynamic interactions within ego networks comprising family, peers, mentors, and caregiving relationships. These networks demonstrate CAS properties, including adaptability, interconnectivity, and variability. Minor relational changes, such as the emergence of stigma, erosion of trust, or introduction of peer support, can generate nonlinear and disproportionate effects on health behaviors.

Individuals adapt their behaviors in response to social feedback, creating iterative feedback loops that may strengthen resilience or increase vulnerability (Cohen & Wills, 1985; Umberson & Karas Montez, 2010). This adaptive process is fundamental to complex systems, as new behavioral patterns arise from local interactions. Individual networks are situated within and shaped by broader organizational, community, and policy systems, exemplifying the CAS principle of nested, multilevel systems and contextual dependencies. Inequities arise when power imbalances or resource limitations within individual networks result in unequal access to support, resources, and information, reflecting the CAS principle of emergent outcomes. To fully understand these networks, it is essential to examine social ties, map feedback loops, identify key opinion leaders and connectors, and trace the diffusion of behaviors within individual-level networks.

Linking Network-Informed Complex Evaluation to Individual-Level Theories

Table 2.2 provides a conceptual mapping of individual-level theoretical perspectives using network analysis, connecting major theories to their associated measurements and network indicators. The table demonstrates how constructs such as social support, social positioning, and exposure to innovation are operationalized through

Table 2.2 Individual-level theories interpreted through network analysis

Theory	Focus	Measurements	Network indicators
Social support theory	Embedded supportive resources within personal networks	Ego network composition; types of social ties; perceived and received support	Ego network size; proportion of supportive alters; ego network density; support network diversity
	Network access and potential buffering capacity	Structure and reach of the ego network	Effective network size; structural constraint; access to nonredundant alters; isolation risk
Social positioning theory	Relational position and influence within social structures	Network location; positional advantage within the network	Degree centrality; betweenness centrality; eigenvector centrality
	Inclusion, exclusion, segregation, and stratification in networks	Group membership patterns and relational similarity	Homophily; assortativity; E–I index; patterns of same-group and cross-group ties
Diffusion of innovations	Exposure to innovations through social networks	Proximity to adopters; peer influence pathways	Number of adopting neighbors; network distance to early adopters
	Adoption dynamics over time	Temporal exposure to innovations within evolving networks	Cumulative exposure to adopters; adoption thresholds; timing to adoption relative to network peers

Note This table reflects the author's synthesis of individual-level theoretical perspectives and their operationalization through social network analysis, informed by literature on social support, social positioning, and diffusion of innovations (e.g., Bourdieu, 2018; Centola, 2010; Cohen & Wills, 1985; Gottlieb, 1981; Harré & van Langenhove, 1999; House, 1983; McPherson et al., 2001; Rogers, 1981; Valente, 2010).
Source Author

observable network structures and relational patterns. This mapping underscores the importance of network-informed approaches in translating abstract theoretical concepts into empirically measurable relational configurations.

Social Support Theory at the Individual Level

Social support theory asserts that social relationships function as embedded resources that enhance health by providing emotional, informational, and instrumental support, as well as by mitigating the adverse effects of stress (Cohen & Wills, 1985; Gottlieb, 1981; Hall & Wellman, 1985; House, 1983). Empirical evidence demonstrates that these supportive resources are not merely individual-level attributes but are fundamentally structured within social networks. The availability, structure, and quality of social ties are critical determinants of access to health-related support and influence individuals' coping capacities when facing stressors (Gottlieb, 1981; Heaney & Israel, 2008).

SNA operationalizes these theoretical concepts by linking social support theory to measurable network properties. Supportive resources are assessed through ego network composition, which encompasses the number and types of social ties that provide emotional, informational, and instrumental support, as well as the density and redundancy of these relationships. Structural indicators—such as ego network size, network constraints, and effective size—measure network access and buffering capacity by evaluating the breadth of available support, the degree of structural limitations from interconnected ties, and access to nonredundant support sources. These metrics facilitate rigorous assessment of whether individuals occupy network positions that enable adequate support during stress or, conversely, increase the risk of social isolation and limited coping resources. This analytic framework identifies individuals or groups with sparse, highly constrained, or excessively redundant networks, which may diminish buffering capacity even when social ties exist. Furthermore, it guides the development of interventions that increase the quantity of social support and optimize network configurations to improve access to diverse, practical support.

Social Positioning Theory at the Individual Level

Social positioning theory asserts that individuals' relative locations within socially organized systems determine their access to voice, influence, and opportunity, independent of the specific resources exchanged through social ties. The theory conceptualizes social life as constituted by positioning processes, whereby individuals are organized into differentiated roles, statuses, and locations within communities and institutions (Harré & van Langenhove, 1999; Lawson, 2022). These positions generate structural consequences by conferring distinct rights, obligations, and capacities for action. As a result, they shape whose perspectives are acknowledged, whose actions are valued, and whose participation is marginalized. Substantial research has demonstrated that demographic and social attributes, such as race, gender, language, disability status, and social class, systematically influence these positioning processes, resulting in persistent patterns of inclusion, exclusion, and stratification across social domains (Bourdieu, 2018; Phelan et al., 2010).

With network-informed evaluation, social positioning theory redirects attention from the mere existence of social ties to the relational positions individuals occupy within networks. The NCE framework operationalizes this perspective by utilizing SNA to assess how demographic characteristics and institutional contexts predict positional advantages or disadvantages. Network measures such as degree centrality, betweenness centrality, and eigenvector centrality identify individuals who are most frequently consulted for opinions, who serve as brokers connecting otherwise disconnected groups, and who acquire influence through proximity to other highly central actors. These positions shape access to information flows, agenda-setting capacity, and opportunities for leadership or recognition (Burt, 1992; Freeman, 1979).

Social positioning theory contends that inequality is sustained not only by individual attributes but also by patterns of relational inclusion and exclusion. The NCE framework investigates these dynamics using measures (e.g., homophily, assortativity, and the external–internal index) to assess whether ties are concentrated within socially similar groups or bridge differences in status, race, gender, or role. Elevated levels of homophily and network segmentation signal structurally embedded barriers to cross-group interaction, restricting exposure to influential actors and reinforcing peripheral positions for marginalized groups (McPherson et al., 2001). From a social positioning perspective, these patterns demonstrate how community structures are organized, with access to valued positions regulated by formal and informal mechanisms of gatekeeping, norms, and institutionalized expectations (Lawson, 2022).

Diffusion of Innovation at the Individual Level

Diffusion of innovations theory describes how new ideas, practices, or interventions disseminate through social systems over time. Social exposure, perceived attributes of the innovation, and individual adoption thresholds influence this process (Rogers, 1981; Rogers et al., 2014). The theory asserts that diffusion is inherently relational, as the likelihood of adoption depends on social connections, information flow within networks, and the timing and intensity of exposure to adopting peers. Empirical studies indicate that social networks shape not only awareness of innovations but also normative pressure, information credibility, and perceptions of risk and legitimacy, all of which influence adoption dynamics across populations. Network pathways, such as the shortest path to early adopters, are critical in understanding how innovations spread through social ties.

In network-based evaluation frameworks, diffusion of innovations theory identifies patterns of exposure and the relational pathways through which innovations spread. The NCE framework applies SNA to assess individuals' proximity to adopters and their embeddedness within diffusion pathways. The key indicators include the shortest path distance to innovators or early adopters, the number and characteristics of adopting alters, and the overall network distance to influential nodes. These measures reveal differences in exposure to innovation-related information and social influence, enabling the identification of individuals who are structurally positioned to encounter innovations early, compared with those who are more distant and less likely to adopt without targeted intervention (Valente, 2010).

Diffusion theory also examines the temporal dynamics of adoption, recognizing that individuals vary in their readiness to adopt and often require cumulative exposure to reach a behavioral threshold. The NCE framework incorporates longitudinal network measures to assess cumulative exposure, observed adoption thresholds, and the timing of adoption relative to peers. These indicators allow evaluators to differentiate among early, intermediate, and late adopters, identify tipping points where adoption accelerates within subgroups, and determine whether diffusion occurs through contagion, reinforcement, or clustered uptake (Centola, 2010; Rogers et al., 2014).

Network-Informed Complex Evaluation at the Organizational Level

At the organizational level, the NCE framework draws on established theories of change, implementation, governance, and structuration to explain how health equity is shaped within and across institutions. By leveraging network analysis, the NCE framework translates abstract theoretical concepts such as organizational readiness for change, implementation context, network governance, and structuration into measurable network constructs. The following overview clarifies these connections and offers a foundation for translating theory into measurable network constructs at the organizational level.

Organizational Level as a Complex Adaptive System

As illustrated in Fig. 2.1 and Table 2.1, organizations exemplify CAS characteristics through the dynamic, interdependent interactions among staff, leadership, and partner organizations. These interactions continuously generate and modify practices, norms, and service delivery patterns. A defining CAS principle—nonlinearity—is evident in how minor changes, such as shifts in leadership, funding, or workforce composition, can trigger organizational adaptation, producing outsized and sometimes unpredictable effects on policies and services (Damschroder et al., 2009; Weiner, 2020).

Organizations are highly adaptive, respond to client, regulatory, and external pressures, and coevolve alongside broader systems of funding, accreditation, and workforce development. This adaptation occurs through feedback loops, allowing organizations to learn, self-organize, and reconfigure routines in response to changing environments. Institutional histories and governance structures further shape organizational responses, demonstrating the CAS principle of path dependence and historical contingency.

Linking Network-Informed Complex Evaluation to Organizational-Level Theories

Table 2.3 operationalizes organizational-level theoretical perspectives through network analysis by linking major theories to corresponding measurements and network indicators. It shows how concepts such as organizational readiness for change, interorganizational governance, and routine enactment can be examined via observable network structures and relational dynamics. These structures encompass patterns of advice and trust among staff, whole-network configurations across organizations, and interaction networks that coordinate workflow. This mapping demonstrates that organizational processes and governance arrangements can be analyzed as measurable relational patterns within network-based evaluations.

Organizational Readiness for Change at the Organizational Level

Organizational readiness for change refers to a collective psychological state among organizational members, characterized by a shared commitment to implementing change and collective efficacy in its execution (Weiner, 2020). From a network perspective, readiness is therefore more than the aggregation of individual attitudes or formal leadership endorsement; it can emerge through organizational patterns of interaction, trust, and influence that shape how members understand and support change. Research on organizational readiness further indicates that implementation is shaped not only by resources but also by motivational readiness, staff attributes, and organizational climate, such that weaknesses across these dimensions can impede organizational change (Lehman et al., 2002; Weiner, 2020).

The NCE framework operationalizes the relational foundations of readiness by employing network analysis to examine advice-seeking and trust networks within organizations. These networks show who exchanges change-related information, whose expertise is considered credible, and who serves as an informal leader. These elements are essential for mobilizing collective action during program implementation. Indicators, including advice-seeking patterns, trust ties among staff, and the presence of informal leaders, allow evaluators to determine whether readiness is broadly distributed or concentrated among a limited subset of actors.

Interorganizational Network Governance at the Organizational Level

Interorganizational network governance theory examines how collective action among autonomous organizations is coordinated through distinct governance forms, including shared governance, lead-organization governance, and network-administrative organization governance (Provan & Kenis, 2008). These arrangements differ systematically in the distribution of authority, decision-making, and accountability, which influence coordination, efficiency, legitimacy, and equity. The literature

Table 2.3 Organizational-level theories interpreted through network analysis

Theory	Focus	Measurements	Network indicators
Organizational readiness for change	Relational foundations of readiness	Advice and trust networks among organizational members	Patterns of advice-seeking; trust ties among staff; high-centrality actors in advice or trust networks
	Distributed agency and influence	Central actors and positional influence in organizational networks	Degree, betweenness, and eigenvector centrality of change champions and skeptics; network centralization or dispersion of influence
	Emergent readiness dynamics	Temporal evolution of relational ties and influence structures	Shifts in centrality over time; changes in advice or trust ties; diffusion or convergence of readiness perceptions
Interorganizational network governance	Governance structure	Whole-network structure and configuration among organizations	Network centralization; network density; presence of hubs; core–periphery structure
	Coordination and control mechanisms	Subgroup, coalition, and brokerage structures among participating organizations	Cliques; cohesive subgroups; dense connectivity among highly central organizations
	Fit between structure and context	Structural alignment between governance form and coordination processes	Alignment of governance form (centralized, shared, lead organization) with coordination patterns and collaborative performance
Structuration theory	Routine enactment of organizational practices	Interaction networks embedded in daily coordination processes	Meeting, communication, and workflow networks; repeated coordination patterns

(continued)

Table 2.3 (continued)

Theory	Focus	Measurements	Network indicators
	Bottlenecks and vulnerability in coordination	Flow structures and positional dependence	Bottleneck positions; high-betweenness actors; delays or disruptions in workflow handoffs
	Equity and resilience in routine practices	Differential access to information and participation in coordination processes	Unequal participation in decision-making networks; disparities in information flow; concentration of workload or decision authority

Note This table reflects the author's synthesis of organizational-level theoretical perspectives and their operationalization through social network analysis, informed by literature on organizational readiness for change, interorganizational network governance, and structuration theory (e.g., Colizza et al., 2006; Giddens, 1984; Lehman et al., 2002; Provan & Kenis, 2008; Provan & Milward, 1995; Weiner, 2020).
Source Author

indicates that no single governance form is universally optimal; instead, effectiveness depends on the alignment between governance structure and contextual factors such as network size, trust, goal consensus, and task complexity (Provan & Kenis, 2008).

Building on this governance perspective, the NCE framework operationalizes governance structure by employing whole-network social network analysis to examine network configuration, utilizing indicators such as network centralization, hub-and-spoke arrangements, and core–periphery structures. These measures determine whether coordination and influence are concentrated within a dominant organization or distributed among network members. NCE further evaluates coordination and control mechanisms through subgroup analyses, identifying cliques, cohesive subgroups, and rich-club connectivity. Rich-club connectivity describes patterns in which highly connected organizations preferentially form ties among themselves (Colizza et al., 2006). Although these configurations can enhance strategic coordination among powerful actors, they may also marginalize smaller or less resourced organizations.

NCE underscores the importance of aligning governance structure with contextual factors by linking structural indicators to performance outcomes, including resource acquisition, service integration, and client impact. Research has demonstrated that interorganizational effectiveness relies not only on individual organizational capacity, but also on the structure and management of networks as systems (Provan & Milward, 1995). By systematically applying network metrics, evaluators can identify bottlenecks, dependency risks, and misalignments between governance forms and stated equity or coordination objectives. This approach yields actionable insights for governance redesign and network improvement.

Structuration Theory at the Organizational Level

Structuration theory offers a dynamic view of how organizational structures are continually reproduced and transformed through everyday practices. The central concept, the duality of structure, asserts that organizational rules, routines, and resources shape action, while those actions, in turn, sustain or modify the structures that guide future behavior (Giddens, 1984). In organizational contexts, this perspective focuses analytic attention on routine interactions, including meetings, workflows, handoffs, and collaborative problem-solving, as primary sites where structure is enacted and change becomes possible.

The NCE framework translates structuration processes into measurable constructs by applying social network analysis to map interaction networks that reflect routine enactment, such as meeting participation, workflow connections, and repeated coordination patterns. These networks illustrate how work is accomplished and frequently reveal informal structures that differ from formal organizational charts. Indicators, including interaction frequency and stability, enable evaluators to assess whether routines are resilient, overly centralized, or dependent on a small number of individuals.

Building on structuration theory's attention to the reproduction and transformation of organizational practices, NCE examines potential bottlenecks and vulnerabilities via positional and flow-based measures such as betweenness centrality and bottleneck analysis. Nodes with high betweenness may indicate critical coordination roles but can also represent single points of failure where overload or disruption could affect the entire organization. NCE applies this analysis to issues of equity and resilience in organizational routines by examining who takes part in decisions, where information flows are uneven, and where workload or authority is concentrated. Monitoring these patterns over time allows evaluators to determine whether organizational routines perpetuate inequities or evolve to support more inclusive, resilient, and adaptive organizational forms.

Network-Informed Complex Evaluation at the Community Level

At the community level, the NCE framework operationalizes key theories of social change by integrating social network analysis to clarify how relationships, influence, collaboration, and participation shape health outcomes. Through this integration, abstract concepts such as the diffusion of innovations, social capital, collective impact, and empowerment are translated into measurable patterns within community networks. The following overview clarifies these connections and illustrates how NCE can guide evaluation at the community level.

Community Level as a Complex Adaptive System

As illustrated in Fig. 2.1 and Table 2.1, communities exhibit CAS characteristics through the interplay of historical legacies and ongoing interactions that give rise to trust, solidarity, and exclusion (Holland, 1992, 1995; Sampson, 2012). Key CAS principles are observed at this level: communities exhibit nonlinearity, as small-scale initiatives can trigger ripple effects across broader systems, producing often unpredictable and transformative outcomes (Byrne & Callaghan, 2014). Crucially, health outcomes at the community level are not isolated phenomena; instead, they are deeply interconnected with other domains, including housing, education, the environment, and public safety (Diez Roux, 2007). This reflects the CAS principle of interdependence, in which changes in one sector can produce intended and unintended consequences across the system. For evaluation scholars, assessing communities as CASs demands attention to both network structures and the lived experiences of community members. SNA offers a powerful lens for mapping patterns of collaboration, pinpointing hidden brokers, highlighting marginalized groups, and uncovering potential network actors that may reinforce stigma or misinformation (Burt, 2004; Provan et al., 2005; Valente, 2010).

Linking Network-Informed Complex Evaluation to Community-Level Theories

Table 2.4 presents the operationalization of community-level theoretical perspectives through network analysis by mapping major theories to their corresponding measurements and network indicators. It highlights how concepts such as diffusion processes, social capital, and cross-sector collaboration can be examined through observable network structures and relational dynamics within communities. Through this mapping, the table illustrates how community-level processes can be analyzed as measurable relational patterns.

Diffusion of Innovations at Community Level

Diffusion of innovations theory explains the dissemination of new ideas, practices, or technologies within communities as a function of social exposure, communication pathways, and normative influences embedded in social systems (Rogers, 1981; Rogers et al., 2014). At the community level, diffusion does not follow a linear or uniform trajectory. Instead, adoption occurs through relational mechanisms such as social contagion, reinforcement, and threshold dynamics, producing nonlinear patterns, such as tipping points, cascades, and clustered uptake (Valente, 2010). Community norms, trust in information sources, and the influence of opinion leaders

Table 2.4 Community-level theories interpreted through network analysis

Theory	Focus	Measurements	Network indicators
Diffusion of innovations	Exposure and spread of behaviors	Relational proximity to adopters in community networks	High-centrality opinion leaders; number or proportion of adopting alters; network distance to adopters
	Network contagion and adaptation	Diffusion patterns across network structures	Clustering of adopters; sequential or staged diffusion across connected groups
	Communication pathways	Communication networks; bridging ties, and brokerage structures	Communication ties among community actors; bridging paths between clusters; bottlenecks in diffusion pathways
Social capital theory	Network cohesion and connectivity	Overall structure of community interaction networks	Network density; network size; component structure and connectedness
	Bonding and bridging resources	Composition and diversity of ties	Bonding, bridging, and linking ties; cross-group connections; structural holes
	Trust and reciprocity	Relational exchange patterns	Reciprocal ties; mutual support relationships; repeated exchanges
Collective impact	Cross-sector collaboration structure	Interorganizational network structure and configuration	Central coordinating organizations (backbone organizations); network centralization in coordination

(continued)

Table 2.4 (continued)

Theory	Focus	Measurements	Network indicators
	Alignment and coordination	Flow of collaboration across sectors	Frequency and direction of collaborative ties; coordination pathways
	Distributed agency	Role differentiation, brokerage, and leadership distribution among participating organizations	Central versus peripheral organizations; brokerage roles; centralization or redundancy of leadership roles

Note This table reflects the author's synthesis of community-level theoretical perspectives and their operationalization through social network analysis, informed by literature on diffusion of innovations, social capital, and collective impact (e.g., Hanleybrown et al., 2012; Kania & Kramer, 2013; Kawachi & Berkman, 2000; Lin, 2001; Putnam, 2000; Rogers, 1981, 2014; Szreter & Woolcock, 2004; Valente, 2010; Woolcock, 1998).
Source Author

are essential in determining whether innovations diffuse widely, remain localized, or fail to spread.

The NCE framework uses network analysis to operationalize community-level diffusion by examining how exposure and behavioral spread occur through relational proximity to adopters. Key indicators include the presence and position of opinion leaders, the number of alternatives adopted within individuals' networks, and the shortest-path distance to early adopters or innovators. These measures capture variation in exposure to innovation-related information and social influence, distinguishing community members who are structurally positioned to adopt early from those who are more isolated or peripheral.

NCE also examines network contagion and adaptation by analyzing adoption patterns in relation to network structure. Indicators such as the clustering of adopters, sequential or staged adoption across connected groups, and the emergence of adoption waves reveal whether diffusion occurs within tightly knit subgroups, across bridges between clusters, or through the broader community. Furthermore, NCE assesses communication pathways by identifying key communication ties, bridging paths between clusters, and bottlenecks that constrain diffusion. These analyses allow evaluators to identify leverage points to accelerate the spread of health-promoting practices, such as engaging opinion leaders, strengthening bridging ties, and redesigning communication strategies to address structural barriers within community contexts.

Social Capital Theory at the Community Level

Social capital theory emphasizes the value embedded within social networks, demonstrating how trust, reciprocity, and cooperation facilitate collective action and promote population health and well-being (Kawachi & Berkman, 2000; Lin, 2001). At the community level, social capital is conceptualized as a relational property of social structures rather than solely as an individual resource, shaping access to information, support, and opportunities. Differentiating among bonding, bridging, and linking social capital provides insight into how various network structures can produce both cohesion and exclusion, foster resilience, and perpetuate inequality (Putnam, 2000; Szreter & Woolcock, 2004; Woolcock, 1998).

The NCE framework operationalizes network cohesion and connectivity through whole-network measures, including network density, size, and overall connectedness. These indicators assess the extent to which community members are embedded in shared relational structures that support trust-building, coordination, and mutual aid. Dense networks foster strong norms and collective efficacy, whereas sparse or fragmented networks may limit information flow and collective response capacity.

NCE distinguishes bonding and bridging resources by analyzing the composition and type of ties. Indicators such as bonding versus bridging ties, cross-group connections, and the presence of structural holes reveal whether social capital is concentrated within homogeneous groups or distributed across diverse social boundaries. Although bonding capital reinforces solidarity and mutual support, excessive reliance on inward-facing ties can increase exclusion and limit access to external resources. Conversely, bridging and linking ties connect communities to new information, services, and institutional power, but these ties are often unevenly distributed across social groups.

Collective Impact at the Community Level

The collective impact framework posits that large-scale social change is more likely when diverse stakeholders align around a shared agenda, engage in mutually reinforcing activities, maintain continuous communication, and receive support from backbone organizations that facilitate coordination (Hanleybrown et al., 2012; Kania & Kramer, 2013). At the community level, collective impact initiatives operate as CASs characterized by distributed agency, interdependence, and ongoing adaptation rather than centralized control.

The NCE framework operationalizes cross-sector collaboration by employing social network analysis to examine interorganizational networks within collective impact initiatives. Indicators such as the presence and positioning of backbone organizations, degree of centralization, and core–periphery structure reveal how coordination and influence are distributed among partners. These measures link to the collective impact framework by distinguishing networks that rely on a single coordinating entity from those with more distributed leadership and redundancy.

NCE assesses alignment and coordination by analyzing the flow of collaboration, including the frequency and direction of collaborative ties, as well as the pathways through which information, resources, and decision-making circulate. These indicators reveal whether communication is continuous and bidirectional, as emphasized by the collective impact framework, or fragmented and isolated across sectors. NCE evaluates distributed agency by examining role differentiation and positional patterns, such as the balance between central and peripheral organizations and the degree of leadership role redundancy or concentration. This analysis allows evaluators to identify structural vulnerabilities, such as overreliance on a single backbone organization or missed opportunities for shared leadership. By tracking these network patterns over time, NCE facilitates adaptive learning, strengthens cross-sector partnerships, and enhances the capacity of collective impact initiatives to advance health equity at the community level.

Network-Informed Complex Evaluation at the Policy Level

The NCE framework applies established policy theories to understand health equity at the policy level. By integrating network analysis with the advocacy coalition framework (Weible & Carter, 2024; Zahariadis, 1995) and policy network theory (Enroth, 2011; Rhodes, 1997), NCE equips evaluators to map, measure, and influence the dynamics of policy arenas. Through this integration, network-informed evaluation highlights how determinants of health, such as housing protection, wages, education funding, and civil rights enforcement, are shaped by coalition politics, agenda-setting, and structural access (Baumgartner & Jones, 1993). The overview below synthesizes these theoretical linkages and translates them into measurable network constructs at the policy level.

Policy Level as a Complex Adaptive System

Figure 2.1 and Table 2.1 illustrate that the policy-level functions as a CAS. Knoke (2011) defines a policy network as "a bounded set of actors and one or more sets of relations that connect these actors" (p. 210). Within such networks, public and private actors are linked by relational ties that enable the exchange of information, expertise, trust, and political resources (Kenis & Schneider, 1991). Policy networks are characterized by dynamic, interdependent interactions among diverse actors, including advocates, agencies, and legislators, each pursuing specific interests and employing distinct resources and strategies. These interactions reflect the fundamental principles of CAS. Policy change often occurs nonlinearly; incremental legislative amendments, advocacy initiatives, or shifts in public sentiment can result in significant and unpredictable reforms (Baumgartner & Jones, 1993). Adaptation and emergence are central features of policy systems viewed as CASs, as policies are continually revised in response to public input, judicial decisions, electoral outcomes, and broader socioeconomic developments. These iterative feedback mechanisms ensure that policy both shapes and is shaped by the broader system in which it exists (Ansell & Geyer, 2017; Room, 2011).

For evaluation scholars, viewing policy systems as CASs requires attention to both structural configurations and relational dynamics. Social network analysis provides a robust methodological framework for mapping influence, identifying coalition leaders or veto players, and clarifying the channels through which power and information circulate. This approach also reveals whose perspectives are amplified or marginalized within policy processes (Knoke, 2017; Provan & Kenis, 2008; Rhodes, 2006). Integrating CAS principles with network analysis enables evaluators to identify persistent inequities, pinpoint leverage points for more inclusive governance, and advance equity-driven policy transformation.

Linking Network-Informed Complex Evaluation to Policy-Level Theories

Table 2.5 operationalizes policy-level theoretical perspectives through network analysis, linking major theories to specific network measures. It illustrates how concepts such as advocacy coalitions, policy networks, and access to decision-making arenas can be analyzed through observable network structures and relational dynamics among policy actors. These include patterns of coalition formation and alignment, brokerage and boundary-spanning roles connecting actors and venues, and the distribution of influence within policy networks. This mapping demonstrates that policy processes and governance relationships can be examined as measurable relational patterns within network-based evaluations.

Advocacy Coalition Framework at the Policy Level

The advocacy coalition framework (ACF) conceptualizes policy change as a long-term, collective process shaped by the interactions of competing and cooperating advocacy coalitions within a policy subsystem (Jenkins-Smith & Sabatier, 1994; Jenkins-Smith et al., 2018). These coalitions consist of individuals and organizations from governmental and non-governmental sectors who share core policy beliefs and coordinate actions over extended periods to influence policy agendas, decisions, and implementation. The ACF posits that policy outcomes emerge from coalitional dynamics, including belief alignment, resource mobilization, strategic coordination, and access to institutional venues, rather than from the actions of isolated actors.

The NCE framework operationalizes coalition composition and alignment by employing social network analysis to map coalition structures. Indicators such as

Table 2.5 Policy-level theories interpreted through network analysis

Theory	Focus	Measurements	Network indicators
Advocacy coalition framework	Coalition composition and alignment	Coalition structure and cohesion based on shared policy beliefs	Number and diversity of actors within coalitions; cohesive subgroups aligned by policy beliefs
	Cross-coalition brokerage	Coalition ties; broker positions; bridging actors	Actors linking coalitions (betweenness or brokerage positions); frequency and strength of cross-coalition ties
	Access to decision venues and agenda pathways	Boundary spanning and venue connectivity (including two-mode actor–venue networks where applicable)	Boundary spanners connecting coalitions to decision venues; network distance to agenda-setting actors or venues; multiplex venue participation indicating potential to leverage policy windows
Policy network theory	Structure of policymaking relationships	Overall structure and configuration of policy actor networks	Network density; size and connectedness of policy networks
	Distribution of influence	Positional advantage; centrality and influence distribution	Centrality of actors (degree, betweenness, eigenvector as appropriate); concentration or dispersion of influence (network centralization)
	Access and exclusion in policymaking	Brokerage; structural holes; stakeholder clustering	Brokers connecting otherwise disconnected stakeholder groups; structural holes and gaps in representation; peripheral or isolated stakeholders; clustered subgroups indicating policy subsystem segmentation

Note This table reflects the author's synthesis of policy-level theoretical perspectives and their operationalization through social network analysis, informed by literature on the advocacy coalition framework and policy network theory (e.g., Burt, 2004; Jenkins-Smith & Sabatier, 1994; Jenkins-Smith et al., 2018; Knoke, 2001, 2011; Rhodes, 2006).
Source Author

the number and diversity of actors, the presence of cohesive subgroups, and clustering by shared policy beliefs provide evidence of coalition robustness and internal coordination. These measures enable evaluators to determine whether coalitions are broad-based and cross-sectoral, or narrow and fragmented, and to assess the structural conditions that influence the capacity for sustained and coordinated policy engagement.

ACF scholars emphasize the importance of cross-coalition interactions for policy learning and negotiated change. The NCE framework captures these dynamics by analyzing intercoalition ties and brokerage positions via measures such as betweenness centrality and the frequency of cross-coalition interactions. These indicators identify actors who occupy structural positions that connect competing coalitions, facilitate information exchange, and broker compromise in uncertain contexts without presuming direct influence. The NCE framework further operationalizes access to decision venues and agenda pathways, a core mechanism in the ACF, by mapping boundary-spanning relationships between coalitions and policy venues. Rather than presuming policy impact, NCE provides systematic evidence of differential access and structural opportunities within the policy process.

Policy Network Theory at the Policy Level

Policy network theory investigates the relational structure of policymaking by analyzing how interactions among governmental and non-governmental actors shape information flow, coordination, and access to decision-making processes (Rhodes, 2006). Policy network analysis identifies key actors, including governmental and non-governmental organizations, interest groups, and individuals, within policymaking institutions to explain the structure of their interactions (Knoke, 2011). Five primary types of interorganizational relations characterize policy networks: resource exchange, which establishes and maintains interorganizational connections; information transmission, which encompasses scientific and technical data as well as policy advice and opinions; asymmetrical power relations, which shape interests within policy domains; boundary penetration, where multiple actors coordinate to achieve shared objectives; and sentimental attachments, which foster mutual assistance among actors (Knoke, 2001, 2011). Network analysis examines the social relationships among network members, the overall network structure, and the impacts at both the individual and organizational levels.

The NCE framework utilizes whole-network metrics, including network size, density, and overall connectedness, to operationalize relationships within policymaking systems. These metrics assess whether policy systems are integrated or fragmented, centralized or dispersed, and identify structural features that influence coordination capacity, policy learning, and responsiveness. Policy network theory further examines the distribution of structural advantages within these systems. The NCE framework measures positional characteristics through centrality metrics adapted to the policy context to determine whether coordination and visibility are concentrated among a few actors or more widely distributed. Additionally, the framework employs social network analysis to investigate access and exclusion in policymaking processes. For instance, brokerage measures and the identification of structural holes highlight areas where stakeholder groups are weakly connected or excluded from central policy discussions (Burt, 2004).

Example: Reconceptualizing the BeSD Framework from a Network Perspective

The Behavioral and Social Drivers (BeSD) framework, developed by the World Health Organization (WHO, 2022), provides a comprehensive model for understanding engagement in vaccination and other health-related behaviors. The framework identifies four interrelated domains: thinking and feeling, social processes, motivation, and practical issues. Each domain can be analyzed using network and complexity perspectives. This systemic approach aligns with CAS principles and highlights the structural and relational factors that shape program outcomes. The following section, along with Table 2.6, demonstrates how BeSD domains can be conceptualized as relational processes within a complex system and operationalized through network mechanisms. This perspective supports network-informed evaluation of the emergence, interaction, and evolution of behavioral, social, motivational, and practical drivers across individual, community, organizational, and system levels.

At the individual level, the BeSD domain of thinking and feeling operates within ego networks comprising family members, peers, and health workers. Individuals act as agents whose behaviors are shaped by and shape others in the network through ongoing interactions. Ego networks are dynamic, with relationships and influence pathways evolving. These networks are entangled, as individuals participate in multiple overlapping social contexts, and are scale-independent, since similar trust and influence dynamics occur across households, peer groups, and provider–client relationships. From an evaluation perspective, network analysis is essential for understanding how individual BeSD outcomes result from relational exposure, reinforcement, and feedback, rather than from isolated attitudes.

At the community level, BeSD social processes, including social norms, stigma, inclusion, and provider recommendation, function as collective phenomena within a CAS. Community members, leaders, and providers act as interdependent agents whose behaviors are governed by community rules, such as conformity to perceived norms and responsiveness to respected authorities. Repeated interactions generate emergent normative patterns that may either support or inhibit vaccination. Community systems are entangled, with norms shaped by interpersonal relationships, institutional signals, media narratives, and historical experiences. Network-informed evaluation enables analysis of these social processes as evolving relational patterns, clarifying how norms stabilize, fragment, or shift in response to interventions or contextual changes.

At the organizational level, BeSD's practical issues, such as availability, affordability, accessibility, respectful service, and readiness, reflect the adaptive behavior of service delivery networks. Facilities, outreach teams, supervisors, and partner organizations act as agents whose behaviors are governed by rules of coordination, accountability, resource utilization, and professional norms. These rules are implemented through routine interactions, including referrals, supervision, information sharing, and collaborative problem-solving. Organizational BeSD systems are dynamic, with

Table 2.6 Network- and complexity-informed mapping of the WHO BeSD framework

BeSD domain	Level of analysis	Network focus (what is measured)	Example Hypothesis	Key network constructs	NCE Use
Thinking and feeling (perceived benefits, safety, and trust)	Individual (Ego network)	Trust, advice, and affective-support relationships; credibility of advice	Individuals embedded in larger, more diverse, and trusting networks demonstrate higher confidence, self-efficacy, and perceived behavioral control	Tie strength; size; density; constraint	Assess how confidence and trust diffuse through social ties; identify isolated or low-trust individuals; track strengthening of supportive ties following demand-generation or trust-building interventions
Social Processes (social norms, provider recommendation)	Individual and community	Peer, community, and provider influence, reciprocity, cohesion, stigma, and inclusion patterns	Peripheral or marginalized individuals (low centrality, high homophily) have reduced exposure to credible norms and fewer trusted recommendations	Degree & betweenness centrality, brokerage, homophily/assortativity, E–I index	Diagnose inequities in influence and information flow; design inclusion strategies; monitor diffusion of provider and peer recommendations across subgroups
Motivation (intention, willingness to act)	Individual network	Exposure to early adopters, reinforcement through peers, and social proof	Proximity to early adopters and trusted peers accelerates the formation of intentions, the willingness to act, and the adoption of preventive behaviors	Exposure indices, shortest path length, temporal thresholds	Identify key influencers and early adopters; guide phased or peer-led rollouts; evaluate speed, reach, and saturation of behavioral diffusion

(continued)

Table 2.6 (continued)

BeSD domain	Level of analysis	Network focus (what is measured)	Example Hypothesis	Key network constructs	NCE Use
Access and use (time, availability, respect)	Individual and community	Resource sharing, support exchange, instrumental support, reciprocity, cooperative problem-solving	Reciprocity and triadic closure foster cooperative strategies that overcome time, cost, and access constraints while reinforcing respect-based norms	Reciprocity, triadic closure, temporal motifs, network stability	Detect the emergence of cooperation and norm stabilization; monitor erosion of trust or cooperation; adapt outreach, supervision, or service design
Availability (service presence, hours, staffing, logistics)	Organizational and interorganizational	Coordination network density and governance fit across facilities and sectors	Systems with distributed, reciprocal governance structures exhibit faster response times, fewer bottlenecks, and more equitable service availability	Coordination centralization, density, core–periphery structure	Diagnose coordination gaps; guide the design of shared or network-administrative governance; monitor the responsiveness of scheduling and supply chains
Affordability (costs, transport, opportunity costs)	Organizational & Outer Setting	Cross-sector linkages with non-health actors (transport, schools, employers, local authorities)	Systems with diverse cross-sector partnerships reduce user costs and expand access through multisectoral support	E–I index, participation coefficients, bridging centrality	Track inclusion of non-health actors; evaluate the effectiveness of multisectoral strategies in reducing financial and opportunity barriers

(continued)

Table 2.6 (continued)

BeSD domain	Level of analysis	Network focus (what is measured)	Example Hypothesis	Key network constructs	NCE Use
Accessibility and convenience (distance, waiting time, user flow)	Health system network	Adaptive coordination among facilities, outreach posts, and community health workers (CHWs)	Shorter network paths between service nodes improve access, reduce waiting times, and increase system adaptability	Average path length, modularity, flow efficiency	Assess referral and outreach efficiency; monitor adaptive realignment of service locations, hours, and delivery modalities
Respectful service and dignity (experience, trust)	Organizational (frontline)	Peer, supervisory, and routine interaction networks embedding dignity norms	Cohesive peer and supervisory networks institutionalize respectful and equitable service norms through daily routines	Reciprocity, triadic closure, temporal motifs	Assess staff cohesion and supervision structures; detect stabilization or erosion of respectful-care norms over time
Organizational responsiveness and readiness (learning, adaptation)	Organizational	Feedback loops, learning ties, advice networks, and adaptive learning capacity	Facilities with dense networks of trust and advice adapt faster and respond more effectively to identified access barriers	Advice/trust density, betweenness, temporal evolution	Monitor readiness and responsiveness to feedback; identify leverage points for system learning, supervision, and continuous improvement

Note Table 2.6 presents the author's network- and complexity-informed interpretation of the WHO's BeSD framework (WHO, 2022). It provides an analytic crosswalk between the BeSD framework and a network-informed complex evaluation perspective. It neither reinterprets nor revises the BeSD framework, nor suggests that network measures fully capture the entire range of behavioral determinants encompassed by the framework. Rather, the table translates BeSD domains into relational and system-level mechanisms that can be empirically examined using established network constructs and evaluation methods. This approach offers a structured method for investigating how behavioral drivers are embedded within and influenced by dynamic, multilevel interaction patterns. The table exemplifies how to operationalize theoretical concepts through network analysis and functions as a methodological scaffold for evaluating BeSD within complex systems contexts.
Source Author

roles and relationships adapting to policy changes, resource constraints, and population needs. These systems are highly entangled, as service delivery depends on interdependent actors across sectors, and are transformative because minor changes in coordination or trust can lead to significant changes in service availability or quality. Emergent outcomes, such as sustained respectful care or persistent access bottlenecks, arise from networked interactions rather than from any single organization. Network-informed evaluation allows examination of practical issues as emergent properties of organizational relationships and routines, rather than as static constraints.

At the policy level, BeSD operates within governance, financing, and regulatory frameworks that establish conditions for individual, community, and organizational agents. Policy actors adhere to rules governing incentives, accountability, and compliance, while organizations and communities modify their behaviors accordingly. System behaviors, such as equity in access, responsiveness to feedback, and sectoral fragmentation, arise from the coevolution of policy decisions and implementation realities. These systems are scale-independent, with coordination challenges and trust dynamics recurring at local, regional, and national levels. They are interconnected, as policies interact with social norms, organizational capacity, and political contexts. Moreover, these systems are emergent, with both intended and unintended effects developing over time. Network-informed evaluation thus traces the propagation of policy signals and reveals how feedback loops influence system behavior.

This book integrates the BeSD framework with NCE as an example to support understanding and evaluation of health-related behaviors within complex systems. The BeSD domains are operationalized using network perspectives and applied through chapter activities, illustrative examples, and case-based exercises to demonstrate how behavioral and social drivers emerge from relational processes.

Chapter Summary

This chapter advanced the NCE framework by elaborating its theoretical foundations and operationalizing them across the multiple levels of the SEM. Building on the conceptual critique presented in Chap. 1, this chapter established NCE as an integrated synthesis of SEM, CAS theory, and SNA. This integration moves evaluation beyond static and reductionist paradigms toward a dynamic, relational, and adaptive systems perspective that can better inform the evaluation of contemporary health programs.

The chapter demonstrates that health inequities cannot be understood as isolated or purely individual phenomena. Rather, they emerge from patterned interactions among individuals, organizations, communities, and policy actors within interconnected social systems. These relational structures shape the distribution of resources, authority, and opportunities over time, influencing both program implementation and health outcomes. Within this framework, relationships serve as central analytic elements through which evaluators examine collaboration, coordination, and influence across social–ecological levels.

To translate this theoretical integration into practical evaluation strategies, this chapter applies CAS principles within each level of the SEM. It introduces network constructs as analytical tools for mapping and interpreting flows of information, influence, and material resources across networks. Furthermore, the chapter identifies theoretical perspectives relevant to NCE at each social–ecological level and illustrates their application through a network-informed evaluative framework. By integrating theoretical synthesis with methodological guidance, this chapter establishes the conceptual and analytical connection between the normative foundations presented in Chap. 1 and the structured network-informed evaluation approach developed in Chap. 3.

Reflection Questions

1. After engaging with the theories and frameworks presented in this chapter, which critical questions or uncertainties remain? How do these unresolved issues shape priorities for future research, methodological innovation, or evaluation practices?
2. What new questions, opportunities, or avenues for evaluation inquiry have emerged regarding methodological skills, theoretical knowledge, or advocacy for equity and systems change within the evaluation field?
3. Reflecting on a recent evaluation project, how might integrating the NCE framework reveal previously overlooked dynamics or patterns? How has this theoretical synthesis enhanced your ability to identify emergent properties, feedback loops, or power structures?

Applied Activities

Scenario: A citywide vaccination campaign was implemented to increase adult immunization rates within a socioeconomically diverse urban community. The campaign operated in a complex environment characterized by significant variation in vaccination rates across neighborhoods. Lower uptake was particularly pronounced in communities affected by historical marginalization, limited access to healthcare, and entrenched institutional mistrust. These disparities underscore the need for strategies that address the social and structural determinants of health in urban settings. The campaign engaged a wide range of stakeholders, including public health clinics, federally qualified health centers, faith-based organizations, neighborhood associations, community health workers, informal community leaders, and city health department officials. This multisectoral approach aimed to leverage both formal and informal networks to reach populations with varying levels of trust in the healthcare system and differing access to resources.

Initial outcome data demonstrated moderate increases in overall vaccination rates citywide. However, uptake remained uneven, with persistent disparities in racialized and low-income communities. Vaccine misinformation disseminated through informal community networks undermined public health messaging. The influence of faith leaders was significant but varied: some actively promoted vaccination, while others maintained neutral or skeptical positions, leading to heterogeneous community responses. Furthermore, structural barriers such as limited clinic hours, inadequate transportation, and stringent documentation requirements continued to restrict access to vaccination services in specific neighborhoods.

Activity: This case presents a fundamental evaluation question: How do relational structures across ecological levels facilitate or restrict health behavior within a complex adaptive system? Vaccination uptake is not merely an individual choice; it results from interpersonal trust relationships, organizational partnerships, structural access conditions defined by SDOH, and norm diffusion and feedback mechanisms within the dynamics of complex adaptive systems. In this activity, develop a network-informed evaluation strategy to analyze how these relational structures affect vaccination uptake across the system.

1. Identify at least two drivers influencing vaccination decisions, including but not limited to:
    - Trust in information sources
    - Social influence within faith-based or neighborhood networks
    - Practical access constraints (e.g., transportation, clinic hours)
    - Institutional credibility

For each driver, specify the following:

- At which SEM level it operates
- Whether it reflects relational (network) or structural (SDOH) determinants
- How it may interact with other levels in a CAS framework

2. Using a network-informed evaluation lens, map actors at the following levels:
    - Interpersonal level: trusted messengers, family ties, and peer networks
    - Organizational level: clinics, faith-based institutions, and health departments
    - Community level: neighborhood associations and informal leaders

For each level, specify the following:

- Indicate flows of the information, resources (e.g., mobile clinics, transportation), and influence (norm-setting, endorsement)
- Explain how network position (e.g., central connectors, bridges across groups) operationalizes theoretical constructs such as social capital, diffusion, and institutional trust

3. Select one driver, such as trust in faith leaders or access barriers. Analyze how the current network structure:

- Amplifies or dampens positive norms
- Reinforces or mitigates misinformation
- Concentrates or distributes influence
- Facilitates or constrains equitable access

In CAS terms, consider:

- Feedback loops, such as whether increased uptake strengthens endorsement
- Nonlinearity, including whether small shifts in trusted nodes produce large changes
- Emergent patterns, such as clusters of high or low uptake

4. Propose one adaptive intervention grounded in network theory, for example:
    - Strengthening bridges between skeptical clusters and trusted health actors
    - Diversifying trusted messengers within marginalized neighborhoods
    - Embedding mobile vaccination services within central community hubs

Explain the following:

- How altering network ties may shift diffusion patterns
- How the intervention addresses SDOH barriers
- How it promotes equity by redistributing influence or access
- How it supports adaptation within a complex system

References

Ansell, C., & Geyer, R. (2017). 'Pragmatic complexity' a new foundation for moving beyond 'evidence-based policy making'? *Policy Studies, 38*(2), 149–167. https://doi.org/10.1080/01442872.2016.1219033

Baumgartner, F. R., & Jones, B. D. (1993). *Agendas and instability in American politics*. University of Chicago Press.

Borgatti, S. P., Everett, M. G., Johnson, J. C., & Agneessens, F. (2024). *Analyzing social networks* (3rd ed.). Sage Publications Ltd.

Bourdieu, P. (2018). The forms of capital. In *The sociology of economic life* (pp. 78–92). Routledge.

Bronfenbrenner, U. (1979). *Ecology of human development: Experiments by nature and design* (1st ed.). Harvard University Press.

Burt, R. S. (1992). *Structural holes: The social structure of competition* (1st ed.). Harvard University Press. https://doi.org/10.4159/9780674029095

Burt, R. S. (2004). Structural holes and good ideas. *The American Journal of Sociology, 110*(2), 349–399. https://doi.org/10.1086/421787

Byrne, D., & Callaghan, G. (2014). *Complexity theory and the social sciences: The state of the art* (First Edition.). Routledge.

Centola, D. (2010). The spread of behavior in an online social network experiment. *Science (American Association for the Advancement of Science), 329*(5996), 1194–1197. https://doi.org/10.1126/science.1185231

Cohen, S., & Wills, T. A. (1985). Stress, social support, and the buffering hypothesis. *Psychological Bulletin, 98*(2), 310–357. https://doi.org/10.1037/0033-2909.98.2.310

Colizza, V., Flammini, A., Serrano, M. A., & Vespignani, A. (2006). Detecting rich-club ordering in complex networks. *Nature Physics, 2*(2), 110–115. https://doi.org/10.1038/nphys209

Damschroder, L. J., Aron, D. C., Keith, R. E., Kirsh, S. R., Alexander, J. A., & Lowery, J. C. (2009). Fostering implementation of health services research findings into practice: A consolidated framework for advancing implementation science. *Implementation Science, 4*(1), 50. https://doi.org/10.1186/1748-5908-4-50

Diez Roux, A. V. (2007). Integrating social and biologic factors in health research: A systems view. *Annals of Epidemiology, 17*(7), 569–574. https://doi.org/10.1016/j.annepidem.2007.03.001

Enroth, H. (2011). Policy network theory. In *The SAGE handbook of governance* (pp. 19–35).

Freeman, L. C. (1979). Centrality in social networks: Conceptual clarification. *Social Networks, 1*(3), 215–239.

Giddens, A. (1984). *The constitution of society: Outline of the theory of structuration*. Polity.

Gottlieb, B. H. (1981). *Social networks and social support*. Sage Publications.

Greenhalgh, T., & Papoutsi, C. (2018). Studying complexity in health services research: desperately seeking an overdue paradigm shift. *BMC Medicine, 16*(1), Article 95. https://doi.org/10.1186/s12916-018-1089-4

Hall, A., & Wellman, B. (1985). Social networks and social support. In S. Cohen & S. L. Syme (Eds.), *Social support and health* (pp. 23–41). Academic Press.

Hanleybrown, F., Kania, J., & Kramer, M. (2012). *Channeling change: Making collective impact work* (pp. 56–78). FSG.

Harré, R., & van Langenhove, L. (1999). *Positioning theory: Moral contexts of intentional action*. Blackwell.

Heaney, C. A., & Israel, B. A. (2008). Social networks and social support. *Health Behavior and Health Education: Theory, Research, and Practice, 4*(1), 189–210.

Holland, J. H. (1992). Complex adaptive systems. *Daedalus, 121*(1), 17–30. http://www.jstor.org/stable/20025416

Holland, J. H. (1995). Hidden order: How adaptation builds complexity.

House, J. S. (1983). Work stress and social support. In *Addison-Wesley series on occupational stress*.

Jenkins-Smith, H. C., & Sabatier, P. A. (1994). Evaluating the advocacy coalition framework. *Journal of Public Policy, 14*(2), 175–203. https://doi.org/10.1017/S0143814X00007431

Jenkins-Smith, H. C., Nohrstedt, D., Weible, C. M., & Ingold, K. (2018). The advocacy coalition framework: An overview of the research program. In *Theories of the policy process* (pp. 135–171).

Kania, J., & Kramer, M. (2013). Embracing emergence: How collective impact addresses complexity.

Kawachi, I., & Berkman, L. (2000). Social cohesion, social capital, and health. In L. F. Berkman & I. Kawachi (Eds.), *Social epidemiology*. Oxford University Press. https://doi.org/10.1093/oso/9780195083316.003.0008

Kenis, P. N., & Schneider, V. (1991). Policy networks and policy analysis: Scrutinizing a new analytical toolbox. In *Policy networks: Empirical evidence and theoretical considerations* (pp. 25–59). Westview Press.

Knoke, D. (2001). *Changing organizations: Business networks in the new political economy*. Westview Press.

Knoke, D. (2011). Policy networks. In *The SAGE handbook of social network analysis* (pp. 210–222). SAGE Publications Ltd.

Knoke, D. (2017). Power networks. In *The Palgrave handbook of political elites* (pp. 539–561). https://doi.org/10.1057/978-1-137-51904-7_34

Lawson, T. (2022). Social positioning theory. *Cambridge Journal of Economics, 46*(1), 1–39. https://doi.org/10.1093/cje/beab040

Lehman, W. E., Greener, J. M., & Simpson, D. D. (2002). Assessing organizational readiness for change. *Journal of Substance Abuse Treatment, 22*(4), 197–209. https://doi.org/10.1016/S0740-5472(02)00233-7

Lin, N. (2001). *Social capital: A theory of social structure and action*. Cambridge University Press.

McPherson, M., Smith-Lovin, L., & Cook, J. M. (2001). Birds of a feather: Homophily in social networks. *Annual Review of Sociology, 27*(1), 415–444. https://doi.org/10.1146/annurev.soc.27.1.415
Mitchell, M. (2009). *Complexity: A guided tour*. Oxford University Press.
Phelan, J. C., Link, B. G., & Tehranifar, P. (2010). Social conditions as fundamental causes of health inequalities: Theory, evidence, and policy implications. *Journal of Health and Social Behavior, 51*(1_suppl), S28–S40. https://doi.org/10.1177/0022146510383498
Plsek, P. E., & Greenhalgh, T. (2001). The challenge of complexity in health care. *BMJ, 323*(7313), 625–628. https://doi.org/10.1136/bmj.323.7313.625
Provan, K. G., & Kenis, P. (2008). Modes of network governance: Structure, management, and effectiveness. *Journal of Public Administration Research and Theory, 18*(2), 229–252. https://doi.org/10.1093/jopart/mum015
Provan, K. G., & Milward, H. B. (1995). A preliminary theory of interorganizational network effectiveness: A comparative study of four community mental health systems. *Administrative Science Quarterly*, 1–33. https://doi.org/10.2307/2393698
Provan, K. G., Veazie, M. A., Staten, L. K., & Teufel-Shone, N. I. (2005). The use of network analysis to strengthen community partnerships. *Public Administration Review, 65*(5), 603–613. https://doi.org/10.1111/j.1540-6210.2005.00487.x
Putnam, R. D. (2000). *Bowling alone: The collapse and revival of American community*. Simon & Schuster.
Rhodes, R. A. (1997). *Understanding governance: Policy networks, governance, reflexivity and accountability*. Open University.
Rhodes, R. A. (2006). Policy network analysis. In *The Oxford handbook of public policy* (Vol. 3, pp. 425–447).
Rogers, E. M. (1981). Diffusion of innovations: An overview. In *Use and impact of computers in clinical medicine* (pp. 113–131).
Rogers, E. M., Singhal, A., & Quinlan, M. M. (2014). Diffusion of innovations. In *An integrated approach to communication theory and research* (pp. 432–448). Routledge.
Room, G. (2011). *Complexity, institutions, and public policy: Agile decision-making in a turbulent world*. Edward Elgar Publishing.
Sampson, R. J. (2012). *Great American city: Chicago and the enduring neighborhood effect*. University of Chicago Press.
Szreter, S., & Woolcock, M. (2004). Health by association? Social capital, social theory, and the political economy of public health. *International Journal of Epidemiology, 33*(4), 650–667. https://doi.org/10.1093/ije/dyh013
Umberson, D., & Karas Montez, J. (2010). Social relationships and health: A flashpoint for health policy. *Journal of Health and Social Behavior, 51*(1_suppl), S54–S66. https://doi.org/10.1177/0022146510383501
Valente, T. W. (2010). *Social networks and health: Models, methods, and applications*. Oxford University Press.
Wasserman, S., & Faust, K. (1994). *Social network analysis: Methods and applications*. Cambridge University Press.
Weible, C. M., & Carter, D. P. (2024). Theories of the policy process: Ways to think about them and strategies for teaching with them. In *Handbook of teaching public policy* (pp. 76–91). Edward Elgar Publishing. https://doi.org/10.4337/9781800378117.00015
Weiner, B. J. (2020). A theory of organizational readiness for change. In *Handbook on implementation science* (pp. 215–232). Edward Elgar Publishing. https://doi.org/10.4337/9781788975995
Woolcock, M. (1998). Social capital and economic development: Toward a theoretical synthesis and policy framework. *Theory and Society, 27*(2), 151–208. https://doi.org/10.1023/A:1006884930135

World Health Organization. (2022). *Behavioral and social drivers of vaccination: Tools and practical guidance for achieving high uptake*. World Health Organization. https://iris.who.int/handle/10665/354459. License: CC BY-NC-SA 3.0 IGO.

Zahariadis, N. (1995). Policy change and learning: An advocacy coalition approach. *Policy Studies Journal, 23*(2), 378–383.

Chapter 3
Development of Network-Informed Complex Evaluation

Introduction

Chapters 1 and 2 established that traditional linear models inadequately capture the complexity and interconnectedness inherent in initiatives aimed at advancing health equity. Network-informed complex evaluation (NCE) addresses this limitation by facilitating program evaluation within real-world system contexts. By integrating complex adaptive systems (CAS) theory, the social–ecological model (SEM), and network science, NCE serves as both a conceptual and a practical framework to strengthen program theory and evaluation methods, thereby enhancing the capacity to design effective interventions in complex, multilevel environments. The chapter is organized around several central questions: *What are the core principles of NCE? How can network constructs be operationalized at the individual, community, organizational, and policy levels within NCE? Which evaluation approach can support NCE implementation and enable evaluators to address the complexities of interconnected systems?*

Principles of Network-Informed Complex Evaluation

This section presents the core principles underlying the NCE approach and explains how these principles align with and extend traditional evaluation standards. As shown in Fig. 3.1, the NCE framework organizes evaluation principles into four layers, each building on the previous one.

- *Foundations:* This layer draws upon systems and social–ecological traditions to justify the application of network-informed evaluation in complex environments. Evaluators face a decision point about which systems or social–ecological models to choose, shaping how complexity is interpreted and applied. This choice ensures

L. Zhang, *Network-Informed Complex Evaluation*,
https://doi.org/10.1007/978-3-032-27495-3_3

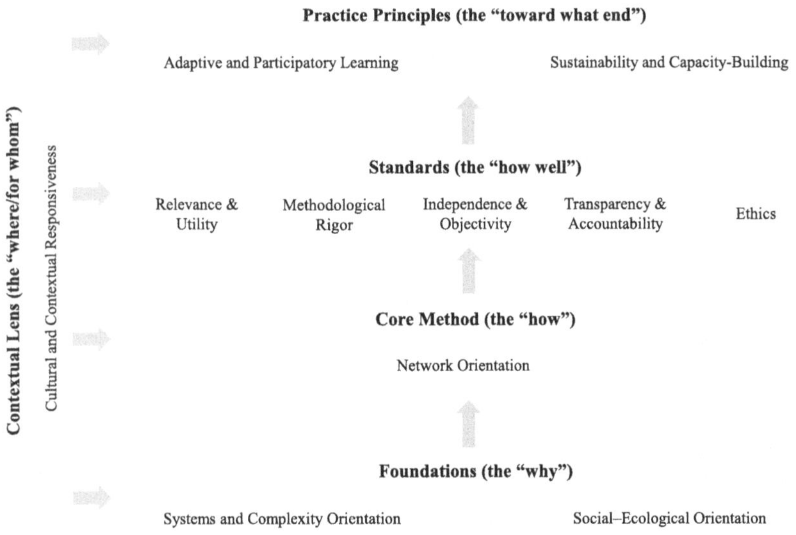

Fig. 3.1 Core principles for network-informed complex evaluation (NCE). *Source* Author

that evaluations align with the broader social and ecological context, enhancing the relevance and applicability of the findings.

- *Core Method:* Emphasizing network orientation shifts the focus from isolated evaluations to the analysis of how interconnected relationships within and across social–ecological levels influence outcomes. A critical decision at this stage involves determining which relational data to collect initially, directly linking theory to practice. Prioritizing the most impactful connections enables evaluators to uncover essential insights that inform evaluation designs and facilitate collaboration with stakeholders.
- *Standards:* This layer ensures evaluations are conducted with rigor, transparency, independence, and ethical integrity. For evaluators, prioritizing standards that govern the rigor and ethical considerations of the evaluation fosters confidence and trust in their work. This alignment with established standards provides confidence in evaluation results and supports stakeholder trust and informed decision-making.
- *Practice Principles:* This upper layer focuses on the evaluation's purposes, highlighting adaptive learning and sustainability as primary objectives. Evaluators determine how to embed adaptive learning to enhance the program's long-term effectiveness.
- *Contextual Lens:* Cultural and contextual responsiveness is integrated throughout all levels, addressing where and for whom evaluations are conducted. Emphasizing such adaptation ensures evaluations accurately represent their environments, promoting meaningful engagement and actionable insights.

Systems and Complexity Orientation

The foundational principle of the NCE is its system- and complexity-oriented approach. Complexity theory asserts that systems consist of interdependent, adaptive, and dynamic elements whose interactions produce outcomes that cannot be predicted or understood by analyzing components in isolation. Outcomes of complex systems emerge from dynamic interactions among system elements rather than from isolated examination of individual components (Byrne & Callaghan, 2014, pp. 1–8). Evaluators must move beyond reductionist input–output models and adopt approaches sensitive to broader, interdependent, and continuously adapting environments in which interventions operate. Evaluation should recognize that interventions are influenced by dynamic relationships, feedback loops, and contextual contingencies that often resist simplistic, linear explanations.

Patton (2011) extends this argument by asserting that, within complex environments, evaluators should facilitate continuous adaptation, promote innovation, and support developmental learning. In this context, evaluation is reconceptualized as an ongoing, generative process that fosters real-time sense-making and iterative decision-making in the face of uncertainty and emergence (Patton, 2011, pp. 124–146). Rogers (2008) reinforces this perspective by noting that causal pathways in complex interventions are rarely linear; rather, they involve multiple, reciprocal, and emergent chains of causation that change over time.

These scholarly perspectives indicate that understanding and evaluating complex initiatives requires a reassessment of both logic models and traditional evidence standards. This approach emphasizes the recognition of evolving patterns, interdependencies, and emergent properties within dynamic systems. Adopting a systems and complexity perspective is fundamental to the NCE methodology, as it is essential for producing robust evaluations that inform practice and support learning amid the complexities of contemporary interventions.

Social–Ecological Orientation

A core principle of NCE is its integration of social–ecological perspectives, which recognize that real-world outcomes are shaped by the dynamic interplay among individuals, relationships, organizations, communities, and policies. Bronfenbrenner (1979) emphasized that "the ecology of human development involves the scientific study of progressive, mutual accommodation between an active, growing human being and the changing properties of the immediate settings in which the developing person lives, as this process is affected by relations between these settings, and by the larger contexts in which the settings are embedded" (p. 21). Likewise, McLeroy et al. (1988) argued that health outcomes are influenced by multiple levels, including intrapersonal, interpersonal, institutional, community, and public policy factors.

Building on these traditions, NCE requires evaluators to examine how networks function across SEM levels and to identify opportunities for system-wide impact. For example, in addressing the opioid overdose crisis, a network-informed evaluation would go beyond mapping connections among patients, emergency responders, and treatment providers at the individual and organizational levels. It would also assess coordination among cross-sector coalitions, city agencies, and policymakers at the community and policy levels to ensure the rapid deployment of naloxone and support for those at highest risk. By illuminating not only who is connected but also how and where collaboration succeeds or breaks down, NCE provides actionable insights to strengthen coordination, address systemic gaps, and improve outcomes. This multilevel, networked approach is essential for tackling complex challenges such as opioid overdose, where the broader context of relationships, organizational practices, and policy environments significantly shapes individual actions.

Network Orientation

NCE employs a network-oriented approach, emphasizing that relationships and connections are central to program outcomes. This perspective rests on the foundational insight that, in social network research, the primary unit of analysis is the relationship between individuals rather than the individual alone (Borgatti et al., 2024). Valente (2010) further explains that networks provide the pathways through which behaviors, attitudes, information, and resources flow and, as such, they can be seen as the infrastructure for the spread of innovations, diseases, health behaviors, and so on (pp. 3–4). By mapping key relational structures such as trust, collaboration, and influence, NCE shows how these connections function as mechanisms of change and levers for program impact. This approach advances the tradition of theory-driven evaluation (Chen, 1990) by clarifying how causal mechanisms are embedded within the network of relationships that comprise a system.

A network perspective also deepens the commitment to equity. NCE challenges evaluators to examine patterns of connection and exclusion by systematically asking: Who is connected? Who is left out? What barriers prevent inclusion? These questions make equity an active, actionable practice within network evaluation. For example, in the opioid overdose crisis, a community health worker may be excluded from decision-making as agencies and stakeholders respond to rising overdoses. As the sole support in a community with significant health needs, this worker faces structural barriers to contributing insights, including limited access to collaborative forums and minimal direct communication with policymakers. This exclusion not only restricts community health workers' ability to offer valuable perspectives but also perpetuates imbalances in resource allocation and responsiveness to urgent public health needs. By illuminating these points of exclusion, NCE prompts concrete actions, such as reallocating resources or revising program guidelines, to foster greater inclusion and ultimately strengthen system effectiveness.

Standards

A core strength of NCE is its direct alignment with the Centers for Disease Control and Prevention's (CDC, 2024) rigorous evaluation standards: relevance and utility, rigor, independence and objectivity, transparency, and ethics. NCE translates each standard into actionable practice, ensuring that these guiding principles are embedded across all aspects of evaluation, as detailed below.

Relevance and Utility

Within NCE, relevance and utility require tailoring evaluation outputs to stakeholders' needs and decision-making timelines. The utilization-focused evaluation tradition asserts that evaluations should be designed for "intended use by intended users" (Patton, 2008, p. 37). NCE evaluators ensure that network maps and relational metrics are not merely technical outputs, but are presented in accessible formats for decision-makers, including narrative summaries, visualizations, and workshops that address strategic and policy implications. Relevance also requires that evaluation questions and data reflect local priorities, cultural norms, and policy environments rather than relying on metrics selected for convenience. This approach enables evaluators to generate outputs that are clear, timely, and actionable for intended users.

Methodological Rigor

Rigorous, credible, and methodologically pluralistic evaluations are essential for fostering stakeholder trust, particularly in assessments involving complex relational dynamics. Credibility depends not only on technical accuracy but also on transparent alignment among methodological choices, the nature of the evaluand, and the informational needs of intended users. The Centers for Disease Control and Prevention (CDC, 2024) states that "evaluations should produce findings that interest holders can confidently rely upon while also providing clear explanations of limitations." Transparency about strengths and limitations is essential for the integrity of evaluation. Methodological pluralism further strengthens this credibility by linking multiple lines of evidence. Weiss (1998) highlights the importance of employing multiple lines of evidence, asserting that convergence across diverse data sources enhances explanatory depth and evidentiary robustness. In complex contexts, reliance on a single method risks producing partial or distorted understandings; integrating complementary quantitative and qualitative approaches allows evaluators to reveal distinct dimensions of program processes and outcomes.

System-oriented scholars caution that adherence to methodological monism risks oversimplifying the complex, interconnected realities of social systems. Williams and Hummelbrunner (2010) contend that no single approach is universally applicable; instead, systems thinking supports the intentional selection and combination of methods based on contextual fit, evaluative purpose, and system dynamics. From this perspective, methodological appropriateness, rather than adherence to a fixed hierarchy of methods, constitutes the primary criterion for rigor. In alignment with these principles, NCE employs a context-responsive, methodologically pluralistic approach, customizing evaluation designs according to program characteristics, evaluation questions, available resources, stakeholder priorities, and feasibility considerations.

Independence and Objectivity

The principles of independence and objectivity are widely recognized as central to credible evaluation practices. The CDC (2024) emphasizes that evaluations should be conducted as independently and objectively as possible, protected from political or other undue influences. Within NCE, this principle is operationalized through attention to bias and positionality. Evaluators are expected to disclose their perspectives, funding sources, and potential conflicts of interest, allowing stakeholders to assess how the findings may have been shaped.

Transparency and Accountability

Transparency is equally vital. As CDC (2024) highlights, evaluations should be transparent across all phases, from planning to implementation to reporting, with decision-making processes clearly documented. NCE builds on this principle by requiring evaluators to document how major methodological choices are made, including the collection and definition of network data, the handling of missing responses, and the dissemination of findings. Accountability ensures that evaluators remain answerable to program participants and stakeholders affected by their work. Within NCE, accountability may involve creating public evaluation plans that outline research questions, network definitions, data sources, limitations, and dissemination strategies. Evaluators may also engage stakeholders through methods such as public forums, meetings, or webinars to present interim findings, gather feedback, and make necessary adjustments.

Ethics

Although ethics is sometimes viewed as distinct from rigor and transparency, it is fundamentally intertwined with the quality and legitimacy of evaluation practices. As emphasized by CDC (2024), "[e]valuations should be conducted to the highest ethical standards to maintain trust in the process and products. Evaluations should be fair, just, and should consider contextual factors that could influence the findings or their use." NCE integrates ethical considerations at every stage of the evaluation process—from the initial sampling of relational data, to the protection of confidentiality within network structures, to the securing of informed consent, and to the careful dissemination of findings to prevent harm. Ethical practice also includes respecting stakeholder perspectives, minimizing unnecessary burden, and ensuring that evaluation activities are conducted in ways that support trust and responsible use of findings.

Adaptive and Participatory Learning

Participatory and developmental evaluation scholarship establishes evaluation as a mechanism for learning, use, and adaptation rather than merely a retrospective judgment. Empirical evidence demonstrates that stakeholder engagement improves both the technical rigor and practical utility of evaluation. Cousins and Whitmore (1998) state that "stakeholder participation in evaluation will enhance evaluation relevance, ownership and thus utilization" (p. 6). Their concept of practical participatory evaluation emphasizes the "fostering of evaluation use," grounded in the premise that evaluation should support programmatic, policy, or organizational decision-making. The literature broadly conceptualizes utilization to include "instrumental," "conceptual," and "symbolic" forms of use, extending its influence beyond discrete decisions to the wider community of users and decision-makers.

Developmental evaluation adds a complementary dimension, particularly suited to complex and evolving contexts. Patton (2011) characterizes developmental evaluation as supporting real-time feedback, rapid adaptation, and continuous learning, integrating evaluation into the innovation process rather than treating it as an external entity. In environments characterized by uncertainty and nonlinear change, fixed designs and end-of-cycle assessments risk obsolescence; adaptive learning processes are essential for maintaining relevance.

NCE positions its practice within this intellectual tradition. Adaptive and participatory learning serve as core organizing principles of the model rather than supplementary elements. The model asserts that evaluation is most effective when it is iterative, collaborative, and action-oriented. Rather than treating evaluation as an external judgment delivered at the end of a program cycle, NCE conceptualizes it as an ongoing dialogue in which evidence is continuously integrated into decision-making. Program staff, community members, and decision-makers engage throughout the evaluative process by shaping questions, interpreting network data, and reflecting on implications for action. Regular, structured opportunities to revisit findings and examine emerging patterns create feedback loops that facilitate adjustment and recalibration over time. NCE institutionalizes participatory and developmental principles instead of merely adopting them rhetorically. By embedding co-creation, responsiveness, and iterative learning into the routine governance of networked initiatives, NCE advances the participatory and developmental tradition and illustrates how evaluation can function as a mechanism for accountability, collective sense-making, and strategic adaptation through network-informed evaluation approaches.

Sustainability and Capacity-Building

Fitzpatrick et al. (2004) assert that "[a]n important use of evaluation is its role in educating others, not simply about the program being evaluated, but also about alternative means for decision-making" (p. 177). They further contend that evaluation can empower stakeholders by fostering active engagement, building evaluation skills, and deepening their understanding of the programs in which they are invested. Similarly, Fetterman and Wandersman (2005) maintain that empowerment evaluation fundamentally seeks to improve program outcomes by actively involving stakeholders in the processes of planning, implementation, and self-assessment. By equipping participants with evaluative tools and skills, this approach strengthens their ability to monitor and improve their programs, thereby increasing the likelihood of achieving meaningful, sustained success. Patton (2008) likewise emphasized the importance of evaluation capacity-building, arguing that evaluative learning should persist and evolve beyond a single study to strengthen both individual and organizational learning over time.

NCE emphasizes sustainability and capacity-building, recognizing that long-term program success relies on stakeholders' continued ability to assess and adapt their efforts. In the NCE framework, capacity-building is conceptualized as a continuous, stakeholder-driven process that involves engagement at all evaluation stages, including context assessment; the development of network-informed program theory during the input stage; evaluation design during the process stage; and the facilitation of interpretation of evaluation outputs during the product stage. Sustainability is regarded as an ongoing process sustained through repeated interactions and shared learning that promote adaptability, collective ownership, and mutual accountability. Embedding these principles within the evaluation process enhances both immediate and long-term capacity for evaluative thinking and action, ensuring that learning and improvement persist beyond individual evaluation projects.

Cultural and Contextual Responsiveness

Cultural and contextual responsiveness is a foundational requirement of NCE, reflecting the recognition that practical evaluation must be attuned to the lived realities and social identities of those involved. Hood et al. (2015) contend that culturally responsive evaluation recognizes the fundamental influence of culture and context on both how programs are implemented and how evaluation is conducted, emphasizing that these factors are central to shaping evaluation practice. Mertens (2008) further emphasizes that evaluators are responsible for addressing issues of discrimination, oppression, and inequity. These insights are brought to the forefront in NCE, where network structures often mirror underlying cultural norms and power relations. For instance, in immigrant communities, informal support systems may function alongside or replace formal service networks. NCE ensures that evaluators do not overlook such culturally embedded dynamics by adapting traditional data collection instruments to capture the full spectrum of relational patterns. By recognizing and validating these structures, NCE enables evaluations to authentically represent the diversity of voices and experiences within a given context.

To ensure that cultural considerations are embedded throughout the evaluation process, NCE engages stakeholders to collaboratively define culturally specific tie types prior to data collection. This participatory strategy not only respects and leverages local expertise but also enhances data validity by ensuring the evaluation is sensitive to the evolving dynamics of each context. In this way, engaging stakeholders in this process operationalizes NCE's commitment to contextual responsiveness, ultimately strengthening both the rigor and the relevance of evaluation findings.

Network Terminology in Complex Evaluation

A core strength of NCE is its ability to tailor evaluations to different network types. Individual networks encompass family or peer support systems and are assessed through tie strength and network density. Organizational networks focus on collaboration and referral pathways and are evaluated via metrics such as centrality and betweenness. Community networks, such as coalitions or advocacy groups, are analyzed through modularity and participation to assess engagement. Policy networks connect agencies and advocacy groups, with metrics such as degree centrality and influence scores highlighting key actors and their impact. The following section outlines the foundational network concepts and measures that support the NCE framework.

Network Concepts in Network-Informed Complex Evaluation

Network concepts are central to analyzing how relationships, structures, and interactions shape outcomes in complex systems. Within the NCE framework, these concepts facilitate the interpretation of multilevel relational dynamics that define complex programs. Precise definition and operationalization of network concepts, including actors, ties, groups, relations, and levels of analysis, enable evaluators to identify opportunities for resource transmission, assess constraints or opportunities for individual actors, and determine the collective mechanisms by which networks influence effectiveness, equity, and sustainability. The foundational concepts described below are critical for the application of NCE in complex contexts.

Actor

Social network analysis (SNA) examines the connections among social units and the outcomes that arise from these relationships. These social units, referred to as *actors*, may include individuals, corporate entities, or collective social groups (Wasserman & Faust, 1994, p. 17). Within the NCE framework, actors may include program staff, participants, agencies, or communities, depending on the analytical level and evaluation objectives. Identifying actors establishes the foundation for mapping relational structures and analyzing the distribution of influence, resources, or information within a system.

Ties

In network analysis, *ties* refer to the interactions that connect actors. Common types of ties include behavioral interactions, such as communication or information exchange; physical connections, such as co-residence; associations or affiliations, such as event attendance or organizational membership; formal relations, such as authority; and transitions between places or statuses, such as social or physical mobility (Wasserman & Faust, 1994, p. 18). Within the NCE framework, ties may represent referrals, collaborations, information sharing, or resource exchanges. The nature, strength, direction, and frequency of ties are essential for analyzing the flow of information and resources within the system. The selection of ties for analysis is determined by the program's theory of change, evaluation questions, and network boundary specifications.

Groups

A *group* consists of all actors among whom ties are measured. According to Wasserman and Faust (1994), a group "consists of a finite set of actors who for conceptual, theoretical, or empirical reasons are treated as a finite set of individuals on which network measures are made" (p. 19). Limiting analysis to a finite set of actors is essential in network analysis, as it requires precise specification of network boundaries, sampling, and group definitions. For example, if vaccination service coordination is county-based, the NCE evaluator may restrict the group to county agencies to maintain relevance and manageability. In the NCE framework, groups may be defined at the individual, organizational, community, or policy levels, depending on program theory and evaluation objectives.

Relation

A *relation* refers to a specific type of contact or connection between a pair of actors, representing a joint dyadic property that sustains their association. Relations may be directed, with one actor initiating and another receiving, such as advice-seeking, or undirected, where mutuality exists, such as joint decision-making (Knoke & Yang, 2008, p. 7). Within the NCE framework, relations may occur at the interpersonal level, including collaboration, discussion, or advice among employees. At the level of collective entities, relations may involve resource exchange, communication, service coordination, or collaboration between organizations. The types of relations measured in network evaluation are determined by the specific objectives of the evaluation project.

Social Network

A *social network* consists of a finite set of actors and the relations defined among them (Wasserman & Faust, 1994, p. 20). Within the NCE framework, the social network perspective emphasizes the structure of relations and their implications for individual or group behavior and attitudes. Networks may be analyzed at multiple scales, including individual (ego), organizational, community, or policy levels. Selecting the appropriate level of analysis is essential in NCE to ensure that network measures align with program theory and produce findings that are relevant and actionable.

Network Variables in Network-Informed Complex Evaluation

NCE applies network analysis to examine how relationships shape intervention processes and outcomes within complex systems. A central analytic distinction in network analysis is between relational variables, which describe observed ties among actors, and positional (structural) variables, which describe actors' locations within the broader network configuration of those ties. *Relational variables* capture patterns of interaction, exchange, or communication among actors. In contrast, *positional variables* are derived from the overall configuration of ties within a network and indicate how actors, organizations, or institutions are situated relative to others in the system (Burt, 1980; Valente, 2010, pp. 55–57). While these two types of variables are often empirically related, they differ in their construction, the dimensions of social structure they represent, and the evaluation questions they help address. Table 3.1 presents a conceptual classification of common relational and positional network constructs across levels of analysis relevant to complex evaluation.

Individual-Level Network Variables

At the individual level, relational variables describe the structure of an individual's ego network, defined as the set of direct ties surrounding a focal actor. Measures such as personal network size, density, tie strength, reciprocity, and multiplexity characterize the immediate relational environment in which individuals are embedded. Ego

Table 3.1 Core relational and positional concepts of network structure across levels of analysis

Level	Relational	Positional
Individual	Personal network size; personal network density; tie strength; reciprocity; multiplexity; trust	Central or peripheral position; degree centrality; betweenness centrality; closeness centrality; prestige; structural constraint
Organizational	Collaboration frequency; information sharing; resource exchange; multiplex interorganizational ties; partnership stability	Organizational centrality (degree, betweenness, eigenvector); brokerage roles; structural equivalence; boundary-spanning positions
Community	Network density; connectedness; reachability; relational cohesion; cross-group ties	Clique membership; subgroup differentiation; bridging positions; network centralization
Policy	Consultation ties; coalition participation; policy communication networks; intergovernmental coordination	Policy actor prestige; centralization of influence; hierarchical partitioning; agenda-setting positions

Note Author's conceptual synthesis of relational and positional network constructs across levels of analysis, informed by Burt's (1980) distinction between relational and positional approaches to network analysis and subsequent developments in network analysis (e.g., Valente, 2010). Relational measures are classified according to their conceptual interpretation as properties of interaction patterns, regardless of the level at which they are computed.

network size is typically quantified as the number of named contacts, while density indicates the proportion of those contacts who are themselves connected. Multiplexity refers to ties that serve multiple roles, such as advice, friendship, or support, indicating stronger obligations and greater potential for coordinated action. In evaluation research, these measures assess mechanisms such as social support, normative reinforcement, and peer-to-peer diffusion. Relational variables are commonly used to examine how interventions function at the interpersonal level, including peer influence, social support, and informal information diffusion.

Positional variables at the individual level describe how a person is situated within the broader network beyond their immediate ties. Measures such as centrality, prestige, betweenness, and structural constraint position individuals within the overall system and capture dimensions of prominence, brokerage, and dependence. Centrality indicates the extent to which an individual is well connected within the network, while prestige reflects the degree to which an individual is the object of ties from others who are themselves prominent. Betweenness identifies actors who lie on the shortest paths between others, indicating potential brokerage roles. Structural constraint measures the redundancy of an individual's network and the limitations on access to novel resources. These positional measures are particularly relevant for evaluating diffusion-based or peer-led interventions, in which individuals' locations within the network influence exposure, reach, and potential impact. These measures should be interpreted as probabilistic indicators of opportunity and constraint, rather than as deterministic markers of leadership or effectiveness (Valente, 2010), and they therefore suggest where influence is more or less likely to occur.

Organizational-Level Network Variables

When organizations are conceptualized as network actors, the relational–positional distinction remains relevant. Relational organizational variables describe direct interactions among organizations, such as collaboration frequency, information sharing, resource exchange, and multiplex interorganizational ties. These measures are typically derived from surveys in which organizations report joint activities, shared funding, or data exchange. They address evaluation questions about implementation processes, coordination, and partnership functioning. For instance, evaluators may examine whether higher levels of interorganizational collaboration are associated with more consistent service delivery, thereby highlighting how coordination and mutual adjustment shape outcomes.

Positional organizational variables capture how organizations are embedded within interorganizational systems. Organizational centrality indicates prominence or visibility within a network; brokerage reflects an organization's role in connecting otherwise disconnected actors or sectors; and structural equivalence identifies organizations occupying similar roles within the system, regardless of whether they are directly connected. These positional properties often shape access to resources, influence over decision-making, and vulnerability to system disruptions. For evaluators, these variables are particularly useful for understanding why certain organizations emerge as coordinators, gatekeepers, or bottlenecks in complex interventions, clarifying where influence and constraint are concentrated.

Community-Level Network Variables

At the community level, network variables describe meso-level structures that emerge from aggregated individual or organizational ties. Relational community-level variables include network density, connectedness, and reachability, which indicate the extent to which community members can interact directly or indirectly and the extent to which these interactions shape intervention reach. High levels of connectedness are often associated with social integration and collective capacity, whereas excessive density may reinforce exclusionary norms or limit innovation, affecting intervention equity and adaptability. These relational properties are analytically ambivalent; their implications depend on intervention goals and contextual conditions.

Positional community-level variables describe the internal structure of communities. Clique formation, subgroup differentiation, and the presence or absence of bridging structures are identified using subgroup-detection algorithms or connectivity analyses between components. From an evaluative perspective, these structural features are critical for understanding how interventions spread within subgroups and across structural boundaries, shaping differential intervention reach, equity, and sustainability. Interventions may diffuse rapidly within cohesive subgroups but often do not cross structural boundaries unless bridging actors or mechanisms are present.

Policy-Level Network Variables

At the policy level, networks consist of decision-makers, agencies, advocacy organizations, and governance bodies. Relational policy-level variables describe patterns of interaction among these actors, including consultation ties, coalition membership, and information exchange. These variables are commonly used in policy evaluation to examine learning processes, cross-sector coordination, and agenda alignment. They capture the dynamics of interactions among policy actors rather than the formal assignment of authority, and they help identify where collaboration or communication may need attention.

Positional policy-level variables characterize the distribution of influence and authority within governance systems. Metrics, including policy network centralization, policy actors' prestige, and hierarchical partitioning, indicate whether influence is concentrated or dispersed and identify actors in structurally advantaged positions. These variables are essential for understanding how policy environments enable or constrain the implementation, adaptation, and long-term institutionalization of interventions. Consistent with other levels of analysis, policy-level positional measures should be interpreted as indicators of structural opportunity and constraint, not as deterministic predictors of policy influence or outcomes.

Network Measures in Network-Informed Complex Evaluation

NCE utilizes a set of network measures to evaluate relational structures, interaction patterns, and system dynamics that impact program planning, implementation, and outcomes. Within the NCE framework, the selection and application of network measures are guided by the program's theory of change and aligned with stakeholder evaluation priorities. Rather than considering network metrics solely as descriptive analytic tools, NCE conceptualizes them as evaluative indicators that demonstrate how relationships shape resource access, coordination, influence, and system functioning across individual, organizational, community, and policy levels.

Table 3.2 synthesizes commonly used network measures and demonstrates their capacity to inform evaluation questions at multiple levels of complex systems. This table represents a conceptual contribution of the NCE framework by organizing established network measures according to the structural functions they reveal within complex intervention systems and by illustrating how these measures can be interpreted in multilevel evaluation practice. Since not all measures are necessary in every evaluation context, evaluators select metrics aligned with the relational mechanisms and evaluation questions most relevant to the intervention system under study. Table 3.2 should be considered a practical guide rather than a prescriptive checklist, helping evaluators identify and apply network measures that best capture the relational processes critical to program performance, system coordination, and collective outcomes.

Reach, Accessibility, and Network Scope

A primary objective of network-informed evaluation is to assess whether relational structures enable actors to access resources, information, and influence across varying degrees of relational distance. Evaluators analyze the scope of networks, actor reachability, the number of intermediaries connecting actors, and the presence of structural barriers that limit connectivity. These analyses correspond to the structural functions of reach, accessibility, and structural span, which address both the breadth of connectivity and the effort required to traverse the network. This structural function is evaluated using metrics including network size, diameter, path distance, reachability, number of components, and closeness centrality.

- *Size* refers to the number of actors (nodes) in a network or ego network (Carolan, 2014, p. 101; Valente, 2010, p. 129). At the individual level, network size reflects the breadth of a person's immediate support system. Within organizations, it indicates the extent to which staff or partner networks are involved in coordination or information exchange. At the community level, it captures the scope of coalitions or collective structures, while at the policy level, it reflects the scale of governance or advocacy networks. Larger networks may provide access to a broader range of resources and perspectives, but can also increase coordination complexity. For evaluators, network size serves as a foundational indicator of relational capacity and potential reach.
- *Diameter* is defined as the length of the longest geodesic (shortest path) between any two actors in a network (Carolan, 2014, p. 105; Valente, 2010, p. 134). It represents the maximum structural distance separating actors in the system. At the individual level, the diameter of an ego network—including ego, alters, and alter–alter ties—denotes the greatest distance between any pair of alters within that personal network. Within organizations and coalitions, diameter establishes an upper bound on the number of intermediaries that may separate the most distant actors. In policy networks, larger diameters may indicate greater structural span and potential coordination challenges. For evaluators, diameter helps characterize the limits of structural reach within a network.
- *Distance*, commonly measured as *average path length*, refers to the average geodesic distance between all pairs of actors in a network (Carolan, 2014, p. 105; Valente, 2010, p. 135). Networks with shorter average path lengths exhibit greater structural accessibility because actors can reach one another through fewer intermediaries. At the individual level, shorter paths may indicate easier access to support or information. Within organizations and communities, shorter average distances can facilitate coordination and communication across units or groups. In policy networks, shorter distances may support more efficient circulation of policy

information or advocacy frames. For evaluators, average path length provides insight into the accessibility and connectivity of relational systems.

- *Reachability* refers to whether a path exists between pairs of actors in a network and, therefore, whether actors can potentially access one another through direct or indirect ties (Wasserman & Faust, 1994, pp. 132–133). Reachability analysis identifies whether networks function as connected systems or whether structural barriers prevent certain actors from interacting. In network-informed evaluation, reachability is used to assess structural access across individual, organizational, community, and policy networks, and to diagnose potential exclusion or fragmentation within relational systems.
- *Closeness centrality* measures how close an actor is to all other actors in a network based on geodesic distance (Carolan, 2014, p. 156; Freeman, 1979). Actors with high closeness centrality can reach others through relatively few intermediaries and are therefore structurally positioned to access information or resources efficiently (Knoke & Yang, 2008). At the individual level, this proximity may enable more timely access to services or support. Within organizations and communities, actors with high closeness centrality may exhibit enhanced responsiveness or coordination capacity. For evaluators, closeness centrality helps identify actors who are structurally positioned to access or disseminate information efficiently.
- A *component* is a maximal subset of actors in which each actor can reach every other actor through one or more paths, whereas isolates are actors with no ties to others in the network (Wasserman & Faust, 1994, p. 109). Identifying connected components and isolates is essential for diagnosing fragmentation, exclusion, and structural barriers to access. Component structures do not function as direct performance indicators; rather, they reveal whether a network operates as a coherent relational system or as a collection of disconnected groups. For example, at the organizational level, multiple components may represent disconnected teams, departments, or partner organizations, potentially hindering coordination, leading to duplication of effort, and limiting organizational learning.

As displayed in Table 3.2A, measures of reach, accessibility, and structural span across multiple analytical levels assess whether network configurations facilitate access to resources, information, and influence within practical relational distances. At the individual level, network size and reachability indicate the breadth of an ego network and the availability of social, informational, or instrumental support. Diameter and average path length within ego networks quantify the structural distance to the most remote contacts and the influence that extends beyond immediate ties. Limited reachability or the presence of isolates indicates increased vulnerability, whereas higher closeness centrality reflects more efficient access to support and services.

At the organizational level, these measures determine whether staff, units, or partner organizations are structurally positioned for effective coordination. Shorter average distances indicate reduced coordination burdens and faster information flow. By contrast, larger diameters or multiple disconnected components indicate peripheral units or partners with limited access to organizational decision-making.

While network size at this level represents organizational reach, it is essential to assess whether increased size is accompanied by sufficient connectivity to support coordination.

At the community level, reach-related measures define the scope and navigability of coalitions and collaborative infrastructures. Networks with high reachability and short average distances are better equipped to mobilize actors, disseminate practices, and sustain collective action. In contrast, fragmented networks with multiple components or isolated subgroups may limit participation and hinder the diffusion of resources or innovations. At the policy level, reach-related network measures influence the diffusion of agendas and cross-sector coordination. While a large network size may indicate broad stakeholder engagement, extended path lengths, large diameters, or fragmented components may signal increased governance complexity and barriers to inclusive access to policy arenas.

Power, Influence, and Structural Control

Evaluation requires an understanding of how influence and coordination are organized within networks. Key considerations include identifying actors in influential positions, assessing the degree of network dependence on specific actors, and detecting vulnerabilities resulting from concentrated control. These issues correspond to the structural functions of connectivity, concentration, brokerage, and control, which affect both system effectiveness and risk. Here, power is viewed as an emergent property of relational structure rather than as an individual attribute. This structural function is assessed using network centralization, degree centrality, betweenness centrality, eigenvector centrality, constraint, and brokerage roles.

- *Network centralization* measures the extent to which centrality scores are concentrated among a small number of actors relative to others in the network (Carolan, 2014, p. 107; Freeman, 1979). Highly centralized networks concentrate structural importance in a limited number of actors. At the individual level, such configurations may lead to reliance on a single caregiver or gatekeeper, increasing vulnerability to disruption. Within organizations, high centralization may create coordination bottlenecks if key actors are unavailable. In communities, concentrated connectivity may limit broader participation, whereas in policy networks it may enable a small number of institutional actors to dominate agenda-setting. For evaluators, centralization provides insight into structural vulnerability, inclusiveness, and potential equity-related risks.
- *Degree centrality* measures the number of direct ties an actor has to other actors in a network (Carolan, 2014, p. 155; Freeman, 1979). At the individual level, higher degree centrality indicates greater potential access to peers, information, or resources through direct connections. In organizations, staff members or units with high degree centrality are directly connected to many others, potentially facilitating information exchange and coordination across organizational units.

- *Betweenness centrality* identifies actors who lie on the shortest paths between other actors in the network, positioning them as potential brokers or bridges (Carolan, 2014, p. 157; Freeman, 1979; Freeman et al., 1991). These actors mediate connectivity between otherwise disconnected groups and may influence coordination or access to resources. At the individual level, peer navigators or community connectors may occupy such bridging roles. Within organizations and communities, liaison positions often link distinct units or constituencies, such as a staff member connecting service providers and client groups. In policy networks, brokerage actors may facilitate negotiation or coordination across coalitions (Sabatier & Weible, 2014).
- *Eigenvector centrality* measures influence by assigning greater weight to connections with highly connected actors (Bonacich, 1987). Actors with high eigenvector centrality are embedded within influential parts of the network and may therefore possess indirect structural influence beyond their immediate ties. This measure helps evaluators identify actors embedded within influential relational clusters and examine how influence is distributed across network structures.
- *Constraint* measures the extent to which an actor's ties are redundant and concentrated among a small set of interconnected alters, thereby limiting brokerage opportunities (Burt, 1992, 2004; Carolan, 2014, pp. 162–164). Higher constraint values indicate fewer opportunities for bridging and suggest restricted access to diverse information or resources. In evaluation contexts, constraint can help diagnose structural limitations on innovation, coordination, or cross-boundary learning.
- *Brokerage* refers to positions in which actors connect otherwise disconnected groups or categories of actors, thereby facilitating or constraining flows of information, resources, or influence across boundaries (Carolan, 2014, pp. 165–166; Gould & Fernandez, 1989). Brokerage roles may include gatekeepers, representatives, coordinators, or liaisons who mediate interactions between groups. From an evaluative perspective, brokerage highlights boundary-spanning roles that shape coordination, access, and power across individual, organizational, community, and policy networks, such as a liaison linking separate programs or stakeholder groups.

As outlined in Table 3.2B, measures of power, influence, and structural control clarify the distribution of coordination and decision-making capacity within networks and the emergence of vulnerabilities arising from concentrated connectivity. At the individual level, degree centrality and betweenness centrality identify actors who serve as key caregivers, navigators, or brokers. Although these positions facilitate access for others, they also increase dependency and risk if these actors become overburdened or unavailable. Constraint further distinguishes between networks that provide access to diverse, nonredundant resources and those characterized by redundancy that limits brokerage opportunities (Burt, 1992).

At the organizational level, network centralization refers to the extent to which coordination depends on a small number of actors or units. Highly centralized structures may enhance efficiency but can also create bottlenecks and succession risks. Degree and eigenvector centrality identify staff or units with disproportionate influence over information flow, while brokerage roles clarify whether actors facilitate cross-unit integration or act as gatekeepers controlling access. Collectively, these measures inform evaluative judgments regarding organizational resilience, inclusiveness, and vulnerability to disruption.

At the community level, brokers identified through betweenness centrality and brokerage role analysis often connect sectors or constituencies, supporting integration across social or organizational boundaries. However, excessive influence may restrict broader participation or reinforce gatekeeping dynamics. Evaluators assess the balance between coordination efficiency and equitable participation by examining both centralization and brokerage structures. In policy networks, eigenvector centrality highlights actors embedded within influential institutional clusters that shape agenda-setting and negotiation capacity, while brokerage roles clarify whether coordination is achieved through inclusive liaison positions or exclusionary control points. These measures are particularly relevant for evaluating equity, representation, and power asymmetries in governance systems.

Cohesion, Reciprocity, and Relational Stability

Evaluation should assess whether networks foster sustained, trust-based collaboration. Key considerations include the degree of relationship cohesion, the presence of mutual and reinforcing ties, and the existence of stable interaction cores. These aspects correspond to the structural functions of cohesion, mutuality, and relational stability, which support durability and collective capacity. These functions are measured using density, reciprocity, tie strength, clustering (transitivity), and k-core analysis.

- *Density* represents the proportion of realized ties relative to all possible ties in a network (Valente, 2010, p. 129; Wasserman & Faust, 1994, p. 101). Dense networks often facilitate reliable communication and mutual support; however, high density can also increase redundancy or insularity depending on context. In policy networks, extremely high density may indicate limited openness to new actors or ideas. Density, therefore, helps evaluators assess network cohesion while considering constraints on innovation or diversity.
- *Reciprocity* measures the proportion of mutual ties in a directed network, indicating the extent to which relationships are reciprocated between actors (Valente, 2010, p. 130). This metric captures bidirectional exchange and provides insight into the balance of interactions within a network. Higher levels of reciprocity are often associated with more stable and cohesive relational structures because mutual ties reinforce ongoing interaction and obligation (Carolan, 2014, p. 103). At the individual level, reciprocal ties typically represent relationships of mutual support, such as caregiving, mentoring, or collaborative exchange. Within organizations, reciprocity may reflect balanced communication or coordination among staff and units. At community and policy levels, reciprocal ties can indicate mutual

recognition, shared commitment, and relational trust among actors. As an evaluative indicator, reciprocity supports the assessment of relational mutuality and potential stability within interaction networks.

- *Tie strength* refers to the intensity or quality of relationships and is typically measured through indicators such as interaction frequency, emotional closeness, or trust (Granovetter, 1973, 1983). Strong ties often provide emotional and instrumental support at the individual level, facilitate collaboration within organizations, stabilize partnerships across community coalitions, and anchor enduring alliances in policy networks. However, excessive reliance on strong ties may also limit exposure to novel information or opportunities. For evaluators, tie strength helps assess relationship durability and the balance between support and openness.
- *Clustering*, also known as *transitivity*, captures the tendency for an actor's contacts to also be connected with one another, forming closed triads (Valente, 2010, p. 132; Watts & Strogatz, 1998). High clustering reflects localized cohesion and may reinforce trust and shared norms among actors. For evaluators, clustering highlights a network's tendency toward triadic closure and potential insularity.
- *K-core* analysis identifies cohesive subgroups in which each actor maintains at least k ties with other members of the subgroup (Carolan, 2014, p. 118; Seidman, 1983). K-cores represent stable cores of interaction that sustain practices or coordination within networks. In evaluation contexts, k-core analysis can help identify clusters of actors responsible for maintaining sustained collaboration or influence.

As shown in Table 3.2C, measures of cohesion, reciprocity, and relational stability assess whether networks facilitate sustained, trust-based collaboration rather than episodic or fragile interactions. At the individual level, dense, reciprocal, and strong ties provide both emotional and instrumental support, whereas weak or unreciprocated ties may indicate a fragile support system. Clustering can promote trust through triadic closure but may also restrict access to novel information or opportunities, underscoring trade-offs between stability and diversity (Granovetter, 1973).

Within organizations, cohesion facilitates coordination, shared norms, and collective efficacy. Density and reciprocity reflect balanced interactions among staff or units, while k-core analysis identifies stable subgroups that anchor institutional practices. These measures enable evaluators to identify areas where organizational capacity is concentrated and where engagement may be fragile or uneven. At the community level, cohesive networks promote trust and sustained participation within coalitions. However, excessive density or clustering can lead to redundancy and insularity, thereby reducing adaptability and openness to new participants. Evaluators should interpret cohesion in relation to contextual objectives and stages of collaboration. In policy networks, strong, reciprocal ties support long-term alliances and stabilize governance processes. However, dense cores may dominate deliberation and marginalize peripheral actors, raising equity concerns that require evaluative attention.

Structural Differentiation, Segmentation, and Inequality

Equity-oriented evaluation requires examining the internal differentiation of networks. Key considerations include identifying boundaries and silos, and assessing how similarity-based ties affect access and power. These concerns align with the structural functions of differentiation, fragmentation, and patterned inequality, which are analyzed using modularity, homophily, and assortativity. Modularity identifies subgroup partitions, homophily reflects similarity-based tie formation, and assortativity measures systematic mixing patterns.

- *Modularity* quantifies the extent to which a network partitions into communities characterized by dense internal connections and relatively sparse ties between groups (Newman, 2003, 2006). High modularity indicates strong subgroup structures within the network. In organizations, such structures may reflect departmental silos; in communities, they may represent fragmented social groups; and in policy networks, they may correspond to ideological or sectoral coalitions. Modularity supports evaluative analysis of both structural integration and fragmentation.
- *Homophily* describes the tendency for actors to form ties with others who are similar to themselves in attributes such as profession, ideology, or demographic characteristics (McPherson et al., 2001). This tendency shapes access to information and opportunities, contributes to clustering within organizations, reinforces social segmentation in communities, and sustains ideological alignment in policy networks.
- *Assortativity* measures the tendency for actors to connect with others who share similar structural characteristics, such as degree or other attributes (Newman, 2003). Positive assortativity indicates that similar actors preferentially connect with one another, whereas negative assortativity indicates connections between dissimilar actors. This metric helps evaluators examine structural stratification and patterns of inequality within networks.

Table 3.2D demonstrates that measures of structural differentiation, segmentation, and inequality enable evaluators to assess the distribution of access, opportunity, and influence within networks. At the individual level, homophily shapes personal networks by reinforcing similarity-based ties, which can restrict exposure to diverse perspectives or resources and contribute to unequal access. These patterns are particularly significant in evaluations focused on inclusion and equity (McPherson et al., 2001).

At the organizational level, modularity and assortativity reveal departmental or professional silos and stratified interaction patterns. These measures facilitate diagnostic assessments of organizational integration and help identify structural barriers to collaboration. At the community level, segmentation along social, cultural, or sectoral lines can reduce the effectiveness of coalitions and reinforce inequalities in participation or influence. Modularity and homophily enable evaluators to determine whether fragmentation arises from functional specialization or structural exclusion. In policy networks, assortativity uncovers patterns of institutional dominance and marginalization, clarifying how governance structures may privilege certain actors while limiting the influence of others.

Network Complexity, Robustness, and Adaptive Capacity

Evaluators should determine whether networks possess the capacity to adapt to change, disruption, and scaling. Key considerations include the complexity of relational ties and the presence of multiple coordination pathways. These concerns align with the structural functions of robustness, redundancy, and multilevel connectivity. This function is measured by multiplexity, small-world properties, and core–periphery structure.

- *Multiplexity* refers to the presence of multiple types of relationships between the same pair of actors (Verbrugge, 1979). For example, two individuals may simultaneously share advice, friendship, and collaboration ties. Such multiplex relationships can strengthen relational robustness by linking actors across multiple roles and contexts, giving evaluators a clearer basis for assessing the complexity and durability of relational systems.
- *Small-world networks* exhibit both relatively high clustering and short average path lengths (Watts & Strogatz, 1998). These structural properties combine local cohesion with efficient global connectivity, facilitating the circulation of information, practices, or resources across networks and allowing evaluators to assess how efficiently a network supports those flows.
- *Core–periphery structure* describes networks in which a densely interconnected core of actors is surrounded by peripheral actors who are connected primarily to members of the core but maintain relatively few ties with one another (Borgatti & Everett, 2000; Valente, 2010, p. 140). In networks with strong core–periphery organization, peripheral actors rely disproportionately on core actors for access to coordination, information flow, and resources. From an evaluative perspective, this structure highlights both potential system resilience and potential vulnerability when coordination depends heavily on a small set of central actors. Evaluators can therefore use core–periphery analysis to determine whether influence and coordination are broadly distributed across a system or concentrated within a small coordinating core.

Table 3.2E shows that measures of network complexity, robustness, and adaptive capacity indicate whether relational systems possess the structural features required to respond to change, disruption, and scaling demands. At the individual level, multiplex ties connect actors across multiple roles or contexts, enhancing resilience by providing alternative pathways for support and information. At the organizational level, multiplexity supports learning, adaptation, and cross-functional coordination. The presence of small-world and core–periphery structures indicates whether organizations maintain stable cores while permitting flexible peripheral connections, which in turn influences their ability to adapt without sacrificing cohesion. These metrics allow evaluators to assess organizational readiness for change and system-level resilience. At the community level, complex networks promote cross-sector collaboration and the diffusion of innovation by linking actors across domains while preserving cohesive subgroups. In policy systems, multiplex structures strengthen negotiation, learning, and long-term governance capacity by facilitating coordination across institutional contexts. These measures establish a structural basis for evaluating sustainability and adaptability in complex, multilevel systems (Table 3.2).

Approaches to Conducting Network-Informed Complex Evaluation

The NCE approach is based on the Context, Input, Process, Product (CIPP) evaluation model, initially developed by Daniel Stufflebeam. Since the early 1970s, the CIPP model has been extensively refined through both theoretical and applied research (Stufflebeam, 1971, 1983, 2000, 2004; Stufflebeam & Coryn, 2014). As a decision-oriented framework, the CIPP model offers conceptual, hypothetical, pragmatic, and ethical principles that collectively inform evaluation theory and practice (Stufflebeam, 2004). Its primary contribution lies in conceptualizing evaluation as a systematic process for guiding planning, implementation, and improvement.

The NCE approach extends the CIPP model by systematically integrating network and complexity perspectives across all stages of evaluation. This integration strengthens evaluators' capacity to address the relational, adaptive, and dynamic characteristics of complex interventions, particularly those situated within multi-sector coalitions, systems, and networks. The incorporation of a network perspective within each CIPP domain supports the design of context-sensitive inputs, the implementation of adaptive evaluation processes, and the production of outputs that are meaningful and actionable for diverse stakeholder groups within interconnected systems.

As shown in Fig. 3.2, the NCE approach represents a network- and complexity-informed enhancement of the traditional CIPP model. This framework reconceptualizes evaluation as an iterative, nonlinear, and adaptive learning system. By incorporating principles from complexity science and network theory, the NCE approach enables the identification and interpretation of emergent patterns, evolving relationships, and adaptive processes that characterize complex systems. Stakeholder identification and engagement remain central, emphasizing their ongoing and integrative role across all evaluation domains.

Table 3.2 Network measures for network-informed complex evaluation across levels

Network Measure	Evaluation Purpose	Individual Level	Organizational Level	Community Level	Policy Level
A. Reach, Accessibility, and Structural Span Guiding evaluation questions include: • Who is connected to whom within the network, and which actors remain disconnected or peripheral? • How far does access to information, resources, or services extend across the network? • What structural distances or barriers limit coordination, communication, or resource access?					
Network Size	Assess the breadth of access and inclusion	Number of personal contacts associated with access to support, information, or opportunity	Number of staff or partner organizations involved in service delivery	Size and inclusiveness of coalitions or interorganizational networks	Scale and inclusiveness of policymaking or governance networks
Diameter	Assess the maximum network span	Longest geodesic distance indicating limits of personal reach	Farthest communication paths within organizations	Maximum distance across coalition members	Structural span of governance or regulatory networks
Distance (average path length)	Evaluate coordination speed and navigability	Average number of steps required to access support or information	Average communication distance among staff or units	Efficiency of coordination across community actors	Rapidity of information or policy diffusion across venues
Reachability	Assess structural access and connectedness of network pathways	Proportion of reachable contacts within the personal network	Connectivity of internal communication structures	Accessibility of services across community networks	Connectedness of inter-agency or transnational coordination pathways
Closeness centrality	Assess structural proximity and potential for rapid access	Structural proximity enabling timely access to support	Units positioned to reach others across departments rapidly	Actors able to mobilize resources quickly across the community	Actors positioned to disseminate information across policy venues rapidly

(continued)

Table 3.2 (continued)

Network Measure	Evaluation Purpose	Individual Level	Organizational Level	Community Level	Policy Level
Components/ isolates	Diagnose fragmentation, isolation, and structural exclusion	Presence of isolated individuals lacking access	Disconnected teams or partners	Fragmented coalitions or disconnected subgroups	Siloed governance subsystems or venues
B. Power, Influence, and Structural Control Guiding evaluation questions include: • Which actors occupy structurally influential positions within the network? • To what extent does coordination or information flow depend on specific actors or groups? • Where do brokerage, gatekeeping, or concentration of control create potential vulnerabilities or inequities?					
Network centralization	Identify the concentration of structural dependence	Reliance on a single caregiver or gatekeeper	Reliance on key coordinators within organizational networks	Concentration of decision-making	Agenda-setting dominance by institutional actors
Degree centrality	Identify highly connected actors	Number of direct ties providing access to peers or resources	Staff or units with extensive direct connections	Organizations serving as highly connected hubs	Actors or institutions with numerous direct alliances
Betweenness centrality	Identify brokerage and bridging positions	Individuals connecting otherwise disconnected social groups	Liaisons linking departments or external partners	Organizations connecting otherwise disconnected community groups	Actors mediating between policy coalitions or sectors
Eigenvector centrality	Assess influence through connectedness to influential others	Influence derived from ties to well-connected or respected peers	Units connected to other central or prestigious units	Organizations embedded in influential partnership networks	Institutions embedded within highly influential policy networks

(continued)

Table 3.2 (continued)

Network Measure	Evaluation Purpose	Individual Level	Organizational Level	Community Level	Policy Level
Constraint	Assess limits on brokerage and access to novel resources	Degree of redundancy limiting exposure to diverse contacts	Structural constraint limiting external organizational ties	Subgroups lacking bridging connections	Redundancy in policy actors' ties within coalitions or subsystems, limiting their ability to broker across venues or sectors
Brokerage roles	Distinguish types of brokerage roles	Gatekeeping or liaison roles	Boundary-spanning or controlling roles	Sectoral liaisons or gatekeepers	Brokers between policy subsystems
C. Cohesion, Reciprocity, and Relational Stability Guiding evaluation questions include: • How cohesive and durable are relationships among actors in the network? • Do network ties reflect mutual exchange, trust, and sustained collaboration? • Are there stable clusters or cores that support ongoing coordination and collective action?					
Tie Strength	Assess the durability and intensity of relationships	Frequency, emotional closeness, or trust within personal ties	Strength of collaborative relationships	Stability of partnerships among organizations	Durability of alliances among policy actors
Reciprocity	Evaluate mutuality in relationships	Mutual exchange in support or mentoring ties	Balanced reciprocal interactions among staff	Mutual exchange among community partners	Reciprocity within advocacy or governance coalitions
Density	Assess overall cohesion	Proportion of existing ties among possible ties in personal networks	Overall connectivity among staff or units	Cohesion or fragmentation across community networks	Intensity of coordination among institutions
Clustering (Transitivity)	Identify localized cohesion and closure	Tendency for contacts to be connected to one another	Presence of tightly connected subgroups within organizations	Clustering among community organizations	Formation of tightly connected policy subgroups

(continued)

Table 3.2 (continued)

Network Measure	Evaluation Purpose	Individual Level	Organizational Level	Community Level	Policy Level
K-core	Identify structurally cohesive cores	Presence of highly interconnected peer groups	Tightly connected staff sustaining organizational practices	Core organizations sustaining coalition activity	Stable inner cores of policymaking actors
D. Structural Differentiation, Segmentation, and Inequality Guiding evaluation questions include: • Where do structural divisions, silos, or subgroup boundaries emerge within the network? • To what extent do actors predominantly establish ties with others who share similar roles, sectors, or identities? • How are access, participation, and influence distributed among various groups within the network?					
Modularity	Detect segmentation or polarization	Division of personal networks into distinct subgroups	Organizational silos versus integration	Segmented or polarized community networks	Ideological or sectoral divisions in policy networks
Homophily	Assess similarity-based tie formation	Tendency to form ties with similar others	Clustering by role or status within organizations	Segregation by demographic or social characteristics	Alignment by ideology or sector
Assortativity	Examine patterned mixing by attributes	Degree of attribute-based connection patterns	Network mixing reflecting hiring or promotion patterns	Structural stratification within community networks	Attribute-based clustering among policy actors
E. Network Complexity, Robustness, and Adaptive Capacity Guiding evaluation questions include: • To what extent does the network demonstrate resilience to disruptions or the loss of key actors? • Are multiple relational pathways present that enable coordination to persist following the removal of central actors? • Does the network structure balance local cohesion and broader system connectivity effectively to facilitate learning and adaptation?					

(continued)

Table 3.2 (continued)

Network Measure	Evaluation Purpose	Individual Level	Organizational Level	Community Level	Policy Level
Multiplexity	Assess layered relational complexity	Overlapping roles across social relationships	Cross-functional or multi-role relationships	Multiple affiliations across community settings	Interdependencies across policy domains
Core–periphery	Assess vulnerability to actor loss and core dependence	Reliance on core contacts	Dependence on core units	Coalition resilience or dependence on core organizations	Stability or vulnerability of governance systems dependent on core actors
Small-world properties	Assess the balance between local cohesion and global connectivity	Combination of short paths and local clustering	Organizational networks supporting rapid information flow	Community networks balancing cohesion and reach	Interconnected policy systems facilitating diffusion

Note. The table reflects the author's synthesis of established social network analysis measures and their application in evaluation contexts (e.g., Borgatti et al., 2024; Burt, 1992, 2004; Carolan, 2014; Freeman, 1979; Knoke & Yang, 2008; Valente, 2010; Wasserman & Faust, 1994). Network measures are diagnostic rather than prescriptive and should be interpreted in relation to network context, scale, and purpose. Path-based measures (e.g., distance and closeness) are interpreted with consideration of component structure and reachability. Higher or lower values do not inherently indicate better performance; instead, they reflect structural conditions that shape access, coordination, influence, equity, and system resilience across levels.
Source Author

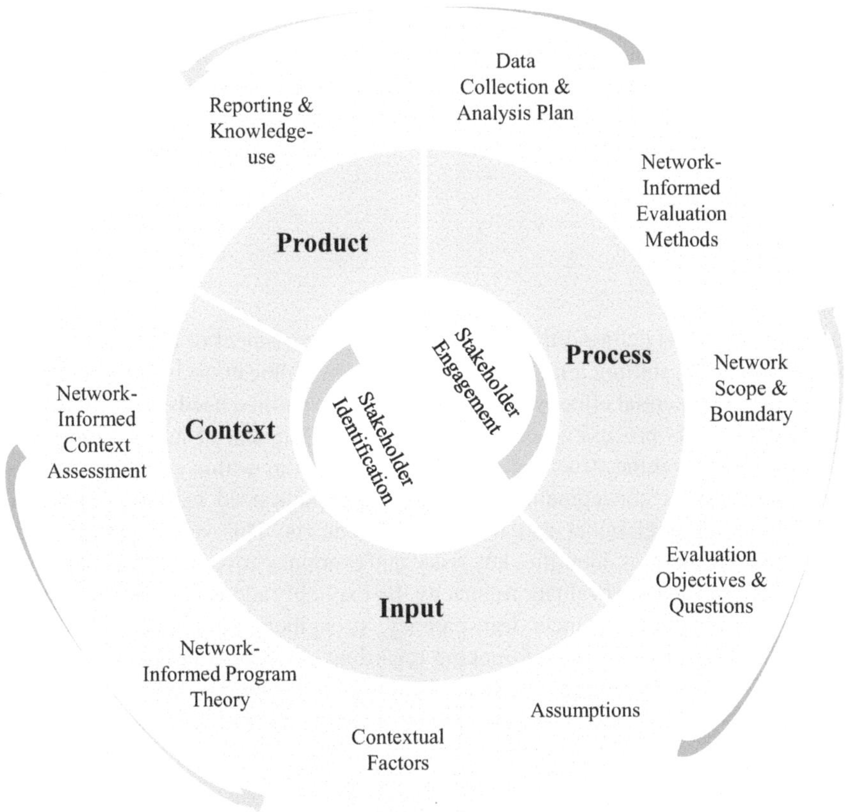

Fig. 3.2 Network-informed complex evaluation (NCE) approach. The NCE approach positions stakeholder identification and engagement as central to evaluation practices and organizes network-informed evaluation activities into four interrelated domains: context, input, process, and product. The circular structure emphasizes the iterative and nonlinear nature of evaluation design, implementation, and application. The figure represents the author's conceptual extension of the CIPP model (Stufflebeam, 2000, 2004), incorporating principles from complexity science and network theory

Context Stage

Stufflebeam (2004) defines context evaluation as the systematic assessment of needs, problems, assets, and opportunities to guide goal setting, priority identification, and judgments regarding program relevance and outcomes. The NCE context stage builds upon this foundation by incorporating a network-informed context assessment that analyzes system conditions, stakeholder needs, and relational dynamics among actors, organizations, and environments. This stage emphasizes understanding network structures, the distribution of power and resources, and the impact of contextual factors on intervention implementation and potential outcomes. A network-informed evaluability assessment delineates goals, network boundaries, governance structures, and evaluative capacities to ensure that evaluation inquiries remain feasible, credible, and appropriate within complex environments. Chapter 4 details the procedures for conducting a network-informed context assessment, including methods to assess the appropriateness and feasibility of NCE.

Input Stage

Stufflebeam (2004) defines input evaluation as the assessment of alternative strategies, action plans, staffing arrangements, and resource allocations to determine their feasibility and potential effectiveness in addressing identified needs. The NCE input stage expands this process by emphasizing the development of network-informed program theory and the structural design of interventions within complex systems. Program theory is conceptualized as a set of hypothesized causal mechanisms embedded within relational and institutional contexts. This stage systematically articulates assumptions, identifies key risks, and examines governance arrangements alongside constraints on evaluation capacity. By explicitly addressing these elements, the NCE input stage enhances transparency, strengthens theoretical plausibility, and facilitates informed decision-making regarding evaluation design and resource allocation. Chapter 5 outlines the steps for designing program theory, considering contextual factors, and assessing evaluation assumptions from a network-informed perspective.

Process Stage

Stufflebeam (2004) defines process evaluation as the assessment of implementation to support program improvement and assist users in interpreting performance and outcomes. Building on this foundation, the NCE approach advances this stage by developing comprehensive, network-informed evaluation plans that address the relational and temporal complexities inherent in networked systems. Chapter 6 outlines the procedures for conducting network-informed evaluation within complex networked systems. Key activities include formulating evaluation objectives and questions, defining the network's scope and boundaries, selecting methods to capture relational dynamics, and designing data collection and analysis plans to monitor interaction patterns and system changes over time. Techniques such as network mapping, visualization, and pattern recognition clarify the evolving roles, relationships, and configurations within the system. These visual and narrative methods complement quantitative analyses by facilitating collaborative sense-making and enhancing stakeholders' understanding of the interactions among structure, process, and meaning in evolving networks. Continuous stakeholder engagement during the process stage fosters shared interpretation, adaptive learning, and the integration of evidence into real-time decision-making.

Product Stage

Stufflebeam (2004) defines the product stage as providing information to guide decisions regarding program continuation, modification, adaptation, or termination, with an emphasis on formative purposes. The NCE approach implements this stage by producing user-centered evaluation products tailored to the needs and decision contexts of network stakeholders, as described in Chapter 6. These products serve as dynamic learning resources that support continuous monitoring, improvement, and accountability within complex systems. The approach emphasizes collaborative interpretation, participatory action planning, and systematic monitoring of progress. Furthermore, robust feedback mechanisms enable ongoing adaptation and learning across the network, reinforcing evaluation as a continuous inquiry process rather than a final assessment.

The NCE approach functions across the four interconnected CIPP domains as a continuous, iterative cycle of inquiry, reflection, and improvement. By integrating the decision-oriented logic of the CIPP model with insights from network and complexity theories, this framework establishes a complex adaptive evaluation method. Its cyclical structure conceptualizes evaluation as a collaborative process involving learning, sense-making, and adaptation within evolving systems. This integration allows the NCE approach to produce context-sensitive, actionable findings through a structured yet flexible evaluation cycle that prioritizes stakeholder engagement, theory-informed analysis, and network-based evidence. Chapter 4 discusses network-informed context assessment, Chapter 5 presents the strategies for supporting stakeholders in defining network-informed program theory, and Chapter 6 describes network-informed evaluation design and reporting strategies.

Chapter Summary

This chapter developed the methodological architecture of NCE by translating its conceptual foundations into a structured approach to evaluation practice. Building on the theoretical integration of CAS, SEM, and SNA, the chapter articulated the guiding principles that inform network-informed evaluation and introduced network typologies relevant to complex social systems. Drawing on SEM and CAS perspectives, the chapter emphasized the need to evaluate interventions across interacting intrapersonal, interpersonal, organizational, community, and policy levels, highlighting emergence, nonlinearity, and contextual interdependence as defining features of real-world systems.

The chapter further examined ethical considerations specific to network-informed evaluation, including confidentiality, transparency, power asymmetries, and cultural responsiveness, positioning equity as a central methodological commitment. The application of network analysis clarified how relational structures influence intervention processes and outcomes. By analyzing network features such as ties, clusters, centrality, density, and modularity, evaluators can assess the circulation of resources, information, and influence within and across system levels. Additionally, the chapter distinguished relational mechanisms from positional structures, demonstrating alignment between evaluation questions and appropriate network concepts and analytic measures.

Additionally, the chapter reinterprets the CIPP evaluation model through a network-informed perspective. Context is reframed as the assessment of relational drivers, stakeholder readiness, and ethical conditions; input as the articulation of network-informed program theory and governance arrangements; process as a participatory, methodologically rigorous evaluation design; and product as network-informed evaluation reports, adaptive system learning, and knowledge sharing. By integrating conceptual foundations with methodological guidance, Chapter 3 establishes the practical framework that informs the applied approaches presented in Chapters 4–6.

Reflection Questions

- How could applying NCE evaluation principles, such as systems and complexity orientation, network orientation, and contextual responsiveness, change the planning, implementation, or interpretation of evaluations within a specific field? Identify a recent or ongoing project where these principles might have yielded different insights or outcomes.
- Reflect on a traditional evaluation model you have used, such as the logic model. How could integrating network measures (e.g., centrality, density, brokerage) enhance your analysis or increase the utility of your findings? What challenges might emerge when operationalizing these network measures, and how could you address them?
- This chapter highlights adaptive and participatory learning as fundamental NCE principles. How can iterative feedback, co-learning with stakeholders, and flexible adaptation be deliberately integrated into evaluation practice to improve understanding of the networked system inherent in the program?

Applied Activities

Scenario: This scenario describes a newly established citywide coalition aimed at improving equitable access to adolescent mental health services. The coalition includes public schools, community mental health clinics, youth-serving nonprofit organizations, faith-based institutions, city health officials, and Medicaid administrators. It was formed in response to rising rates of youth anxiety, depression, and suicide, particularly in historically marginalized neighborhoods experiencing persistent access barriers and fragmented services.

Despite a strong commitment to collaboration among coalition members, the relational infrastructure remains uneven. Referral pathways between schools and clinics are inconsistent, information-sharing practices vary, and certain organizations hold disproportionate influence in decision-making forums. Youth representation in governance processes is limited, and cultural responsiveness differs among service providers. Funding streams are fragmented, and Medicaid eligibility criteria impact access to care. The coalition is uncertain whether persistent access disparities primarily stem from weak coordination, uneven trust, concentrated decision-making authority, or structural policy constraints. Rather than focusing solely on service utilization or symptom reduction, the evaluation should examine how relational structures, governance arrangements, and systemic constraints affect the coalition's capacity to provide equitable access to mental health services.

Activity: Using the NCE methodological framework presented in this chapter, design a network-informed evaluation for this coalition. Data collection or analysis is not required. The emphasis should be on demonstrating conceptual alignment among evaluation questions, ecological levels, and network concepts, and on clarifying how relational and positional dynamics may explain persistent inequities in adolescent mental health access. Structure your analysis in the following stages.

1. Assess the coalition's relational and structural context.

    - Analyze potential feedback loops among schools, clinics, youth-serving organizations, and policy actors. Identify conditions under which changes in Medicaid eligibility or funding might reconfigure referral patterns and service capacity.
    - Conceptually map intervention dynamics across ecological levels (intrapersonal, interpersonal, organizational, community, policy). Identify where key behavioral drivers, including trust, norms, and perceived support, are embedded within relational structures.
    - Examine the distribution of influence and participation. Identify actors likely to occupy central or brokerage positions, and organizations at risk of peripheralization.
    - Consider the ethical implications of mapping power and influence, including confidentiality, transparency, and potential consequences of disclosing positional inequalities.

2. Clarify how relational structures are expected to support equitable access to adolescent mental health care.
   - Identify the types of relationships most critical to equitable access, including referral, information-sharing, resource exchange, and governance.
   - Explain the theoretical rationale for how these ties are expected to reduce fragmentation and improve coordination.
   - Distinguish between:
     - Relational mechanisms (interaction processes including trust, reciprocity, and information flow), and
     - Positional structures (structural locations including centrality, brokerage, and peripheralization that shape opportunity and constraint regardless of intention).
   - Discuss how these mechanisms and structures may promote or hinder the coalition's equity objectives by specifying their expected effects.
3. Interpret network dynamics and system consequences by specifying the conditions and structural patterns the evaluation should identify.
   - Under what conditions might concentration of influence improve coordination efficiency while also reproducing inequity?
   - Where are structural bottlenecks most likely to emerge across ecological levels?
   - How might feedback loops amplify adaptive learning or entrench silos and disparities?
   - What structural configurations would indicate progress toward more equitable inclusion of youth voices and culturally grounded organizations?

References

Bonacich, P. (1987). Power and centrality: A family of measures. *The American Journal of Sociology, 92*(5), 1170–1182. https://doi.org/10.1086/228631

Borgatti, S. P., & Everett, M. G. (2000). Models of core/periphery structures. *Social Networks, 21*(4), 375–395.

Borgatti, S. P., Everett, M. G., Johnson, J. C., & Agneessens, F. (2024). *Analyzing social networks* (3rd ed.). Sage.

Bronfenbrenner, U. (1979). *The ecology of human development: Experiments by nature and design* (1st ed.). Harvard University Press.

Burt, R. S. (1980). Models of network structure. *Annual Review of Sociology, 6*(1), 79–141. https://doi.org/10.1146/annurev.so.06.080180.000455

Burt, R. S. (1992). *Structural holes: The social structure of competition*. Harvard University Press.

Burt, R. S. (2004). Structural holes and good ideas. *The American Journal of Sociology, 110*(2), 349–399. https://doi.org/10.1086/421787

Byrne, D., & Callaghan, G. (2014). *Complexity theory and the social sciences: The state of the art* (First Edition.). Routledge. https://doi.org/10.4324/9780203519585

Carolan, B. V. (2014). *Social network analysis and education: Theory, methods & applications*. Sage.

Centers for Disease Control and Prevention. (2024). *CDC evaluation standards*. https://www.cdc.gov/evaluation/php/evaluation-framework/about-evaluation-standards.html

Chen, H. T. (1990). *Theory-driven evaluations*. Sage.

Cousins, J. B., & Whitmore, E. (1998). Framing participatory evaluation. *New Directions for Evaluation, 80*, 5–23. https://doi.org/10.1002/ev.1114

Fetterman, D. M., & Wandersman, A. (Eds.). (2005). *Empowerment evaluation principles in practice*. Guilford Press.

Fitzpatrick, J. L., Sanders, J. R., & Worthen, B. R. (2004). *Program evaluation: Alternative approaches and practical guidelines*. Pearson.

Freeman, L. C. (1979). Centrality in social networks conceptual clarification. *Social Networks, 1*(3), 215–239.

Freeman, L. C., Borgatti, S. P., & White, D. R. (1991). Centrality in valued graphs: A measure of betweenness based on network flow. *Social Networks, 13*(2), 141–154. https://doi.org/10.1016/0378-8733(91)90017-N

Granovetter, M. S. (1973). The strength of weak ties. *American Journal of Sociology, 78*(6), 1360–1380.

Granovetter, M. (1983). The strength of weak ties: A network theory revisited. *Sociological Theory, 1*, 201–233. https://doi.org/10.2307/202051

Gould, R. V., & Fernandez, R. M. (1989). Structures of mediation: A formal approach to brokerage in transaction networks. *Sociological methodology* (pp. 89–126). American Sociological Association.

Hood, S., Hopson, R. K., & Frierson, H. (2015). *Continuing the journey to reposition culture and cultural context in evaluation theory and practice*. Information Age Publishing.

Knoke, D., & Yang, S. (2008). *Social network analysis* (2nd ed.). Sage.

McLeroy, K. R., Bibeau, D., Steckler, A., & Glanz, K. (1988). An ecological perspective on health promotion programs. *Health Education Quarterly, 15*(4), 351–377. https://doi.org/10.1177/109019818801500401

McPherson, M., Smith-Lovin, L., & Cook, J. M. (2001). Birds of a feather: Homophily in social networks. *Annual Review of Sociology, 27*(1), 415–444. https://doi.org/10.1146/annurev.soc.27.1.415

Mertens, D. M. (2008). *Transformative Research and Evaluation*. Guilford Press.

Newman, M. E. (2003). Mixing patterns in networks. *Physical Review E, 67*(2), Article 026126. https://doi.org/10.1103/PhysRevE.67.026126

Newman, M. E. (2006). Modularity and community structure in networks. *Proceedings of the National Academy of Sciences, 103*(23), 8577–8582. https://doi.org/10.1073/pnas.0601602103

Patton, M. Q. (2008). *Utilization-focused evaluation* (4th ed.). Sage.

Patton, M. Q. (2011). *Developmental evaluation: Applying complexity concepts to enhance innovation and use*. Guilford Press.

Rogers, P. J. (2008). Using programme theory to evaluate complicated and complex aspects of interventions. *Evaluation, 14*(1), 29–48. https://doi.org/10.1177/1356389007084674

Sabatier, P. A., & Weible, C. (Eds.). (2014). *Theories of the policy process*. Westview Press.

Seidman, S. B. (1983). Network structure and minimum degree. *Social Networks, 5*(3), 269–287. https://doi.org/10.1016/0378-8733(83)90028-X

Stufflebeam, D. L. (1971). *The relevance of the CIPP evaluation model for educational accountability*. Ohio State University

Stufflebeam, D. L. (1983). The CIPP model for program evaluation. In *Evaluation models: Viewpoints on educational and human services evaluation* (pp. 117–141). Springer Netherlands.

Stufflebeam, D. L. (2000). The CIPP model for evaluation. In D. L. Stufflebeam, G. F. Madaus, & T. Kellaghan (Eds.), *Evaluation models. Evaluation in education and human services* (Vol. 49). Springer. https://doi.org/10.1007/0-306-47559-6_16

Stufflebeam, D. (2004). The 21st-century CIPP model: Origins, development, and use. In M. C. Alkin (Ed.), *Evaluation roots* (pp. 245–266). Sage. https://doi.org/10.4135/9781412984157.n16
Stufflebeam, D. L., & Coryn, C. L. S. (2014). *Evaluation theory, models, and applications* (2nd ed.). Jossey-Bass.
Valente, T. W. (2010). *Social networks and health: Models, methods, and applications*. Oxford University Press.
Verbrugge, L. M. (1979). Multiplexity in adult friendships. *Social Forces, 57*(4), 1286–1309. https://doi.org/10.1093/sf/57.4.1286
Wasserman, S., & Faust, K. (1994). *Social network analysis: Methods and applications*. Cambridge University Press.
Watts, D. J., & Strogatz, S. H. (1998). Collective dynamics of 'small-world'networks. *Nature, 393*(6684), 440–442. https://doi.org/10.1038/30918
Weiss, C. H. (1998). *Methods for studying programs and policies*. Wiki-Devel. Sugarlabs. Org.
Williams, B., & Hummelbrunner, R. (2010). *Systems concepts in action: A practitioner's toolkit* (1st ed.). Stanford University Press. https://doi.org/10.1515/9780804776554

Chapter 4
Context Assessment in Networked Systems

The Critical Role of Context Assessment in Network-Informed Complex Evaluation

A comprehensive understanding of program context is essential for evaluators. Wholey et al. (2010) demonstrated that factors including multicultural environments, stakeholder characteristics, data availability, and operational constraints influence evaluation processes and outcomes (pp. 10–11). Fitzpatrick et al. (2004) emphasize the risks of neglecting context, noting that program failures often result from misalignments between intended plans and actual conditions, such as lack of consensus on goals, challenges in data collection, and ambiguities regarding the evaluation's purpose (pp. 182–183). Stufflebeam (2000) identifies the primary function of context assessment as determining the needs of the target group, which informs goal setting and provides a basis for outcome judgment. The Context, Input, Process, Product (CIPP) framework considers context assessment foundational for aligning evaluation activities with program objectives, stakeholder priorities, and the broader operational environment (Stufflebeam & Coryn, 2014). Within the Network-Informed Complex Evaluation (NCE) framework, rigorous context assessment is particularly critical because programs often emerge from complex interactions, such as collaboration, influence, and resource flows, rather than from discrete, isolated activities. Consequently, context assessment serves as a strategic entry point and a guiding mechanism for determining whether, why, and how a network perspective should shape the design and implementation of evaluation.

The NCE context assessment fulfills both diagnostic and prospective functions. It evaluates the significance of relational dynamics, including partnerships, information exchange, and referral networks, to determine whether a networked evaluation approach is justified and feasible from ethical and practical perspectives. Valente (2010) argues that network analysis is most appropriate when patterns of interaction, rather than individual attributes, drive programmatic change (p. 3). Accordingly, the NCE context assessment integrates needs and evaluability assessments, with

L. Zhang, *Network-Informed Complex Evaluation*,
https://doi.org/10.1007/978-3-032-27495-3_4

an explicit focus on connections, system boundaries, and readiness for relational inquiry. This approach exceeds basic feasibility by requiring evaluations to be practical, ethical, and reflective of the complexities inherent in dynamic systems. Rogers (2008) similarly advises evaluators to move beyond linear logic models and consider the evolving, systemic nature of interventions. These perspectives underscore the necessity of rigorous NCE context assessment to ensure that network methodologies are applied only when relevant, impactful, and contextually appropriate. This process is guided by critical questions such as the following:

- Is the application of a network lens necessary and justified in this context? Assess whether stakeholder relationships or interactions fundamentally influence program outcomes, or whether linear or individual mechanisms can sufficiently explain them.
- Are stakeholders and organizations prepared and willing to participate in a relational evaluation? Evaluate their readiness to share sensitive network data and to act upon the evaluation findings.
- Are sufficient resources, technical expertise, and ethical safeguards in place to conduct and utilize a network-informed evaluation responsibly? Examine whether these supports are available and adequate for the evaluation.
- Are personnel and financial resources adequate to meet the demands of the evaluation? Consider whether adjustments can be made to align available resources with the evaluation's complexity.

Furthermore, a systematic context assessment ensures that NCE methodologies are implemented with strategic intent, prioritizing contextual relevance, methodological alignment, and stakeholder utility. The following dimensions illustrate its critical role:

- *Identifying the Need for NCE.* A network lens is not warranted in every evaluation context. Inappropriate application of network analysis can result in methodological mismatches, inefficient resource allocation, and diminished stakeholder engagement. Borgatti et al. (2024) argue that network analysis is most effective when outcomes are shaped by relational structures such as influence, collaboration, or information diffusion. Similarly, Valente (2010) observes that network approaches provide explanatory power when interactions, rather than individual variables, drive change. Context assessment acts as a safeguard, ensuring that network methodologies are used only when strategically justified. For example, applying network analysis without a clear rationale can lead to unnecessary survey efforts, wasted resources, and stakeholder fatigue, ultimately reducing engagement.
- *Ensuring Relevance and Fit.* Methodological rigor depends on careful assessment of contextual fit. When program outcomes depend on interorganizational collaboration, diffusion processes, or coordinated stakeholder engagement, NCE offers analytical frameworks designed to address these complex challenges. Conversely, if individual-level or linear causal models sufficiently explain outcomes, network methods may introduce unnecessary complexity and diminish explanatory clarity.

- *Defining Scope, Boundaries, and Stakeholders.* Rigorous evaluation requires explicit delineation of system boundaries and identification of relevant actors, relationships, and levels of analysis. Employing socioecological frameworks enables evaluators to determine whether to focus on individuals, organizations, communities, or policy actors. Clear boundary specification reduces ambiguity, enhances methodological rigor, and minimizes the risk of collecting irrelevant relational data.
- *Fostering Stakeholder Engagement and Readiness.* Early and substantive stakeholder engagement is critical for effective context assessment. Eliciting stakeholder priorities, concerns, and experiences enables evaluators to identify relational challenges, such as referral gaps, coordination failures, and imbalances of influence. This collaborative approach enhances both the legitimacy and practical utility of the evaluation (Patton, 2008) while also building trust, fostering buy-in, and increasing the likelihood that findings will be implemented (Cousins & Whitmore, 1998). Co-design conversations in the initial stages directly influence the application of findings, as stakeholders are more likely to support and act on insights they help develop. This connection between early engagement and subsequent application underscores the value of investing in meaningful stakeholder collaboration. Additionally, context assessment determines whether stakeholders and organizations possess the necessary resources, technical capacity, and commitment to participate in relational evaluation (Stufflebeam & Coryn, 2014).
- *Addressing Complexity and Ethics.* Network evaluations present distinct ethical challenges, including threats to participant confidentiality, exposure to power asymmetries, and the risk of further marginalizing vulnerable actors (Borgatti & Molina, 2005). Proactive context assessment is essential for identifying and managing these issues. By systematically evaluating the network's relational and structural dimensions, evaluators can anticipate ethical risks and implement safeguards from the outset.
- *Theoretical and Practical Anchoring.* Robust context assessment grounds NCE evaluations in both theoretical rigor and practical relevance. By linking systems and complexity theories to real-world scenarios, network-informed approaches translate abstract concepts into actionable strategies. This process enables evaluators to trace the development and interaction of innovation, influence, and resilience across multiple system levels, resulting in evaluation designs that are both conceptually robust and operationally meaningful.
- *Applying a Multilevel Lens.* Adopting a multilevel perspective is essential for comprehensive evaluation. By systematically posing guiding questions at the individual, organizational, community, and policy levels, evaluators can reveal the equity implications embedded in network boundaries and structures. For example, asking, "Who gains voice if boundaries are redrawn?" prompts critical analysis of who benefits from current configurations and who may be advantaged or disadvantaged by changes. This reflection also identifies whose voices remain unheard, even after boundaries shift, ensuring that equity remains central to methodological decision-making.

Conducting Network-Informed Context Assessment

Network-Informed Context Assessment (NICA) is an evaluability assessment instrument designed to determine whether a program, policy, or system is suitable for NCE. Network-informed evaluation approaches are particularly appropriate in contexts where outcomes emerge from interorganizational relationships, collaboration, and information diffusion rather than from the actions of a single organization. In such settings, relational dynamics, such as coordination among agencies, referral pathways, partnership structures, and patterns of influence, play a critical role in shaping program implementation and outcomes. NCE therefore focuses on the analysis of relational structures and interaction patterns among actors, drawing on concepts from complex systems evaluation and social network analysis. Conceptually, the NICA checklist integrates insights from two influential traditions in evaluation theory: the Context dimension of the CIPP evaluation model (Stufflebeam, 2000; Stufflebeam & Coryn, 2014) and the emphasis on intended use central to utilization-focused evaluation (Patton, 2008).

Table 4.1 presents the NICA checklist, which operationalizes these concepts into a practical diagnostic tool for assessing readiness for network-informed evaluation. The checklist evaluates key dimensions, including conceptual relevance, stakeholder readiness, network boundary feasibility, data availability, organizational and technical capacity, and ethical safeguards. Evaluators rate each item on a four-point readiness scale based on document review, stakeholder interviews, and preliminary system mapping. These scores help determine whether conditions are appropriate for conducting an NCE and identifying areas requiring preparatory work. The following sections describe each checklist domain in detail and provide guidance on interpreting and applying the results during evaluation planning.

Section A: Needs and Opportunity Analysis

Fitzpatrick et al. (2004) emphasize that evaluators should first develop a clear and comprehensive understanding of the rationale behind the evaluation request, its intended objectives, and the key questions to be addressed. This foundational step, supported by Wholey et al. (2010) and Scriven (1991), ensures that the evaluation reflects genuine program needs and stakeholder priorities and establishes coherent evaluative logic and an appropriate scope. Needs and opportunity analysis begins with the systematic identification of the core problems, needs, or opportunities motivating the evaluation. Evaluators must determine whether program outcomes are primarily influenced by relational mechanisms such as collaboration, coordination, information diffusion, or collective decision-making, rather than by individual characteristics alone. Network analysis is most suitable when changes result from interaction patterns among actors rather than solely from individual characteristics. Rogers (2008) highlights the importance of aligning evaluation methods with intervention

Table 4.1 Network-informed context assessment checklist

Purpose: This instrument assesses whether a program, policy, or system is conceptually appropriate, practically feasible, and ethically suitable for Network-Informed Complex Evaluation (NCE)

Scoring Scale (per item):
- **1 = Low readiness** (major barriers present)
- **2 = Limited readiness** (partial evidence; significant gaps remain)
- **3 = Moderate readiness** (most elements present; manageable risks)
- **4 = High readiness** (strong evidence; ready to proceed)

Category	Item	Score (1–4)	Evidence Examples
Section A. Needs and Relevance (7 items)			
A1. Network Relevance	A1a Relational mechanisms: Are program outcomes driven by relational processes such as collaboration, referrals, diffusion, or coordination?		Evidence of shared service delivery, cross-agency referrals, policy coalitions, or information-sharing networks
A1. Network Relevance	A1b Limitations of traditional evaluation: Would a conventional evaluation overlook important relational dynamics?		Prior evaluations focused on individuals or organizations without examining partnerships or interorganizational coordination
A1. Network Relevance	A1c Stakeholder perception of interdependence: Do stakeholders view cooperation and partnerships as essential to program success?		Stakeholder interviews, coalition statements, or meeting minutes emphasizing collaborative success factors
A2. Alignment with Program Theory	A2a Relational program theory: Does the program's theory of change explicitly include relational mechanisms?		Theory of change or logic models depicting collaboration, referrals, influence, or collective action
A2. Alignment with Program Theory	A2b Network processes in outcomes: Are network constructs (e.g., trust, influence, shared leadership) central to the program's expected outcomes?		Strategic plans or program documents referencing trust, coordination, or collective impact
A3. Contextual Fit	A3a System complexity: Does the program operate within a complex system involving multiple organizations or sectors?		Presence of coalitions, service networks, cross-sector collaborations, or multi-agency partnerships

(continued)

Table 4.1 (continued)

Category	Item	Score (1–4)	Evidence Examples
A3. Contextual Fit	A3b External drivers: Do external drivers (e.g., funders, policymakers, or environmental factors) emphasize collaboration or system coordination?		Funding requirements for partnerships, cross-sector initiatives, or policy mandates
Section B. Intended Use and Decision Pathways (6 items)			
B1. Intended Users	B1a Identified decision-makers: Have the intended users of the evaluation been clearly identified?		Named audiences such as funders, policymakers, program leaders, coalition partners, or community stakeholders
B1. Intended Users	B1b Stakeholder participation in evaluation planning: Have stakeholders contributed to defining the evaluation's priorities?		Stakeholder workshops, advisory committees, or planning meetings
B2. Intended Uses	B2a Network-related decisions: Will the evaluation inform decisions related to collaboration, referrals, or partnership strategies?		Evaluation terms of reference include collaboration, network strengthening, or coordination objectives
B2. Intended Uses	B2b Decision urgency: Are the evaluation findings needed to inform imminent strategic or policy decisions?		Funding renewals, policy windows, strategic planning cycles, or organizational decision timelines
B3. Utility Alignment	B3a Added value of network analysis: Do stakeholders expect network analysis to generate insights beyond those obtainable through conventional evaluation approaches?		Stakeholders identify gaps in understanding partnerships, interorganizational relationships, or system coordination
B3. Utility Alignment	B3b Accessible reporting formats: Are plans in place to communicate findings in accessible formats appropriate for intended users?		Network maps, dashboards, plain-language reports, stakeholder presentations, or policy briefs

(continued)

Table 4.1 (continued)

Category	Item	Score (1–4)	Evidence Examples
Section C. Stakeholder Landscape and Engagement (6 items)			
C1. Stakeholder Mapping	C1a Multilevel stakeholder identification: Have stakeholders been identified across the individual, organizational, community, and policy levels?		Stakeholder maps, coalition membership lists, organizational directories, or partnership rosters
C1. Stakeholder Mapping	C1b Inclusion of marginalized actors: Are marginalized or less powerful actors included in the evaluation design?		Representation of grassroots organizations, minority-led groups, or community voices
C2. Willingness and Engagement	C2a Willingness to share relational data: Are stakeholders willing to participate in relational data collection?		Stakeholder agreement to report collaborations, referrals, or partnerships
C2. Willingness and Engagement	C2b Participation barriers: Have potential barriers to participation been identified?		Concerns related to confidentiality, survey burden, organizational capacity, or political risk
C3. Buy-In and Co-Ownership	C3a Co-design of evaluation: Have stakeholders participated in co-designing the evaluation?		Co-creation workshops, collaborative evaluation planning sessions, or stakeholder advisory groups
C3. Buy-In and Co-Ownership	C3b Commitment to using findings: Is there evidence that stakeholders intend to use evaluation results?		Leadership statements, governance agreements, or funder mandates
Section D. Boundaries and Data Feasibility (7 items)			
D1. Boundary Specification	D1a Boundary clarity: Can the network boundary be defined (coalition membership, service providers, agencies)?		Coalition membership lists, service provider registries, or formal partnership agreements
D1. Boundary Specification	D1b Boundary relevance: Are the defined boundaries meaningful for evaluation purposes?		Network boundaries align with program goals, evaluation purposes, or evaluation questions

(continued)

Table 4.1 (continued)

Category	Item	Score (1–4)	Evidence Examples
D1. Boundary Specification	D1c Boundary consensus: Is there stakeholder consensus regarding network membership?		Consistent boundary definitions across stakeholder interviews
D2. Data Sources	D2a Availability of relational data: Are relational data sources available (referral logs, rosters, surveys, admin data) for network analysis?		Referral logs, administrative data, prior network surveys, organizational rosters, or client tracking systems
D2. Data Sources	D2b Expected response rates: Are anticipated response rates sufficient to support reliable network analysis?		Anticipated participation $\geq$ 60% of organizations or $\geq$ 50% of individuals
D3. Data Access and Agreements	D3a Data-sharing agreements: Are data-sharing agreements in place or feasible to establish?		Existing memoranda of understanding (MOUs), data-sharing agreements, or collaboration agreements
D3. Data Access and Agreements	D3b Legal or institutional constraints: Are there legal or institutional barriers to accessing relational data?		Data governance policies, ethics requirements, institutional restrictions, or privacy regulations
Section E. Organizational and Technical Readiness (9 items)			
E1. Leadership Support	E1a Leadership endorsement: Do organizational leaders support the use of network analysis in the evaluation?		Leadership statements, strategic priorities, or resource commitments supporting network analysis
E1. Leadership Support	E1b Sensitivity readiness: Are leaders prepared to respond to potentially sensitive findings from network analysis?		Willingness to address weak partnerships, structural gaps, power imbalances, or system bottlenecks
E2. Evaluation Culture	E2a Collaborative learning culture: Does the organization promote collaborative learning and systems thinking?		Organizational mission statements, learning strategies, prior coalition initiatives, or continuous improvement practices
E2. Evaluation Culture	E2b Evidence-informed practice: Are staff familiar with evidence-based decision-making?		Staff training, prior evaluation experience, or history of evaluation use

(continued)

Table 4.1 (continued)

Category	Item	Score (1–4)	Evidence Examples
E3. Technical Capacity	E3a SNA expertise availability: Are technical skills available for social network analysis?		Staff or consultants with experience in social network analysis methods
E3. Technical Capacity	E3b Analytical software availability: Are appropriate software and secure data management systems available?		Access to software such as R, Gephi, UCINET, or other network analysis platforms, along with secure data management infrastructure
E3. Technical Capacity	E3c External expertise access: Is external expertise available to support the evaluation, if needed?		Partnerships with universities, research organizations, consultants, or technical assistance providers
E4. Resources and Timing	E4a Financial resources: Are adequate financial resources available for network data collection and analysis?		Evaluation budgets covering data collection, analysis, visualization, and dissemination
E4. Resources and Timing	E4b Timeline feasibility: Is the evaluation timeline realistic for capturing relational dynamics?		Data collection schedules aligned with collaboration cycles, program implementation, or policy timelines
Section F. Ethical and Equity Considerations (6 items)			
F1. Consent and Confidentiality	F1a Transparent consent procedures: Are consent processes transparent about relational data collection?		Consent forms describing relational data collection, nomination procedures, confidentiality protections, and potential risks
F1. Consent and Confidentiality	F1b Data protection protocols: Are confidentiality and data protection protocols robust and compliant with relevant data governance standards?		Procedures for anonymization, secure data storage, controlled data access, and compliance with relevant privacy or ethics requirements
F2. Risks and Mitigation	F2a Power imbalance risks considered: Have potential risks associated with revealing network structures (e.g., power imbalances, isolates, or central actors) been identified and addressed?		Risk assessment documents or mitigation plans

(continued)

Table 4.1 (continued)

Category	Item	Score (1–4)	Evidence Examples
F2. Risks and Mitigation	F2b Dissemination protocols: Are protocols established to govern access to and dissemination of network maps and evaluation findings?		Restricted dissemination policies, data-sharing protocols, anonymization procedures, or stakeholder agreements
F3. Equity and Inclusion	F3a Equity-sensitive evaluation design: Does the evaluation design promote equity and avoid reinforcing existing inequities or stigmatizing individuals or groups?		Inclusive evaluation design processes, equity assessments, fairness reviews, or stakeholder consultation
F3. Equity and Inclusion	F3b Inclusive interpretation of results: Are stakeholders engaged in interpreting and validating the evaluation findings?		Community workshops, stakeholder feedback sessions, participatory interpretation meetings, or validation activities

Domain-level summary table			
Domain	# Items	Possible Score Range	Domain Purpose
A. Needs & Relevance	7	7–28	Assesses the conceptual appropriateness of a network perspective
B. Intended Use and Decision Pathways	6	6–24	Assesses the intended use and decision relevance of the evaluation
C. Stakeholder Landscape and Engagement	6	6–24	Assesses stakeholder readiness for participation and engagement
D. Boundaries and Data Feasibility	7	7–28	Assesses the feasibility of defining and measuring network boundaries and relationships
E. Organizational and Technical Readiness	9	9–36	Assesses organizational capacity, leadership support, technical expertise, and available resources

(continued)

Table 4.1 (continued)

Domain-level summary table			
F. Ethical and Equity Considerations	6	6–24	Assesses ethical safeguards and equity considerations for network-informed evaluation practice
Total	41	41–164	Overall readiness for Network-Informed Complex Evaluation

Note This table presents the Network-Informed Context Assessment (NICA) checklist developed by the author. The checklist integrates the context dimension of the CIPP evaluation model (Stufflebeam, 2000; Stufflebeam & Coryn, 2014), the emphasis on intended use in utilization-focused evaluation (Patton, 2008), and the principles from complex systems evaluation and social network analysis.

Proposed Readiness Thresholds (Total Score: 41–164): These thresholds are proposed interpretive guidelines developed by the author to support practical application of the Network-Informed Context Assessment (NICA). They are intended to guide evaluative judgment and should be interpreted alongside contextual information and professional expertise.

132–164 (High readiness): The program or system is well positioned for a Network-Informed Complex Evaluation (NICE). Proceed with full implementation.

99–131 (Moderate readiness): The program or system demonstrates adequate readiness but may require targeted risk mitigation (e.g., pilot testing, capacity building, or refinement of the evaluation scope).

66–98 (Low readiness): Important readiness gaps are present. Capacity building, preparatory work, or refinement of the evaluation design is recommended before attempting a full NCE evaluation.

≤65 (Very low readiness): Substantial readiness gaps limit the feasibility of a full Network-Informed Complex Evaluation. Priority should be given to strengthening foundational conditions before implementation.

Evaluator's Recommendation Template

Total Score: ____/164

Readiness Category: [High/Moderate/Low/Very Low]

Priority Readiness Gaps: ________________________________

Recommended Mitigation or Preparatory Steps: ____________________________

complexity, recommending the selective use of network-based approaches when relationships and interconnections within a program are critical to its functioning and outcomes.

Section A, presented in Table 4.1, outlines a structured approach to assess whether a network-based evaluation is conceptually appropriate and necessary by examining the program's characteristics, theory of change, and operating context. The initial analytical step, network relevance (A1), determines whether key program outcomes depend on interorganizational or interpersonal relationships and whether traditional evaluation methods may overlook critical dynamics such as partnerships, coalitions, referral pathways, or influence relationships. This evaluation includes analyzing relational mechanisms (A1a), identifying essential network dynamics that conventional designs may omit (A1b), and assessing stakeholder perceptions of interdependence and cooperation as crucial contributors to program success (A1c). Evidence for this assessment is drawn from program documentation, prior evaluations, and stakeholder consultations to establish whether relational processes are central to both implementation and outcomes.

Subsequently, evaluators assess alignment with the program theory (A2) by determining whether relational constructs are explicitly incorporated into the program's theory of change. Relevant documents, including logic models, theories of change, and strategic plans, are reviewed to identify assumptions concerning collaboration, coordination, or collective action, thereby ensuring conceptual consistency between the program's intended functioning and a network-informed evaluation approach. Finally, contextual fit (A3) is evaluated by situating the program within its broader system environment, including multi-actor service systems, policy networks, and cross-sector collaborations, as well as external factors such as funding requirements, policy mandates, and environmental conditions, which may enhance the relevance of network perspectives. Through systematic integration of these factors, evaluators determine whether a network-oriented evaluation is suitable for addressing the program's needs, contextual conditions, and system complexities.

Section B: Intended Users and Uses

Fitzpatrick et al. (2004) assert that "evaluation is intended to enhance our understanding of the value of whatever is evaluated" (p. 176) and highlight the evaluator's responsibility to facilitate two-way communication, ensuring that stakeholders understand both the evaluation process and its potential uses and implications. This approach is consistent with utilization-focused evaluation, which emphasizes designing evaluations for "intended use by intended users" (Patton, 2008, p. 37).

As presented in Table 4.1, Section B expands the conceptual assessment from Section A by specifying the intended users of network-informed evaluation findings, their anticipated applications, and the decision pathways targeted by the evaluation. The initial analytical step involves identifying and engaging intended users (B1), including confirming whether key decision-makers have been identified (B1a) and whether they have contributed to shaping evaluation priorities (B1b). Evaluation plans must explicitly name the primary audiences and define their roles in decision-making processes. Early engagement of intended users ensures that the evaluation addresses relevant questions and produces findings that are both meaningful and actionable.

The subsequent analytic dimension addresses intended uses (B2) and utility alignment (B3). Evaluators assess whether the anticipated applications of network insights are clearly documented and linked to specific decisions, such as strengthening referral pathways, reallocating resources, enhancing cross-organizational coordination, or modifying implementation strategies (B2a). The analysis also examines whether evaluation activities are scheduled to align with key decision points, including funding renewals, strategic planning cycles, or policy windows (B2b), thereby maximizing the practical utility of the findings. Finally, Section B evaluates whether stakeholders recognize the added value of network-informed evaluation in generating insights unavailable through conventional data systems (B3a) and whether reporting and visualization methods, such as network maps, dashboards, or plain-language summaries, are designed to ensure accessibility and interpretability for diverse stakeholder groups (B3b).

Section C: Stakeholder Landscape and Engagement

Bryson and Patton (2015) define stakeholders as "individuals, groups, or organizations that can affect or are affected by an evaluation process or its findings" (p. 31). Within network-informed evaluation, the credibility, ethical integrity, and utility of findings rely on the systematic identification and engagement of stakeholders at individual, organizational, community, and policy levels. The willingness and readiness of each stakeholder group to participate, share relational data, and engage with evaluation findings should be systematically assessed. Building trust and mutual understanding is critical—evaluators are expected to clearly communicate expectations, address confidentiality concerns, and maintain transparency throughout the evaluation process. Early and inclusive stakeholder engagement is widely recognized as fundamental for ensuring the legitimacy and utility of evaluation, as it fosters buy-in and facilitates the uptake of findings (Cousins & Whitmore, 1998).

As outlined in Table 4.1, Section C examines the stakeholder landscape and the engagement conditions necessary to conduct a network-informed evaluation. The analysis begins with stakeholder mapping (C1), which assesses whether key actors have been systematically identified across multiple system levels, including individual, organizational, community, and policy domains. Evidence of stakeholder mapping, such as stakeholder analyses, coalition rosters, membership lists, or formal mapping exercises, helps ensure that relevant perspectives are represented in the evaluation. Particular attention is given to the inclusion of marginalized, less powerful, or historically underrepresented actors (C1b). Their meaningful participation is essential to accurately represent network structures and prevent analyses that inadvertently privilege dominant organizations or actors. By ensuring inclusive stakeholder identification, evaluators strengthen both the representativeness and ethical integrity of the evaluation design.

This section further evaluates stakeholder willingness and capacity for engagement (C2), emphasizing participants' preparedness to support relational data collection and other evaluation activities. It involves assessing stakeholders' willingness to report collaborative relationships or referral patterns (C2a) and identifying potential barriers to participation, including confidentiality concerns, political sensitivities, or evaluation burden (C2b). Additionally, Section C examines stakeholder buy-in and co-ownership (C3) by assessing the extent to which stakeholders can meaningfully engage in co-designing evaluation priorities and demonstrate commitment to applying the findings. Evidence of co-design processes, such as collaborative planning workshops or advisory groups (C3a), alongside explicit commitments to using evaluation results in decision-making (C3b), indicates greater readiness for network-informed evaluation and increases the likelihood that insights will facilitate learning and system improvement.

The criteria in Section C provide a framework for determining whether the stakeholder landscape is sufficiently understood, inclusively represented, and actively engaged to support network-informed evaluation. Building on this framework, Table 4.2 presents a multilevel stakeholder landscape for network-informed evaluation in complex systems, spanning individual, organizational, community, and policy levels. The table identifies key stakeholder categories, their roles within networks, their relevance to relational analysis, and critical engagement considerations.

Section D: Network Boundaries and Data Availability

Clearly specifying network boundaries constitutes a foundational methodological step in network evaluation. It is necessary to determine whether the network is defined by coalition membership, referral partnerships, policy actors, or other relevant criteria. Once boundaries are established, the availability and adequacy of data sources, such as rosters, administrative records, or survey instruments, must be assessed to ensure sufficient coverage. Without clear boundaries and reliable data, network evaluations risk producing biased or incomplete findings (Laumann et al., 1989).

As outlined in Table 4.1, Section D examines the practical and methodological feasibility of conducting a network-informed evaluation by assessing whether network boundaries can be clearly defined and whether sufficient, accessible, and ethically usable relational data are available. Because network analysis depends on well-specified boundaries and adequate relational data, this section focuses on foundational conditions that influence the validity, reliability, and interpretability of network findings. The first analytical focus is boundary specification (D1), which assesses whether the network of interest can be delineated for evaluation. This includes determining whether boundaries can be defined using clear criteria such as coalition membership, service provider participation, organizational affiliation, geographic scope, or service-area coverage (D1a). The analysis also assesses whether the proposed boundaries align with the program's goals and the population served (D1b), ensuring that the network definition reflects the program's substantive context rather than merely administrative convenience.

Evaluators also assess whether stakeholders demonstrate reasonable consensus regarding network membership (D1c). Ambiguity in membership can compromise the interpretation of network measures; therefore, comparing stakeholder perspectives helps identify inconsistencies or contested definitions. Section D further investigates the availability and feasibility of relational data sources (D2), including whether existing administrative records, referral logs, stakeholder rosters, or network surveys

Table 4.2 Stakeholder landscape for network-informed complex evaluation

System level	Stakeholder category	Primary roles in NCE	Relevance to NCE	Key engagement considerations
Individual	Program staff, frontline practitioners, service providers	Implement services; coordinate referrals; exchange information; enact collaborative practice across organizational boundaries	Provide relational data on coordination, trust, knowledge exchange, and information flow; reveal informal networks	Address confidentiality, participation burden, power asymmetries, and informed consent; clarify network nomination procedures
Individual	Clients, beneficiaries, community members (when appropriate)	Receive services; navigate systems; act as connectors	Illuminate service pathways, barriers to access, user navigation, and lived experiences of network functioning	Employ participatory and trauma-informed approaches; ensure privacy, voluntary participation, and culturally appropriate engagement
Organizational	Partner organizations; coalition members; service agencies	Coordinate services; formalize partnerships; share resources; implement collective action	Reveal interorganizational structures, collaboration patterns, brokerage roles, cohesion, and network fragmentation	Secure organizational commitment; clarify network boundaries; and establish data-sharing agreements
Organizational	Organizational leadership (executive directors, managers)	Set priorities; authorize participation and data-sharing; allocate resources, and support use of evaluation findings	Influence governance, sustainability, decision-making, and organizational responsiveness to findings	Prepare leaders for potentially sensitive findings; establish expectations regarding interpretation and use
Community	Community-based organizations; grassroots groups; advocacy organizations	Represent community interests; mobilize resources; advocate for underserved populations	Ensure equity, inclusion, and representation of marginalized actors; enhance network inclusiveness	Promote equitable participation; avoid overrepresentation of well-resourced organizations; recognize community knowledge and local leadership
Community	Community leaders and informal influencers	Shape community norms, trust, and informal coordination; connect otherwise disconnected actors	Reveal informal influence structures, trusted relationships, and community brokerage not captured through formal organizational networks	Apply culturally responsive and relationship-based engagement strategies; acknowledge local power dynamics

(continued)

Table 4.2 (continued)

System level	Stakeholder category	Primary roles in NCE	Relevance to NCE	Key engagement considerations
Policy/Systems	Funders; government agencies; policymakers	Establish policy priorities, funding mechanisms, accountability requirements, and system-level incentives	Illuminate structural conditions, policy environments, resource dependencies, and external influences on network performance	Align evaluation timelines with policy cycles; clarify expectations regarding evidence use and reporting
Policy/Systems	System conveners or backbone organizations	Coordinate cross-sector efforts; support shared infrastructure; convene stakeholders; coordinate collective action	Serve as network hubs for data collection, coordination, knowledge mobilization, interpretation of findings, and adaptive learning across the system	Clarify governance arrangements; maintain transparency; and manage potential conflicts of interest

Note This table presents the author's original synthesis of the multilevel stakeholder landscape for network-informed complex evaluation. It conceptualizes stakeholder roles, relational relevance, and engagement considerations across individual, organizational, community, and policy levels within complex systems.
Source Author

provide the necessary information to construct the network (D2a), and whether anticipated response rates are sufficient for reliable network analysis (D2b). Finally, the section addresses data access and governance conditions (D3), evaluating the feasibility of establishing data-sharing agreements (D3a) and identifying any legal or institutional constraints that may restrict access to relational data (D3b). These factors determine whether the network can be measured in a way that supports rigorous and ethically responsible evaluation.

Section E: Organizational and Technical Readiness

A comprehensive assessment of organizational preparedness for network evaluation is critical, with particular attention to leadership support, organizational culture, staff capacity, and technical expertise in social network analysis. Preskill and Boyle (2008) emphasize that building evaluation capacity within organizations is fundamental to effective evaluation processes and the sustained application of findings. Provan and Milward (1995) highlight the importance of organizational conditions, including staff involvement and commitment, while demonstrating the methodological demands associated with rigorous network assessment. Valente (2010) further highlights the importance of specialized knowledge in social network analysis to generate meaningful and actionable evaluation outcomes.

As outlined in Table 4.1, Section E assesses whether the organizational conditions, technical capacity, and resources necessary to support a network-informed evaluation are in place. Because network-informed evaluation can reveal sensitive relational dynamics and requires specialized analytic expertise, its successful implementation depends not only on methodological rigor but also on leadership commitment, an organizational culture that values evaluation, and adequate operational capacity. Within this section, the first analytical focus concerns leadership support (E1), which assesses whether organizational leaders explicitly endorse network-informed evaluation and demonstrate readiness to engage with its findings. Evidence may include formal leadership statements, signed agreements, or the allocation of staff time and financial resources to evaluation activities (E1a). Equally important is leaders' willingness to act on potentially sensitive findings from network analysis (E1b), such as weak partnerships, coordination gaps, central bottlenecks, or uneven influence among actors. Leadership openness to such insights is a key indicator of whether evaluation results will be used constructively to support learning and system improvement.

Section E also examines the organization's evaluation culture (E2), assessing whether the institution prioritizes collaborative learning, reflection, and system-level perspectives. Indicators include mission statements, strategic plans, or documented histories of coalition-based initiatives that emphasize collaboration and shared learning (E2a). The analysis further considers staff familiarity with evidence-informed decision-making (E2b), supported by prior use of evaluation findings, staff training in evaluation methods, or established organizational learning practices. Technical capacity (E3) is evaluated by determining the availability of skills and tools necessary for network analysis, including expertise in survey design, social network analysis, and data visualization (E3a), as well as access to appropriate analytical software and secure data management systems (E3b). External partnerships with universities or specialized consultants may supplement this expertise (E3c). Finally, resources and timing (E4) are assessed by determining whether sufficient financial and temporal resources are available to support network data collection, analysis, and interpretation. This assessment includes whether evaluation budgets adequately cover network surveys, analysis, and visualization activities (E4a) and whether evaluation timelines align with collaboration cycles, policy processes, or coalition decision points, ensuring that relational dynamics are captured and interpreted with contextual and analytical validity (E4b).

Section F: Ethical Considerations

Network evaluation poses specific ethical challenges, including risks to confidentiality, exposure of power dynamics, and potential stigmatization of marginalized actors (Borgatti & Molina, 2005). Therefore, the development of robust protocols for informed consent, confidentiality, and risk management is critical. Section F addresses the ethical and equity implications of network-informed evaluation, focusing on consent, confidentiality, risk, and inclusion. Network analysis requires the collection and representation of relational data, which may involve eliciting nominations and disclosing sensitive information about collaboration, influence, or exclusion.

As detailed in Table 4.1, Section F addresses the ethical and equity considerations in conducting network-informed evaluations. Network analysis, involving the collection and examination of relational data on interactions among individuals or organizations, presents distinct ethical challenges related to consent, confidentiality, and the potential disclosure of sensitive relationships. This section begins by evaluating consent and confidentiality procedures (F1) to determine whether participants are adequately informed about the nature of relational data collection and the implications of others' identification within the network. It further assesses whether consent processes explicitly specify how relational data will be collected, stored, and reported (F1a), and whether robust data protection measures are implemented to safeguard confidentiality and comply with relevant data governance standards (F1b). Transparent consent and secure data management practices are essential for maintaining participant trust and ensuring the responsible collection and use of network data.

Section F further evaluates risks and mitigation strategies (F2) associated with network-informed evaluation. Given that network analyses may reveal sensitive structural patterns—such as power imbalances, isolated actors, or central bottlenecks—evaluators must determine whether potential reputational, relational, or political risks have been anticipated and addressed through appropriate mitigation measures. This includes identifying potential harms associated with disclosing network positions or structural inequalities (F2a) and establishing clear dissemination protocols that specify who may access network maps or findings and under what conditions (F2b). Additionally, the section examines equity and inclusion (F3) by assessing whether the evaluation design promotes inclusive participation and avoids reinforcing existing inequities. Strategies such as participatory interpretation workshops, community feedback sessions, and collaborative data interpretation processes help ensure diverse stakeholder representation throughout the evaluation and interpretation of findings (F3a–F3b). Addressing these ethical and equity considerations ensures that network-informed evaluation is conducted responsibly, transparently, and with respect for the communities involved.

Network-Informed Complex Evaluation Readiness

Findings from previous steps must be integrated using a structured rubric that evaluates relevance, purpose, stakeholders, data sufficiency, organizational capacity, and ethics within the NCE context, and links each result to the appropriate action. Overall readiness should be categorized into actionable groups: Go (fully ready), Modify (ready with adjustments or pilot), Build (capacity-building required), or No-Go (not evaluable at this stage). This synthesis provides decision-makers with a clear, evidence-based foundation for subsequent actions and facilitates the ethical and practical application of the NCE framework in its appropriate context.

Identifying Stakeholders in a Network-Informed Approach

The identification and analysis of stakeholders are foundational methodological elements in rigorous program evaluation. Evaluation theory demonstrates that both stakeholder selection and the nature of stakeholder involvement significantly affect the relevance, credibility, and use of evaluation findings (Patton, 2008). Stakeholders contribute empirical data, organizational context, program theory, methodological design, and interpretation of results (Bryson & Patton, 2015). Stakeholder identification is not simply a procedural step but a methodological consideration with substantial implications for evaluating validity and utility.

Stakeholder identification is essential during the context assessment stage, which clarifies the program's purpose, theory of change, core components, implementation features, and contextual influences. In complex programs, employing a systematic, relational approach is essential to achieving comprehensive and equitable representation. Building on this need, network analysis offers a theoretically grounded and empirically robust framework for advancing stakeholder identification and mapping in evaluation. As Bryson and Patton (2015) note, "a purpose network (or hierarchy) diagram indicates the various interrelated purposes that the evaluation might serve" (p. 40).

A network-informed approach combines traditional stakeholder analysis with network analysis by identifying stakeholders according to attributes such as role, influence, interest, and relational positions within the evaluative system. This approach extends beyond recognizing only prominent individuals to include key groups and diverse perspectives that might otherwise be overlooked (Borgatti, 2006; Fitzpatrick et al., 2004). In doing so, network-informed stakeholder identification reveals gaps and inequities in engagement. Peripheral or weakly connected stakeholders often represent important communities or sectors affected by the program but are frequently excluded from decision-making processes. Including these actors constitutes both a methodological necessity and an ethical obligation, aligning evaluation with equity-focused and participatory principles and helping to prevent the reinforcement of existing power imbalances (Brandon, 1998; Cousins & Whitmore, 1998; Mertens, 2007).

Network-Informed Stakeholder Identification Criteria

Stakeholder identification and analysis at the context assessment stage are critical for defining the evaluation focus, informing question development, and guiding engagement strategies. This process combines traditional stakeholder analysis with network-informed methods to ensure that identified stakeholders represent both formal organizational roles and complex relational dynamics within the program system. Stakeholders can be assessed using a combination of attribute-based and relational criteria, including the following:

- *Relevance to program design or implementation.* Stakeholders directly involved in program design or implementation possess unique experiential knowledge critical for understanding how programs function in real-world contexts. Their perspectives are indispensable for accurately capturing program mechanisms and identifying feasible, actionable recommendations (Patton, 2008; Weiss, 1998). Including these stakeholders ensures that evaluation findings are grounded in operational realities and more likely to be adopted.
- *Knowledge of program theory, operations, or context.* Stakeholders with deep knowledge of program theory or the organizational context can clarify the logic, assumptions, and contextual factors that underpin program activities. Their input is vital for refining program theory, surfacing contextual moderators, and identifying plausible outcomes (Funnell & Rogers, 2011; Rogers, 2008). In network terms, these stakeholders often serve as information hubs, facilitating cross-boundary understanding and learning.
- *Interest in learning and potential evaluation use.* Evaluation findings are more likely to be adopted when stakeholders are motivated to learn from and apply the results. Utilization-focused evaluation emphasizes the involvement of individuals with a vested interest in the findings, as their engagement enhances commitment to both the evaluation process and the implementation of recommendations

(Patton, 2008). Identifying these stakeholders increases the practical utility of the evaluation.

- *Influence on program decisions or adaptations.* Both formal and informal stakeholders shape program priorities, resource allocation, and the implementation of recommendations. According to network analysis literature, influential stakeholders, whether possessing formal authority or social capital, often serve as gatekeepers or change agents within organizational systems (Prell et al., 2009; Valente & Pumpuang, 2007). Engaging these stakeholders is critical to translating evaluation findings into actionable outcomes.
- *Position within program-related interaction networks.* Relational criteria derived from network analysis provide practical methods for identifying stakeholders occupying influential positions within a program system. Central actors facilitate efficient information dissemination, whereas brokers connect otherwise isolated groups, fostering collaboration and innovation (Borgatti, 2006; Wasserman & Faust, 1994). Although peripheral stakeholders have fewer connections, they may represent marginalized voices or unique perspectives that are critical for advancing equity and inclusivity in evaluation (Lienert et al., 2013).

Network-Informed Stakeholder Identification Steps

Figure 4.1 illustrates a five-step process for network-informed stakeholder identification: defining the evaluative system boundary, specifying relational ties, collecting stakeholder network data, identifying key stakeholders, and triangulating findings through participatory validation. This iterative methodology is continuously refined and informs subsequent evaluation stages, including the input, process, and product stages.

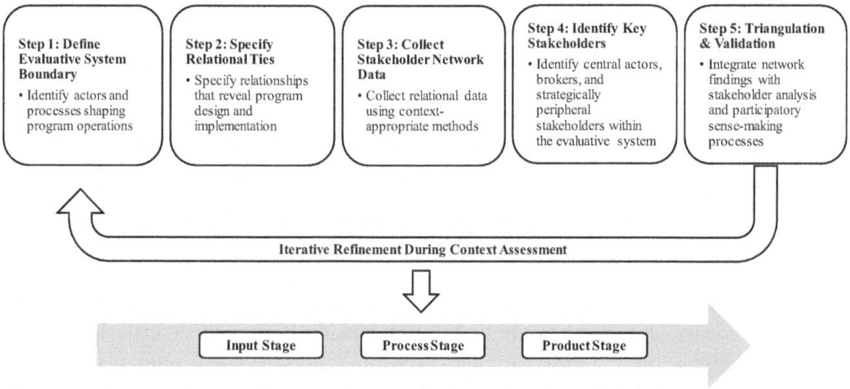

Fig. 4.1 Network-informed approach to stakeholder identification in evaluation. *Source* Author

- *Step 1: Defining the evaluative system boundary.* The initial step is to identify the actors, organizations, and processes that significantly influence program operations. In context assessment, boundaries are determined by the evaluation's substantive focus rather than by formal organizational charts alone. This approach includes implementers, partners, referral entities, funders, community intermediaries, and informal actors whose interactions affect program delivery or uptake. Clearly specifying boundaries enhances transparency, defines the scope of inference, and provides a defensible rationale for decisions about stakeholder inclusion (Bryson & Patton, 2015).
- *Step 2: Specifying relational ties relevant to the program.* The next step is to identify the types of relationships most relevant to understanding the program. During context assessment, evaluators should prioritize relational ties that reveal how the program is designed, implemented, and adapted, such as information-sharing, consultation, activity coordination, and referral relationships. Distinguishing program-relevant ties from broader social connections ensures that network measures capture stakeholders with experiential and interpretive knowledge, which is essential for refining the evaluation focus and questions (Lienert et al., 2013; Wasserman & Faust, 1994).
- *Step 3: Collecting stakeholder network data.* Network data-collection strategies for context assessment must align with the program system's relational dynamics. Roster-based network surveys are suitable for environments with clearly defined boundaries and high trust among participants (Marsden, 2014; Wasserman & Faust, 1994). Conversely, name-generator approaches are recommended for systems characterized by uncertain membership or open boundaries (Marsden, 2014). If survey burden or limited relational trust restricts data collection, qualitative methods such as key informant interviews or participatory network mapping can more effectively capture authentic relational data (Prell, 2011). Framing data collection as a learning opportunity may promote honest responses and improve data validity, especially in informal or cross-organizational settings.
- *Step 4: Identifying stakeholders with high informational and interpretive value.* This step prioritizes identifying stakeholders who can meaningfully inform the context assessment, rather than limiting consideration to individuals with formal authority. Network measures identify central actors with integrative knowledge, brokers who connect distinct segments of the system, and peripheral stakeholders who offer perspectives on frontline implementation and participant experience. Engaging stakeholders from these diverse positions ensures that context assessment reflects both system-level dynamics and operational realities (Borgatti, 2006).
- *Step 5: Triangulation and participatory validation.* Network-informed stakeholder findings should be triangulated with stakeholder analysis criteria, such as program engagement, familiarity with program theory or implementation, interest in learning, and potential contributions to evaluation use. Participatory sensemaking activities, including stakeholder review and interpretation of network findings, enable evaluators to identify missing actors, clarify relationships, and incorporate contextual knowledge that extends beyond the limitations of network

metrics (Lienert et al., 2013; Prell et al., 2009; Reed et al., 2009). This iterative process enhances analytic credibility and fosters early stakeholder ownership, thereby strengthening the foundation for subsequent evaluation use.

Network-Informed Stakeholder Identification Example

Table 4.3 presents an example of network-informed stakeholder identification conducted during the NCE's context assessment stage. The table categorizes stakeholder groups and individual actors based on their program roles, relational connections within the program system, and structural positions within the stakeholder network. Beyond identifying functional roles, the table evaluates stakeholders' program knowledge, influence on program design or implementation, and network positions such as central, broker, or peripheral actors. Integrating these dimensions, the analysis demonstrates how stakeholders contribute distinct knowledge and influence within the evaluative system. This network-informed classification enables evaluators to identify actors who can clarify program theory, facilitate access to information, support data collection, and promote the interpretation and use of evaluation findings across organizational and community contexts.

Utilizing Context Assessment Findings

Within the CIPP evaluation framework, context evaluation facilitates decision-making by systematically identifying needs, defining target populations, clarifying barriers and available resources, and establishing criteria for program improvement and judgment (Stufflebeam, 2000). Its primary value extends beyond describing the program environment to informing subsequent evaluative decisions and guiding evaluation design. In the NCE framework, context assessment is conducted as a multidimensional, network-informed inquiry. By integrating stakeholder analysis and social network perspectives, the NICA produces evidence regarding system readiness, stakeholder configurations, relational dynamics, and evaluability conditions. These insights form the analytic foundation for decisions that shape the input, process, and product stages of evaluation within the CIPP model.

Implications for the Input Stage

Findings from the context assessment inform key decisions at the input stage, including clarifying program goals, refining program theory, and selecting appropriate evaluation strategies (Stufflebeam, 2000). Within the NCE framework,

Table 4.3 Example of network-informed stakeholder identification results

Stakeholder group/actor	Role in program	Primary relationship to program	Program knowledge level	Influence on program design or implementation	Network position*	Potential evaluation contribution
Program Leadership	Strategic oversight and governance	Program design, policy alignment, strategic decision-making	High	High	Central	Clarify program intent, underlying theory, strategic constraints, and decision priorities
Implementation Staff	Day-to-day program delivery	Operational processes, adaptations, and implementation practices	High	High	Central or Broker	Identify core program components, operational realities, and patterns of program adaptation
Partner Organizations	Coordinated service delivery	Cross-organizational collaboration and coordination activities	Moderate–High	Moderate	Broker	Surface coordination dynamics, organizational interdependencies, and system-level interactions
Frontline Providers	Direct participant interaction	Service-delivery experience and participant engagement	High	Low–Moderate	Peripheral	Illuminate participant experience, implementation fidelity, and contextual constraints

(continued)

Table 4.3 (continued)

Stakeholder group/actor	Role in program	Primary relationship to program	Program knowledge level	Influence on program design or implementation	Network position*	Potential evaluation contribution
Community Representatives	Program beneficiaries or advocates	Program relevance, accessibility, and responsiveness to community needs	Low-Moderate	Low	Peripheral	Identify contextual factors, equity considerations, and community-level impacts of program activities
Funders/Sponsors	Resource provision and accountability oversight	Accountability, reporting, and learning priorities	Low-Moderate	Low–Moderate	Peripheral	Clarify evaluation information needs, reporting requirements, and intended uses of evaluation findings

Note This table presents an illustrative example developed by the author to demonstrate network-informed stakeholder identification within the NCE framework. It does not represent data from a specific program or evaluation but is intended to show how stakeholder roles, relational characteristics, and network positions can be integrated to inform evaluation design and use.

*Network position refers to a stakeholder's relational location within the evaluative system, as reflected in patterns of interaction, coordination, or information exchange. *Central actors* maintain numerous connections within the system and often influence information flow and decision-making. *Brokers* link otherwise disconnected groups and facilitate coordination across organizational or sectoral boundaries. *Peripheral actors* typically have fewer direct connections but often provide critical contextual, experiential, or equity-relevant perspectives that may otherwise be overlooked.

network-informed stakeholder identification helps clarify the program's target population, key needs, and the constraints and resources that influence program implementation. These insights support the development of evaluation questions, indicators, and data-collection strategies that reflect the relational dynamics through which programs operate.

Engaging stakeholders occupying central or brokerage positions within the evaluative system enhances evaluation planning. These actors often possess extensive knowledge of program design, implementation history, and system interdependencies. Their involvement enables evaluators to refine program theories, clarify underlying assumptions, and prioritize evaluation questions that accurately represent the program's operational context. As emphasized in utilization-focused evaluation, involving intended users in shaping evaluation design increases the likelihood that findings will be relevant and actionable (Patton, 2008). Thus, context assessment findings guide decisions regarding the responsiveness and feasibility of proposed evaluation inputs relative to identified needs and contextual conditions.

Implications for the Process Stage

Context assessment findings also inform decisions during the process stage by shaping evaluation design, implementation strategies, and ongoing monitoring activities. Network-informed stakeholder mapping identifies relational pathways through which information flows, coordination occurs, and participation is mobilized within the system. Understanding these relational structures enables evaluators to design data-collection strategies that align with existing system dynamics rather than imposing external structures that may disrupt collaboration or limit participation.

During evaluation implementation, stakeholders occupying central or brokerage positions facilitate access to key data sources, promote engagement across organizational boundaries, and assist in interpreting emerging findings within their operational contexts. Continued engagement with network-positioned stakeholders enables evaluators to address challenges such as uneven participation, data quality issues, or changing contextual conditions. This adaptive engagement enhances both the credibility and validity of the evaluation process by ensuring implementation remains responsive to the evolving system environment.

Implications for the Product Stage

Context assessment findings are equally important for informing decisions at the product stage, particularly concerning the interpretation, judgment, and use of evaluation results. Early clarification of stakeholder priorities, information needs, and communication pathways increases the likelihood that evaluation products will be perceived as credible, meaningful, and actionable (Patton, 2008). Network-informed stakeholder analysis also assists evaluators in identifying appropriate channels for communicating findings across diverse audiences.

Stakeholders occupying central or brokerage roles within the network often serve as translators and boundary spanners, facilitating interpretation of findings for different groups and promoting learning and action across organizational or sectoral boundaries. Simultaneously, the intentional inclusion of peripheral stakeholders, particularly those closest to program beneficiaries, ensures that evaluation findings reflect diverse perspectives and address issues of equity, accessibility, and lived experience. Consistent with CIPP theory, context assessment findings establish both the criteria for judging outcomes and the conditions under which evaluation results are most likely to support program improvement.

Chapter Summary

This chapter established context assessment as a foundational component of the NCE framework, identifying it as the analytic step for determining the appropriateness and feasibility of applying network-informed evaluation. Moving beyond a generic situational analysis, the chapter introduced a multidimensional model that integrates stakeholder analysis, needs assessment, system boundary specification, and organizational readiness evaluation. This approach underscores the importance of rigorous context assessment to determine whether relational dynamics are central drivers of program implementation and outcomes before applying network methodologies. By systematically examining contextual alignment, data availability, technical capacity, and ethical feasibility, the chapter clarified the conditions under which network analysis can produce meaningful and responsible evaluative insights.

A central contribution of the chapter is the development of structured tools to operationalize the assessment process. The NCE context assessment checklist and accompanying stakeholder mapping framework assist evaluators in defining network boundaries, identifying relational gaps, assessing organizational readiness, and anticipating risks related to confidentiality, equity, and inclusion. The chapter highlights the importance of early stakeholder engagement, particularly with marginalized or peripheral actors whose perspectives are often underrepresented in evaluation processes. This approach enhances both the legitimacy and methodological rigor of network-informed evaluation. These insights inform subsequent stages of the CIPP evaluation framework and translate complexity-informed principles into adaptive strategies suited to dynamic program environments. Chapter 5 builds on this foundation by advancing the next phase of network-informed evaluation design.

Reflection Questions

- Reflect on a familiar program or evaluation context. Identify key relational or systemic features that would support or oppose using a network-informed evaluation approach, as described in this chapter. How could a context assessment help determine whether NCE is the most suitable framework?
- How can early and inclusive stakeholder mapping and engagement, especially with marginalized or peripheral actors, enhance the rigor, credibility, and equity of your evaluation? What challenges might emerge, and what strategies could address them?
- Which ethical challenges, including confidentiality, power dynamics, and inclusion, are specific to network-informed context assessment? How can organizational readiness and technical capacity be accurately assessed and enhanced to ensure responsible and effective evaluation?

Applied Activities

Scenario: A regional public health initiative was implemented to increase childhood vaccination uptake through strategies informed by the BeSD framework. This initiative targets behavioral determinants, including vaccine confidence, social norms, practical access barriers, and provider–community interactions. Program activities encompass school-based vaccination campaigns, community outreach through trusted local organizations, healthcare provider engagement, and referral pathways that connect families to immunization services. The initiative involves a diverse partnership including public health departments, pediatric healthcare providers, community-based organizations, faith leaders, school systems, and parent advocacy groups. It was developed in response to declining vaccination rates across multiple communities, particularly among populations encountering structural barriers such as limited access to healthcare, transportation challenges, language barriers, and historical distrust of medical institutions.

Despite a shared goal of improving vaccination coverage, the initiative's collaborative structure remains loosely organized. Organizational participation varies, with some partners actively coordinating outreach and referral efforts while others engage sporadically. Information exchange and referral practices among healthcare providers, community organizations, and schools are predominantly informal and inconsistently documented. Incomplete data-sharing agreements hinder tracking of vaccination referrals and follow-up outcomes. Community representation in program governance is limited, particularly among populations most affected by low vaccination coverage. Furthermore, funding streams are short-term and unevenly distributed, and program eligibility criteria differ across service providers, potentially creating access barriers for certain families.

Program leaders are considering commissioning a network-informed evaluation to elucidate collaboration patterns among partners and identify gaps in outreach, referral coordination, and information-sharing. However, it remains uncertain whether relational dynamics—such as trust relationships, coordination among community actors, or information diffusion through social networks—constitute primary drivers of vaccination behavior. Alternatively, behavioral determinants identified within the BeSD framework, including vaccine confidence, perceived social norms, access constraints, and provider communication practices, may exert greater influence on vaccination uptake. Consequently, evaluators must first assess whether the program's context and theory of change justify applying a network-informed approach before conducting a network analysis.

Activity: This activity focuses on the foundational methodological question of this chapter: Under what conditions is the network-informed evaluation methodologically appropriate, contextually feasible, and ethically justified? Using the NCE context assessment checklist (see Table 4.1), evaluators must determine whether relational dynamics represent the primary mechanisms influencing vaccination behavior within the program's theory of change. The assessment should evaluate whether system boundaries can be established and whether adequate organizational, technical, and ethical readiness exists to conduct relational inquiry responsibly. The objective is not to design a comprehensive evaluation but to assess the justification and feasibility of applying network-informed methods in this context.

References

Borgatti, S. P. (2006). Identifying sets of key players in a social network. *Computational and Mathematical Organization Theory, 12*(1), 21–34. https://doi.org/10.1007/s10588-006-7084-x

Borgatti, S. P., Agneessens, F., Johnson, J. C., & Everett, M. G. (2024). *Analyzing social networks.* Sage Publications.

Borgatti, S. P., & Molina, J. L. (2005). Toward ethical guidelines for network research in organizations. *Social Networks, 27*(2), 107–117. https://doi.org/10.1016/j.socnet.2005.01.004

Brandon, P. R. (1998). Stakeholder participation for the purpose of helping ensure evaluation validity: Bridging the gap between collaborative and non-collaborative evaluations. *The American Journal of Evaluation, 19*(3), 325–337. https://doi.org/10.1016/S1098-2140(99)80215-X

Bryson, J. M., & Patton, M. Q. (2015). Analyzing and engaging stakeholders. In K. E. Newcomer, J. S. Wholey, & H. P. Hatry (Eds.), *Handbook of practical program evaluation* (pp. 36–61). Wiley. https://doi.org/10.1002/9781119171386.ch2

Cousins, J. B., & Whitmore, E. (1998). Framing participatory evaluation. *New Directions for Evaluation, 1998*(80), 5–23. https://doi.org/10.1002/ev.1114

Fitzpatrick, J. L., Sanders, J. R., & Worthen, B. R. (2004). *Program evaluation: Alternative approaches and practical guidelines.* Pearson.

Funnell, S. C., & Rogers, P. J. (2011). *Purposeful program theory: Effective use of theories of change and logic models.* Jossey-Bass.

Laumann, E. O., Marsden, P. V., & Prensky, D. (1989). The boundary specification problem in network analysis. *Research Methods in Social Network Analysis, 61*(8), 176–179.

Lienert, J., Schnetzer, F., & Ingold, K. (2013). Stakeholder analysis combined with social network analysis provides fine-grained insights into water infrastructure planning processes. *Journal of Environmental Management, 125*, 134–148. https://doi.org/10.1016/j.jenvman.2013.03.052

Marsden, P. V. (2014). Survey methods for network data. In J. Scott & P. J. Carrington (Eds.), *The SAGE handbook of social network analysis* (pp. 370–388). SAGE Publications Ltd. https://doi.org/10.4135/9781446294413.n25

Mertens, D. M. (2007). Transformative paradigm: Mixed methods and social justice. *Journal of Mixed Methods Research, 1*(3), 212–225. https://doi.org/10.1177/1558689807302811

Patton, M. Q. (2008). *Utilization-focused evaluation* (4th ed.). Sage.

Prell, C. (2011). *Social network analysis: History, theory and methodology*. Sage.

Prell, C., Hubacek, K., & Reed, M. (2009). Stakeholder analysis and social network analysis in natural resource management. *Society & Natural Resources, 22*(6), 501–518. https://doi.org/10.1080/08941920802199202

Preskill, H., & Boyle, S. (2008). A multidisciplinary model of evaluation capacity building. *The American Journal of Evaluation, 29*(4), 443–459. https://doi.org/10.1177/1098214008324182

Provan, K. G., & Milward, H. B. (1995). A preliminary theory of interorganizational network effectiveness: A comparative study of four community mental health systems. *Administrative Science Quarterly*, 1–33. https://doi.org/10.2307/2393698

Reed, M. S., Graves, A., Dandy, N., Posthumus, H., Hubacek, K., Morris, J., Prell, C., Quinn, C. H., & Stringer, L. C. (2009). Who's in and why? A typology of stakeholder analysis methods for natural resource management. *Journal of Environmental Management, 90*(5), 1933–1949. https://doi.org/10.1016/j.jenvman.2009.01.001

Rogers, P. J. (2008). Using programme theory to evaluate complicated and complex aspects of interventions. *Evaluation, 14*(1), 29–48. https://doi.org/10.1177/1356389007084674

Scriven, M. (1991). *Evaluation thesaurus* (4th ed.). Sage Publications.

Stufflebeam, D. L. (2000). The CIPP model for evaluation. In D. L. Stufflebeam, G. F. Madaus, & T. Kellaghan (Eds.), *Evaluation models. Evaluation in education and human services* (Vol. 49). Springer. https://doi.org/10.1007/0-306-47559-6_16

Stufflebeam, D. L., & Coryn, C. L. S. (2014). *Evaluation theory, models, and applications* (2nd ed., Vol. 50). Wiley.

Valente, T. W. (2010). *Social networks and health: Models, methods, and applications*. Oxford University Press.

Valente, T. W., & Pumpuang, P. (2007). Identifying opinion leaders to promote behavior change. *Health Education & Behavior, 34*(6), 881–896. https://doi.org/10.1177/1090198106297855

Wasserman, S., & Faust, K. (1994). *Social network analysis: Methods and applications*. Cambridge University Press.

Weiss, C. H. (1998). *Methods for studying programs and policies*. Wiki-Devel. Sugarlabs. Org.

Wholey, J. S., Hatry, H. P., & Newcomer, K. E. (2010). *Handbook of practical program evaluation* (3rd ed.). Jossey-Bass.

Chapter 5
Program Theory Through a Network-Informed Lens

Network-Informed Complex Evaluation: Why Input Stage Matters

Many of the programs we evaluate are not traditional programs, but networks of relationships through which influence, resources, and decisions flow. Over time, I have come to recognize that the most influential determinants of program outcomes are often found not only in the activities we evaluate but also in the relationships we seldom examine. Contemporary interventions often unfold across interconnected systems involving multiple organizations, sectors, and stakeholders, whose interactions shape program trajectories that conventional evaluation models struggle to capture. Recognizing programs as relational systems requires evaluators to reconsider how program theory is conceptualized and how evaluation designs are constructed.

Theory-driven evaluation provides a foundational approach for this reconsideration. It conceptualizes programs as explicit theories that specify the mechanisms and processes through which change is expected to occur. According to Chen (1990), programs function as hypotheses that link specific actions to anticipated outcomes through defined causal mechanisms. This perspective reframes interventions as structured propositions about their intended effects on social conditions, rather than as mere aggregations of activities. Clearly articulating these propositions is essential for rigorous and credible evaluations, particularly in complex or uncertain environments where underlying assumptions might otherwise remain implicit or unexamined.

Contemporary social, health, and policy interventions operate within environments with multiple interacting components, nonlinear causal pathways, feedback loops, and significant contextual dependencies (Funnell & Rogers, 2011). To address this complexity, evaluation theory must provide conceptual tools that consider interaction effects, emergent properties, and contextual variability. Network-informed complex evaluation (NCE) extends theory-driven evaluation by integrating systems thinking and principles from complexity science. This approach recognizes that outcomes rarely result from isolated program components; rather, they emerge from

L. Zhang, *Network-Informed Complex Evaluation*,
https://doi.org/10.1007/978-3-032-27495-3_5

interactions among actors, organizational capacities, institutional norms, and contextual forces within networks. Consequently, evaluation must assess not only whether change has occurred but also how and why change unfolds within interconnected systems.

Within this theoretical framework, the input stage is particularly significant. Evaluators must first understand an intervention's structural and relational foundations before assessing implementation, outcomes, or impacts. The input stage links evaluation theory to practical decision-making during program planning, a phase in which designs remain flexible and strategic choices can substantially influence future outcomes. The decision-oriented function of input evaluation is illustrated by the CIPP evaluation model, in which Stufflebeam (2000) describes it as a systematic process of identifying, critically examining, and comparing alternative approaches to recommend a course of action. This process enables decision-makers to select strategies that are theoretically robust, feasible, cost-effective, and responsive to contextual constraints.

The input stage of the CIPP model is essential for designing evaluations that are methodologically rigorous and contextually responsive. Stufflebeam and Coryn (2014) define input evaluation as the process of assessing whether proposed strategies are appropriate, feasible, and adequately resourced to achieve meaningful and sustainable outcomes. The NCE framework strengthens this function by incorporating relational mechanisms and network structures into program theory. By examining structural interdependence, governance arrangements, and contextual constraints, the input stage ensures that the evaluation design reflects the realities of complex, multisector systems. The following section outlines the core components of the input stage and provides structured guidance for evaluators and stakeholders seeking to ground their work in robust theory and contextual realities. A complete network-informed program theory template is provided in Appendix A.

Supporting Stakeholders in Clarifying Their Program Theory

Clarifying program theory is a foundational task in network-informed complex evaluation and a central responsibility during the input stage. Chen (1990) defines program theory as "a set of interrelated assumptions, principles, and/or propositions to explain or guide social actions" (p. 40). Program theory specifies how and why an intervention is expected to produce change by describing relationships among activities, mechanisms, contexts, and outcomes. Within a theory-driven evaluation paradigm, programs serve as testable hypotheses about social change, with evaluation processes examining, refining, and generating insights from these hypotheses (Rogers, 2008; Weiss, 1998). Clarifying program theory is especially complex in networked interventions, where causal agency and responsibility are distributed across multiple actors, organizations, and system levels. Evaluators therefore promote conceptual clarity and shared understanding to establish a foundation for coherent implementation and credible evaluation.

In networked initiatives, stakeholders often hold divergent perspectives regarding the problem, the intervention, and the causal pathways linking actions to outcomes. These differences frequently arise from organizational mandates, professional cultures, funding priorities, or power relations within the network (Funnell & Rogers, 2011). If unaddressed, such divergence may result in implicit, fragmented, or contested program theories, compromising implementation coherence and the credibility of evaluation findings. The input stage of evaluation plays a critical facilitative role by establishing structured, participatory processes that enable stakeholders to articulate, interrogate, and align their understanding of program purposes and causal logic (Patton, 2011). This collaborative process enhances conceptual clarity and fosters stakeholder ownership and consensus, both of which are essential for effective action in complex, networked environments.

The evaluation literature emphasizes the importance of participatory approaches in constructing robust program theory. Engaging stakeholders clarifies concepts and improves the utility and application of evaluation findings (Patton, 2011). Logic models and theories of change offer structured visual representations for mapping causal assumptions and timelines (Chen, 2015). For network-informed interventions, these tools require adaptation to depict interacting causal pathways, feedback loops, and organizational dependencies. This adaptation makes program theory more usable for planning, coordination, and evaluation by moving beyond linear models to accurately represent the dynamics of adaptive systems (Pawson & Tilley, 1997; Rogers, 2008).

Chen's (2015) distinction between the program plan and the action plan is particularly pertinent in networked settings. The program plan defines the problem's scope, identifies the target population, and specifies intended outcomes to guide strategic direction. The action plan operationalizes strategy by detailing activities, delivery methods, and implementation strategies to achieve program objectives (pp. 97–98). Within networks, a clear program plan consolidates goals and priorities, while a precise action plan delineates roles, responsibilities, and coordination mechanisms, facilitating coherent action across the network.

The NCE framework offers a structured, network-informed approach to program theory by organizing it into three interdependent components: program scope, action planning, and program effects (see Fig. 5.1). This framework acknowledges that programs operate within dynamic networks of actors, organizations, and contextual influences that shape the pathways and mechanisms through which change occurs. By integrating network concepts, the NCE approach ensures that program scope includes not only the problem and target population but also the relationships, resource flows, and interorganizational linkages critical to the intervention context. Action planning focuses on coordinating roles, facilitating information exchange, and establishing

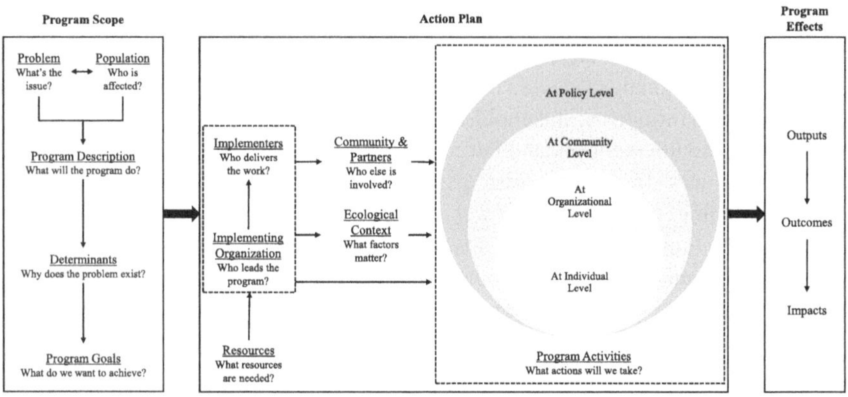

Fig. 5.1 Network-informed program theory: Scope, action plans, and effects. The framework shows how defining the problem, population, and goals leads to an action plan that mobilizes organizations, partners, and resources across multiple levels. Program effects are reflected in outputs, outcomes, and long-term impacts across social-ecological levels. *Note* The author's conceptual framework is built on the theory-driven evaluation model proposed by Chen (2015)

collaborative mechanisms that leverage network structures to achieve program objectives. Program effects are conceptualized as emergent outcomes resulting from interactions among multiple actors and system feedback, rather than as linear consequences of isolated activities. Building on this conceptual foundation, the subsequent section presents practical methods to help stakeholders define network-informed program theory.

Defining Program Scope in Networked Systems

Prior to analyzing how network perspectives expand program scope, it is essential to clarify why scope matters for practical evaluation decisions. Chen (2015) defines program scope as the "stakeholders' statement of program focus and goals" (p. 98), which includes the identified problem, target population, program description, determinants or causes, and program goals (p. 99). A clearly articulated program scope establishes the foundation for planning, communication, and evaluation (Chen, 2015, p. 100). In network-informed evaluation, program scope extends beyond these traditional elements to explicitly incorporate relational and systemic dynamics.

To clarify this extension, the subsequent section, supported by Table 5.1, presents a structured comparison between conventional interpretations of program scope and their network-informed counterparts. The table retains Chen's core components while demonstrating how each element takes on additional significance when analyzed from a relational perspective. Rather than replacing traditional evaluation concepts, the network-informed interpretation enhances them by integrating structural properties, such as density, centralization, modularity, brokerage, reciprocity, and structural

Table 5.1 Network-informed interpretation of program scope

Program scope component	Conventional evaluation interpretation	Network-informed interpretation
Problem Definition	Identified need, service gap, or performance deficit affecting a defined population	Structural conditions within an interorganizational network (e.g., fragmentation, excessive centralization, modular clustering, structural holes, limited bridging ties, inefficient diffusion pathways)
Target Population	Individuals or groups intended to benefit from the intervention	Actors embedded within defined network boundaries, with attention to positional location (central, peripheral, brokerage roles) and differential access to information, resources, and influence
Program Description	Activities and services designed to address the identified problem	Deliberate modification of relational structures and interaction processes (e.g., strengthening referral pathways, activating bridging ties, reducing excessive centralization, formalizing governance mechanisms) to improve system functioning
Determinants/ Causes	Individual, organizational, or contextual factors contributing to the problem	Network-level mechanisms shaping coordination and resource flow, including structural holes, homophily, concentrated centrality, weak reciprocity, low density, and limited cross-sector integration
Program Goals	Desired short- and long-term goals for participants or organizations	Dual goals combining substantive improvements (e.g., coordination, equity, access) with measurable structural targets (e.g., increased connectivity, reduced fragmentation, balanced centrality distribution, improved diffusion efficiency)

Note This table presents the author's network-informed reconceptualization of program scope components based on Chen's program theory framework (1990, 2015). It extends core components by incorporating relational and structural perspectives from social network analysis. Table A1 in Appendix A provides an example of network-informed program scope specification.
Source Author

holes. This comparison clarifies how problems can be reframed as systemic configurations, how network boundaries and positional embeddedness should define target populations, and how determinants and goals may be expressed both substantively and through measurable structural indicators.

Problem Definition or Challenge

In networked contexts, problems often stem from relational dynamics rather than solely from individual or organizational factors. Challenges may arise due to fragmented service systems, siloed communication patterns, excessive centralization, weak interorganizational trust, or inequitable participation in decision-making. Social network analysis (SNA) provides tools to diagnose these structural conditions, using metrics such as density, centralization, modularity, clustering, reciprocity, and average path length (Borgatti et al., 2009; Wasserman & Faust, 1994). For instance, a highly centralized network can create bottlenecks and increase vulnerability to hub failure, whereas fragmented subnetworks may impede information diffusion and coordinated service delivery. Furthermore, high homophily tends to reinforce sectoral silos, limiting cross-sector collaboration. Low reciprocity often indicates weak trust relationships that undermine collective action.

Networks convert problems into identifiable patterns. A network-informed problem definition involves structural diagnosis, including analysis of connection patterns, identification of structural holes, detection of homophily-based segmentation, and evaluation of whether existing relational configurations facilitate or impede desired outcomes. This diagnostic approach shifts the analytic focus from individual deficits to systemic conditions. Rather than questioning the sufficiency of service, stakeholders evaluate whether relational infrastructures enable or constrain coordinated responses. This perspective broadens causal understanding by showing how network structures shape outcomes and better aligns program objectives with the complexities inherent in networked systems.

Target Population

Traditional program theory defines the target population as individuals or groups intended to benefit from the intervention (Chen, 2015, p. 105). Network-informed program theory extends this definition by requiring the specification of network boundaries and identification of key nodes or subgroups. A critical issue is determining who defines these boundaries and what criteria are applied. Typically, boundary specification is a collaborative process in which stakeholders decide inclusion based on the program's aims, existing relationships, and strategic priorities. This process also involves identifying analytically relevant types of ties, such as communication, referral, collaboration, or governance (Laumann et al., 1989). Additionally, the target population may include structurally marginalized actors who occupy peripheral positions and have limited access to information, resources, or influence. Therefore, network-informed evaluation considers not only who is affected by the problem but also how structural position shapes opportunities. By integrating substantive and relational criteria, evaluators enhance the precision and inclusivity of the program scope.

Program Description

The program description details how the intervention seeks to modify relational structures or processes. Programs may aim to strengthen referral pathways, enhance cross-sector collaboration, activate bridging ties, reduce structural fragmentation, or redistribute influence among actors. These efforts constitute network interventions, defined as deliberate attempts to alter relationship patterns to improve system performance (Valente, 2010). Rather than focusing solely on individual behavior change, network-informed program descriptions specify expected shifts in relational configurations and their contributions to desired outcomes. For instance, establishing cross-sector working groups can increase bridging ties and facilitate the diffusion of innovation. Formalizing communication channels may reduce path length and enhance coordination. These structural adjustments represent central components of the program theory.

Determinants/Causes

Identifying determinants that influence outcomes is essential for clarifying program scope (Chen, 2015). Chen (2015) defines determinants as underlying causes, leverage points, or forces directly linked to the production of outcomes. He warns that stakeholders often conflate related terms such as intermediate outcome, mediator, facilitator, barrier, and root cause without conceptual precision, thereby obscuring causal logic (pp. 108–109). Determinants must be explicitly identified because, once activated or modified, they are expected to affect outcomes. Given limited resources, programs cannot address every plausible cause; therefore, they must select a limited number of major determinants that are theoretically defensible and aligned with organizational capacity. This disciplined specification improves causal reasoning and clearly delineates the program's intended influence.

For network-informed interventions, network-level determinants are structural characteristics that shape relational processes and influence outcomes. These characteristics include insufficient bridging ties, excessive homophily, concentrated centrality, low trust density, structural holes, and weak reciprocity. Such features affect diffusion processes, collective action, and resource coordination (Borgatti et al., 2009; Coleman, 1988). For instance, limited bridging ties may restrict access to diverse information, reducing innovation and adaptability. At the same time, excessive centralization may create dependence on a few actors, increasing system vulnerability and reinforcing power imbalances. Similarly, weak reciprocity and low trust density can undermine sustained collaboration and collective efficacy.

Consistent with Chen's (2015) emphasis on explicitly linking determinants to outcomes, identifying network-level structural conditions clarifies the mechanisms through which relational configurations influence program performance. Defining determinants in precise, theoretically grounded terms strengthens internal validity by ensuring interventions target plausible causal drivers rather than diffuse symptoms. This explicit specification enhances theoretical coherence, guides intervention design, and refines the evaluative focus on whether selected structural levers are responsible for observed changes in network and substantive outcomes.

Program Goals

Drawing on Chen's program theory framework, clearly articulating program goals is fundamental to both implementation and evaluation. Chen (2015) distinguishes ultimate goals as broad, long-term social conditions that a program aims to influence, from practical goals, which are achievable targets within available resources and time constraints (pp. 106–107). This distinction is especially important for network-informed initiatives. While stakeholders may aspire to systemic transformations such as equity, integration, or improved population well-being, these aspirations must be translated into concrete, feasible, and measurable goals that define the program's realistic achievements and the outcomes it is intended to produce.

Within this framework, network-informed program goals should include both substantive and relational dimensions. Substantive goals focus on improvements in services or client outcomes, such as enhanced access, reduced disparities, or improved coordination. Relational structural goals specify intended changes in interaction patterns among participating actors, including increased connectivity, reduced fragmentation, greater inclusion of marginalized organizations, or more balanced distributions of influence. To clarify evaluative criteria, it is essential to specify explicit decision thresholds for these network metrics. For instance, a program might define success as achieving at least a 15% increase in network density or a reduction in modularity by 0.10. Establishing such thresholds at the outset guides measurement plans, determines goal attainment, and provides stakeholders with clear progress indicators. Where possible, these thresholds should be tailored using baseline data and informed by stakeholder priorities and relevant empirical benchmarks.

Consistent with Chen's (2015) emphasis on clearly defined outcomes as the foundation of evaluability (p. 107), these relational targets should be operationalized through measurable changes in network properties, such as increased density, reduced modularity, or improved centrality distribution. This approach ensures that collaboration and integration are explicit program goals rather than incidental outcomes. By articulating both substantive and relational goals in measurable terms, stakeholders enhance the evaluability of network-informed interventions. Clear program goals provide observable indicators linked to program theory, guide data collection and analysis, and establish transparent accountability criteria. Consequently, relational transformation becomes embedded within the intervention logic, ensuring that network change is integral to program success.

Defining Action Plan in Networked Systems

Chen (2015) identifies key functions of an action model for evaluators, including facilitating the development or refinement of action plans, clarifying implementation strategies and responsibilities, understanding factors influencing implementation toward program goals, communicating action plans to stakeholders, and preparing evaluation efforts to assess program effectiveness (p. 119). Within the NCE framework, the action plan performs these functions by integrating network constructs into program design, enhancing the operationalization of program theory.

The action plan translates the clarified program scope into coordinated implementation strategies by specifying required technical, human, and financial resources; identifying implementing organizations and actors; delineating partnering organizations; situating activities within their ecological context; and articulating program activities across social-ecological model levels (Chen, 2015, pp. 118–120). Traditional evaluation practices emphasize organizational responsibilities, administrative processes, and procedural sequencing. However, implementation in networked environments occurs in interorganizational systems characterized by distributed authority, structural interdependence, and relational variability.

A network-informed action plan must extend beyond administrative coordination to encompass governance structures, positional influence, and patterns of relational connectivity. Governance arrangements, such as participant-governed networks, lead-organization models, or network-administrative organizations, determine the distribution of authority and the coordination capacity (Provan & Kenis, 2008). The choice of governance model significantly affects program effectiveness; for instance, selecting an inappropriate structure may lead to coordination breakdowns, erosion of trust, or the concentration of power, whereas an appropriate fit enhances adaptability, participation, and system resilience. Implementers often occupy structurally central or brokerage positions that influence information diffusion, cross-sector integration, and resource mobilization. Partnering organizations should be systematically mapped and engaged to address structural holes and strengthen bridging ties. Additionally, ecological context, including policy frameworks, resource distribution, and historical relationships, shapes network evolution and the sustainability of collaboration. Incorporating these relational factors into the action plan improves alignment between program theory and implementation design.

To clarify this extension of Chen's (2015) action model, Table 5.2 presents a structured comparison between conventional interpretations of action plan components and their network-informed counterparts. The table retains Chen's core elements while demonstrating how each gains additional significance when examined from a relational perspective. Rather than replacing traditional implementation planning, the network-informed interpretation enhances it by incorporating governance modes, structural positioning, relational capacity, trust development, boundary spanning, and measurable network signatures that indicate implementation progress. This comparison reinforces the connection between program scope and action planning by illustrating how relational design and structural coordination are essential for operationalizing program theory in complex networked systems.

Table 5.2 Network-informed interpretation of action plan components

Action plan component	Conventional evaluation interpretation	Network-informed interpretation
Resources	Financial, human, and technical inputs required for implementation	Core implementation conditions supporting program integrity and fidelity, including organizational capacity, relational data systems, network analysis tools, facilitation expertise, ethical data governance, and sustained funding for longitudinal network monitoring and adaptive learning
Implementing Organizations and Actors	Organization(s) responsible for delivering program activities and managing personnel	Governance structures as implementation mechanisms shaping authority distribution, coordination capacity, and accountability, alongside recognition of positional influence (e.g., centrality, brokerage) affecting information diffusion and resource mobilization
Partnering Organizations and Community Partners	Collaborating organizations and community partners contributing to program implementation	Structurally embedded actors whose roles, communication patterns, and governance arrangements must be explicitly defined; includes intentional strengthening of bridging ties, bridging structural holes, and attention to power asymmetries to sustain coordinated collaboration
Ecological Context	External environmental factors influencing implementation	Enabling institutional and relational infrastructure within the action model, including policy mandates, governance norms, historical relationships, and resource distribution patterns shaping trust development, authority concentration, network evolution, and collaboration sustainability
Program Activities	Planned activities delivered to achieve program objectives	Theoretically grounded relational interventions specifying what is done, by whom, and under what conditions, with explicitly hypothesized effects on network structure (e.g., increased bridging, shorter average path length, more balanced centrality) across social-ecological levels

Note This table presents the author's network-informed reconceptualization of action plan components based on Chen's program theory framework (1990, 2015). It extends core components by incorporating relational and structural perspectives derived from social network analysis. Table A2 in Appendix A provides an illustrative example of network-informed action plan specification.
Source Author

Resources

Resources represent fundamental elements of the action model rather than peripheral administrative concerns. Chen (2015) emphasizes that programs depend on implementing organizations to allocate resources, coordinate activities, and recruit, train, and supervise personnel (p. 75). The adequacy of technical, human, and financial resources directly influences the quality of implementation. If the implementing organization lacks the capacity to mobilize and sustain these resources, the intervention's integrity and the credibility of outcome claims are compromised. Explicitly specifying required resources improves feasibility, clarifies organizational responsibility, and enhances program evaluability.

In network-informed interventions, resource requirements extend beyond traditional service-delivery inputs. Technical resources include rigorous data-collection instruments, such as relational surveys and integrated administrative data systems; specialized network analysis software; and visualization platforms capable of representing complex structural configurations. Human resources include analysts trained in social network methods, facilitators skilled in stakeholder engagement, and personnel responsible for data governance and ethical oversight. Financial resources must support initial data collection, longitudinal monitoring, iterative feedback cycles, and capacity-building activities across participating organizations. Because network structures evolve over time, sustained funding is essential to capture dynamic structural changes rather than relying on static, one-time assessments.

Adequate resource allocation is essential for robust, ethical, and sustainable network evaluation. Longitudinal structural analysis requires continuity in staffing, analytic expertise, and technological infrastructure. Ethical responsibilities, such as protecting relational confidentiality, managing sensitive positional information, and ensuring informed consent, require deliberate investment. Consistent with Chen's (2015) emphasis on organizational capacity as a determinant of implementation success, articulating resource commitments and aligning them with program phases enhances theoretical coherence, supports implementation fidelity, and strengthens the internal validity of claims concerning network transformation.

Implementing Organization and Implementers

Chen (2015) states that a program depends on organization(s) to allocate resources, coordinate activities, and recruit, train, and supervise implementers (p. 75). Consequently, implementation quality is closely linked to organizational structure and capacity. Clearly identifying the implementing organizations and personnel responsible for service delivery is essential to avoid role ambiguity, diffusion of responsibility, and accountability failures. Furthermore, Chen highlights that programs must ensure implementing organizations have sufficient managerial, technical, and human resource capacities; without these capacities, even well-designed interventions are unlikely to achieve intended outcomes. Thus, organizational arrangements and capabilities are critical components of the action model and require explicit theoretical and evaluative attention.

In interorganizational or networked contexts, implementation analysis must extend beyond individual organizational capacity to encompass governance structures and relational configurations. Governance models—such as participant-governed networks, lead-organization forms, or network-administrative organizations (NAOs)—systematically shape the distribution of authority, coordination mechanisms, and accountability processes (Provan & Kenis, 2008). These structural choices affect decision-making, conflict resolution, and resource flows across the system rather than merely reflecting administrative preferences. Explicit clarification of governance arrangements reduces ambiguity, enhances strategic alignment, and strengthens coherence between the program's structural design and substantive objectives. From a program theory perspective, governance structure functions as a hypothesized mechanism influencing implementation effectiveness. The practical value of positional analysis is demonstrated in real-world implementation; for example, a network analysis during a multisector health partnership identified that critical information was consistently bottlenecked at a single organizational node. By recognizing a key broker whose positional influence had been previously unacknowledged, program leaders formally engaged this actor as a liaison, promptly resolving communication bottlenecks and facilitating timely cross-organizational coordination. This targeted intervention, informed by positional insight, prevented prolonged implementation delays and aligned network resources with program goals.

Implementers in networked programs often occupy structurally significant positions within the relational system. Actors with high centrality may exert disproportionate influence on information diffusion and resource mobilization, while brokers connecting otherwise disconnected clusters facilitate cross-sector learning and coordination. Recognizing these positional dynamics improves implementation planning by identifying leverage points, vulnerabilities, and bottlenecks. Consistent with Chen's (2015) emphasis on aligning organizational capability with program design, integrating network positional analysis into implementation strategies enhances theoretical precision and strengthens internal validity. By linking governance structures, organizational capacity, and relational positions to anticipated implementation processes, evaluators can more effectively assess whether structural arrangements support or constrain the achievement of program outcomes.

Partnering Organizations and Community Partners

Chen (2015) articulates an action model in which associate organizations and community partners are essential components of effective program implementation rather than peripheral contributors. Many programs benefit from, and sometimes require, cooperation between implementing organizations and other entities to ensure feasibility, coordination, and contextual responsiveness. Failure to establish and maintain productive working relationships with relevant partners can hinder implementation and diminish program effectiveness. From a program theory perspective, collaboration represents a structurally necessary condition embedded within the action model rather than a mere informal aspiration.

In network-informed interventions, partnering agencies, community organizations, and key stakeholders essential for building and sustaining network ties must be systematically identified and relationally mapped. Such mapping clarifies patterns of interaction, authority, and resource exchange across the system. Governance mechanisms for regular communication, joint decision-making, and collaborative problem-solving should be explicitly defined to reduce ambiguity and enhance accountability. Clearly articulated coordination structures—formalized through memoranda of understanding, shared protocols, or designated convening bodies—align relational processes with program objectives and reduce fragmentation. This structured approach acknowledges that collaboration requires intentional design rather than reliance on informal goodwill.

An inclusive partnership strategy deliberately addresses relational gaps or structural holes that impede coordination and innovation. Drawing on network theory, bridging disconnected actors enhances information flow and resource integration, while inclusive participation mitigates power imbalances and marginalization. By incorporating diverse perspectives and capacities, programs strengthen both implementation fidelity and adaptive capacity. Consistent with Chen's (2015) emphasis on aligning structural arrangements with intended change mechanisms, articulating partner roles, communication channels, and governance processes enhances theoretical coherence, supports effective coordination, and reinforces the internal validity of claims concerning collaborative impact.

Ecological Context

The ecological context refers to the segment of the environment that directly interacts with and influences program implementation (Chen, 2015, pp. 77–78). Chen (2015) highlights that both micro-level supports, such as family, peer, and immediate organizational environments, and macro-level conditions, including community norms, political climates, and economic structures, can facilitate or impede program success. Contextual support is essential; when critical for achieving outcomes, it must be deliberately incorporated into program design rather than assumed. Therefore, ecological conditions constitute part of the enabling infrastructure of the action model and determine whether intervention mechanisms function as intended.

Network-informed interventions require a systematic description and analysis of the broader social, organizational, community, and policy environments that influence network structures and processes. Contextual factors—including governance norms, resource distribution, historical interorganizational relationships, regulatory frameworks, and prevailing cultural expectations—shape interaction patterns within the network. For example, policy mandates may encourage collaboration or, conversely, maintain competitive funding dynamics that obstruct information sharing. Historical mistrust among organizations can impede reciprocity and collective action, while unequal resource distribution may concentrate power and reinforce existing asymmetries. These contextual conditions influence information flow, trust development, participation equity, and the sustainability of collaborative relationships.

A careful consideration of the ecological context improves the realism, feasibility, and sustainability of the action plan. Explicit assessment of contextual supports and constraints enables program designers and evaluators to reinforce the plausibility of causal assumptions within the program theory. Incorporating contextual analysis into network design ensures that structural interventions, such as increasing bridging ties or redistributing coordination roles, correspond with environmental realities rather than being implemented in isolation.

Program Activities by Social-Ecological Level

The action plan forms the operational core of the action model. Chen (2015) emphasizes that the action model is essential for developing or refining implementation plans, clarifying strategies and responsibilities, identifying critical implementation conditions, communicating intended processes to stakeholders, and preparing for comprehensive evaluation (pp. 73–78). Program activities represent theoretically grounded interventions rather than procedural steps and are designed to activate specific mechanisms that generate desired outcomes. A well-specified action plan explicitly defines tasks, responsible actors, contextual conditions, and expected effects.

Within NCE, the action plan must specify program activities at each level of the social-ecological model and explicitly link each activity to anticipated relational or structural changes within the network. For instance, strengthening referral systems can reduce average path lengths and increase bridging ties, thereby enhancing information flow and service coordination. Coalition mobilization efforts seek to reduce homophily and promote cross-sector integration, expanding collaboration beyond isolated clusters. Knowledge diffusion initiatives—such as shared learning forums or digital communication platforms—can broaden participation and redistribute influence, as reflected by changes in centrality or brokerage patterns. By defining these anticipated "network signatures," program designers translate abstract relational objectives into observable structural indicators.

Linking activities to measurable structural changes operationalizes program theory and enhances adaptive management. By specifying expected relational shifts in advance, evaluators can monitor whether implementation proceeds as theorized and adjust strategies accordingly. This approach aligns with Chen's (2015) emphasis on using the action model to clarify causal assumptions and prepare for rigorous evaluation. Within NCE, embedding network constructs directly into the action plan improves theoretical coherence, facilitates real-time learning, and ensures that implementation progress is assessed not only through outputs but also through empirically verifiable transformations in relational structure.

Defining Program Effects in Networked Systems

The third component of the NCE framework conceptualizes program effects as outputs, outcomes, and impacts, each representing distinct yet interrelated dimensions of change. In network-informed evaluation, these categories move beyond terminological differences to analytically distinguish layers of relational and systemic transformation. Disaggregating program effects in this way enables evaluators to trace the progression from immediate, tangible results (outputs) to observable changes in network structure and function (outcomes), culminating in enduring system-level impacts.

This layered conceptualization aligns with theory-driven evaluation, which requires explicit specification of how proximal program activities generate intermediate changes and ultimately long-term social effects (Chen, 2015; Rogers, 2008; Weiss, 1998). Within the NCE framework, outputs are immediate, observable products of implementation—such as newly established partnerships, formalized referral agreements, or convened cross-sector forums—that reflect relational activation. Outcomes are measurable shifts in network properties, such as increased connectivity, reduced fragmentation, strengthened reciprocity, more balanced centrality distribution, and improved information flow. Impacts involve durable transformations in system functioning, including resilient relational infrastructures, institutionalized collaboration, equitable participation in governance, and sustained cross-sector learning. This differentiation enhances evaluability by linking specific structural indicators to theoretically defined stages of change.

To clarify this relational progression, Table 5.3 presents a structured comparison between conventional interpretations of outputs, outcomes, and impacts and their network-informed counterparts. The table retains traditional distinctions commonly used in evaluation practice while showing how each category acquires additional analytical depth when examined through structural and relational perspectives. Instead of redefining these categories, the network-informed interpretation specifies how each level corresponds to progressively deeper transformations in network configuration and systemic capacity. This comparison reinforces the cumulative logic of program effects and illustrates how relational mechanisms mediate the pathway from immediate implementation results to enduring system change.

Outputs

Outputs are the direct, observable products generated by program activities (Mathison, 2005, p. 287). In network-informed evaluation, outputs include concrete actions such as initiating cross-sector partnerships, formalizing referral agreements, delivering training sessions, facilitating collaborative meetings, and disseminating policy briefs. Each activity produces immediate, verifiable results that serve as empirical evidence of implementation. From a network perspective, outputs represent the

Table 5.3 Network-informed interpretation of program effects

Program effect component	Conventional evaluation interpretation	Network-informed interpretation
Outputs	Direct and observable products generated through program activities	Immediate and verifiable relational activations, including the formation or strengthening of ties (e.g., new partnerships, formalized referral agreements, convened cross-sector forums) that signal initial structural engagement within the network
Outcomes	Short- and medium-term changes resulting from program implementation	Observable and measurable shifts in network structure and relational patterns, such as increased density (connectivity), reduced fragmentation, improved information flow (shorter average path length), strengthened reciprocity, greater integration of peripheral actors, decreased excessive centralization, and the emergence of bridging ties across sectors
Impacts	Long-term and enduring system-level transformations resulting from sustained intervention	Durable structural and systemic transformations, including resilient relational infrastructure, institutionalized collaboration, sustained cross-sector learning, and the diffusion of innovation demonstrated through the longitudinal persistence of network reconfiguration

Note This table presents the author's network-informed reconceptualization of program effects, building on Chen's program theory framework (1990, 2015). It extends the core components by incorporating relational and structural perspectives derived from social network analysis. Table A3 in Appendix A provides an illustrative example of network-informed program effects specification.
Source Author

creation or intensification of relational ties—for example, establishing a partnership forms a new network link, while enhanced communication strengthens existing connections. Thus, outputs function not only as markers of implementation initiation but also as indicators of relational activation, the initial phase of systemic change. By focusing on these tangible products, evaluators can document foundational shifts in network structure that precede broader outcomes and impacts, thereby strengthening the evidentiary basis for subsequent claims of effectiveness.

Outcomes

Chen (2015) defines outcomes as explicitly stated, empirically observable changes that result directly from program implementation. He differentiates outcomes from broader ultimate goals by emphasizing their temporal immediacy, practical attainability, and capacity for rigorous measurement (pp. 106–107). Consistent with Mathison (2005, p. 287), outcomes encompass multiple domains and can be measured at individual, organizational, community, or policy levels.

In network-informed interventions, outcomes refer to concrete, measurable changes in relational and structural patterns. These include short- and medium-term shifts such as increased network density, indicating greater connectivity among actors; reduced fragmentation, reflecting fewer isolated subgroups; improved information flow efficiency, as demonstrated by shorter average path lengths; strengthened reciprocity and trust; expanded inclusion of marginalized or peripheral actors; and enhanced cross-organizational coordination. Additional indicators, such as decreased centralization or the emergence of bridging ties across sectors, provide empirical evidence of the intervention's effectiveness in reshaping network configuration. Network-informed outcomes are theoretically grounded and methodologically assessable, representing changes beyond mere description. By specifying anticipated structural shifts prior to implementation, evaluators transform concepts such as collaboration, integration, and inclusion into operationalized, observable conditions. This emphasis on clarity and measurability, consistent with Chen's (2015) framework, strengthens causal attribution, improves alignment between evaluation and program theory, and enhances the scholarly rigor of claims regarding network-induced change.

Impacts

Impacts refer to enduring, system-level transformations resulting from sustained programmatic, policy, organizational, or technological interventions (Mathison, 2005, p. 194). In network-informed evaluation, impacts manifest as resilient and adaptive relational infrastructures characterized by redundancy, robustness to actor turnover, and the capacity to withstand external shocks. Additional indicators include institutionalized learning processes, more equitable participation in governance structures, and the diffusion of innovation, as demonstrated by policy and community shifts across sectors (Valente, 2010). Methodologically, longitudinal network analyses are crucial for assessing whether observed structural changes persist over time and whether new relational patterns become embedded in organizational routines and practices. Institutionalization is particularly important because it signifies that collaborative capacity for coordinated collective action is maintained independently of cyclical funding or external support. Monitoring these durable changes allows evaluators to substantiate claims of systemic impact and provide robust empirical evidence for the long-term effectiveness of network-based interventions.

Addressing Contextual Factors in Network-Informed Complex Evaluation

Programs operate within complex social, organizational, political, and economic environments that influence both implementation and outcomes. Chen (1990) defines contextual support as micro- and macro-level conditions that facilitate program success. Micro-level support encompasses social, psychological, and material resources that sustain stakeholder engagement, including trust, motivation, skills, and access to resources. Macro-level support comprises organizational norms, institutional cultures, and political and economic processes that shape program priorities, constraints, and opportunities.

Building on this perspective, context can be understood as a multidimensional construct with several interrelated domains, including (a) descriptive and demographic characteristics, such as population size, composition, and diversity; (b) material and economic features, including infrastructure, resources, and indicators of scarcity or abundance; (c) institutional and organizational climate, such as governance structures, decision-making processes, and norms; (d) interpersonal dimensions, reflected in interaction patterns, relationship norms, and social dynamics; and (e) political dynamics, including contested interests, power relations, and distributions of influence and privilege (Mathison, 2005, p. 83). These domains show that context is layered, relational, and dynamic, and evaluators should examine how these domains intersect, overlap, and evolve in response to broader systemic changes.

Why Contextual Factors Matter in Network-Informed Complex Evaluation

In program evaluation, *context* is defined as "the setting within which the evaluand (the program, policy, or product being evaluated) and thus the evaluation are situated" (Mathison, 2005, p. 83). Scholars emphasize that context should not be treated as a secondary factor, particularly in complex programs where outcomes emerge from nonlinear interactions among multiple actors and systems (Fitzpatrick et al., 2004; Rogers, 2008). In such programs, effectiveness depends on how program mechanisms interact with contextual conditions, rather than on program components alone.

Realist evaluation theory further clarifies that program mechanisms operate differently across contexts, leading to variation in outcomes (Pawson & Tilley, 1997). This viewpoint maintains that determining effective strategies requires a thorough and explicit assessment of contextual variables, rather than efforts to control or overlook them. In complex programs, context is inherently dynamic, as organizational restructuring, policy reforms, funding changes, and evolving stakeholder relationships continuously modify the conditions under which programs operate. Wholey et al. (2010) argue that evaluators should account for both the broader human environment and immediate situational factors influencing evaluation planning and use, as these elements affect program implementation, evaluation processes, and the application of findings.

Network-informed evaluation approaches extend these insights by conceptualizing context as fundamentally relational. Rather than viewing context solely as external conditions, a network perspective defines it in terms of patterns of relationships, resource exchanges, and institutional linkages among actors. Provan and Milward (1995) demonstrate that network structures themselves serve as contextual factors influencing program effectiveness. For example, fragmented networks may hinder coordination and information flow, whereas highly centralized networks can enhance efficiency but restrict adaptability and resilience. This approach enables evaluators to examine how relational configurations shape program functioning, moving beyond the perception of context as an uncontrollable factor.

Conceptualizing Contextual Dimensions Through a Network Lens

SNA offers a rigorous methodological framework for examining contextual factors within complex, networked programs. Context typically manifests through relationships such as collaboration, communication, authority, and resource exchange. SNA enables evaluators to map and analyze these relational structures. Key network measures, such as density, centralization, cohesion, and brokerage, reveal patterns of information flow and identify actors who serve as connectors or gatekeepers within program environments. Therefore, SNA operationalizes context as a set of structural and relational conditions that influence program implementation.

Table 5.4 offers a network-informed reconceptualization of contextual factors. Drawing on the multidimensional perspective of context (Mathison, 2005, p. 83), NCE translates key contextual domains into defined network configurations. It proposes propositions to clarify how these configurations may enable or constrain program mechanisms within complex environments. Rather than treating context as an external variable, Table 5.4 positions it as an integral component of program theory, enacted through patterns of relationships, resource exchanges, governance arrangements, interpersonal dynamics, and power relations. This framework serves three complementary purposes. First, it presents a conceptual map that links core dimensions of context to network structures amenable to network analysis. Second, it advances analytic propositions to guide evaluators in identifying relational conditions most significant for participation, coordination, learning, equity, and implementation coherence. Third, it integrates theory-driven evaluation with complexity-informed methods by demonstrating how contextual conditions can be operationalized from a network perspective. The following sections elaborate on each contextual dimension, beginning with descriptive and demographic characteristics.

Table 5.4 Network-informed conceptualization of contextual factors

Contextual dimension	Role in program evaluation	Network-informed conceptualization	Analytic proposition	Network concepts and measures
Descriptive and demographic characteristics	Structural and compositional features that shape participation, representation, and access	Network composition and structural positioning of actors differentiated by role, sector, geography, or social attributes	Greater demographic diversity, combined with cross-group connectivity, is likely to support broader participation and a more balanced distribution of program resources, whereas highly homophilous or segmented networks may constrain participation and learning	Network size; density; homophily indices (e.g., E–I index); community detection; assortativity
Material and economic features	Distribution of financial, material, and informational resources that enable or constrain program functioning	Resource exchange networks structuring access to and control over critical assets	Programs embedded in resource networks with multiple exchange pathways and lower dependency on single actors are more likely to demonstrate sustainability and resilience than those reliant on highly centralized resource flows	Degree centrality (resource provision); in-degree/out-degree; network centralization
Institutional and organizational climate	Governance arrangements, decision-making processes, and organizational norms shaping coordination and accountability	Governance and coordination networks enacted through formal and informal relational structures	Balanced governance and coordination networks are likely to support implementation coherence and adaptive capacity more effectively than weakly coordinated or rigidly hierarchical arrangements	Betweenness centrality; network centralization; multiplexity (formal–informal ties); core–periphery structures

(continued)

Table 5.4 (continued)

Contextual dimension	Role in program evaluation	Network-informed conceptualization	Analytic proposition	Network concepts and measures
Interpersonal dimensions	Relational norms influencing trust, collaboration, communication, and learning	Social interaction networks capturing patterns of collaboration, trust, and influence	Higher levels of cohesion, reciprocity, and trust within interpersonal networks are likely to facilitate the activation of program mechanisms, collective learning, and adaptive implementation	Tie strength; reciprocity; clustering coefficient; transitivity; network cohesion
Political dynamics	Power relations, contested interests, and distributions of influence affecting decision-making and evaluation use	Power and influence networks shaping agenda-setting, brokerage, and control over resources or information	Concentrated influence and brokerage within political networks are likely to amplify power asymmetries and contestation, whereas more distributed influence structures may support broader participation and shared ownership of program outcomes	Betweenness centrality; eigenvector centrality; brokerage roles; network constraint; influence concentration measures

Note This table presents the author's network-informed reconceptualization of contextual factors, drawing on the multidimensional perspective of context in program evaluation (Mathison, 2005). It extends the key contextual dimensions by conceptualizing them as relational structures examined through social network analysis. The analytic propositions outline theoretically grounded expectations regarding how contextual conditions operate within complex program environments and may be examined in future research.

Source Author

Descriptive and Demographic Characteristics as Network Composition and Structure

Descriptive and demographic characteristics of a setting, including the size, composition, and diversity of participating populations (Mathison, 2005, p. 83), can be conceptualized as elements of network composition and structure. In this way, network analysis shifts the focus from aggregate demographic attributes to the positions of individuals and groups within relational systems. For example, demographic diversity is important not only for representation but also for understanding how diverse actors connect or bridge across network subgroups.

Network size, density, and homophily—the tendency for similar individuals to connect—serve as analytical tools to examine how demographic characteristics influence access to information, participation opportunities, and exposure to program resources. The NCE framework reconceptualizes demographic context as fundamentally relational by showing how network composition and structure shape which voices are amplified, whose knowledge is disseminated, and whose participation is either sustained or marginalized within program networks.

Material and Economic Features as Resource Networks

Material and economic contextual features, such as physical infrastructure, financial resources, and indicators of scarcity or abundance (Mathison, 2005, p. 83), can be conceptualized as *resource networks* that structure the flow of tangible and intangible assets. The NCE framework enables evaluators to analyze resource distribution among actors, identify nodes that control critical assets, and examine the formation of dependency relationships, thereby clarifying how context shapes access and influence.

Rather than viewing resources as static inputs, a network perspective emphasizes that access to material and economic supports is mediated through relationships such as funding partnerships, shared infrastructure agreements, and informal exchanges. Organizations occupying central network positions often have privileged access to funding or infrastructure, whereas peripheral actors may face barriers to resource acquisition. These patterns of resource centralization or fragmentation influence program sustainability, equity, and resilience, underscoring the importance of resource networks in contextual analysis. Additionally, resource flows are affected by external factors, including policy changes and broader economic trends, which should be incorporated into the analysis to ensure a comprehensive understanding.

Institutional and Organizational Climate as Governance and Coordination Networks

Institutional and organizational climate, encompassing organizational characteristics, governance structures, decision-making processes, and organizational norms

(Mathison, 2005, p. 83), can be conceptualized as a network of governance and coordination. The evaluation literature identifies governance as a critical determinant of program performance. Governance includes the structures, processes, and relationships through which programs are directed, coordinated, and held accountable, thereby influencing decision-making authority, stakeholder engagement, resource allocation, and the use of evaluation findings (Fitzpatrick et al., 2004; Wholey et al., 2010). Wholey et al. (2010) emphasize that programs operate within broader administrative, political, and interorganizational governance systems that shape program implementation, determine which forms of evidence are considered legitimate, and influence the interpretation and application of evaluation results. Weak or fragmented governance arrangements can undermine program coherence, limit accountability, and reduce the likelihood that evaluation findings will inform decision-making.

Governance challenges are especially pronounced in complex, collaborative programs such as cross-sector initiatives or networked service-delivery systems. In these settings, authority and responsibility are distributed among multiple actors rather than centralized. Provan and Kenis (2008) identify various governance models for networks, each influencing coordination, effectiveness, and accountability differently. These distinctions underscore the importance of examining governance as a multidimensional construct whose structural configurations and functional roles vary across program contexts. Network-focused evaluations must systematically assess not only formal governance structures but also informal influence patterns, coordination mechanisms, and key relationships that shape program operations in practice.

From a network perspective, governance extends beyond official organizational charts and occurs through repeated interactions among individuals and organizations. The NCE framework shifts focus from static structures to dynamic relationships through which authority, coordination, accountability, and influence are exercised. This approach enables evaluators to analyze how decision-making power is allocated, how coordination is centralized or dispersed, and how formal and informal connections jointly influence program delivery. Network patterns reveal organizational norms, such as when specific actors assume coordination roles, when individuals bridge separate groups, or when clusters remain isolated due to weak connections. These patterns establish a context that can either facilitate or impede collective action, adaptability, and consistent program implementation.

Interpersonal Dimensions as Social Interaction Networks

Interpersonal dimensions of context, including interaction patterns, relationship norms, and social dynamics (Mathison, 2005, p. 83), closely align with social interaction networks. Network analysis provides a systematic approach to examining trust, collaboration, communication, and influence as relational phenomena rather than as individual attributes. Employing measures such as tie strength, reciprocity, and cohesion allows evaluators to assess how relational norms facilitate or hinder collaboration, learning, and adaptation within programs. Interpersonal networks influence program implementation by shaping how information is interpreted, how norms are enforced, and how participants respond to program requirements. Therefore, interpersonal context should be understood as a dynamic relational process rather than a static background condition.

Political Dynamics as Power and Influence Networks

Political dynamics, including contested interests, power relations, and distributions of influence and privilege (Mathison, 2005, p. 83), can be conceptualized as networks of power. Network analysis enables evaluators to examine how influence is exercised, how coalitions form, and how actors gain control over decision-making. Rather than assuming that power derives solely from formal roles or positions, a network perspective shows that power operates through brokerage, centrality, and control over critical information or resources. This approach uncovers often-hidden relational structures that sustain privilege or marginalization within program contexts, allowing evaluators to assess how political dynamics influence implementation and the use of evaluation findings.

Addressing Assumptions in Network-Informed Complex Evaluation

Assumptions form the foundation of program theory and evaluation. These implicit beliefs shape expectations regarding the dynamics of social problems, processes of change, and the mechanisms by which program activities generate outcomes. In theory-driven evaluation, assumptions establish the logical framework that links program inputs, activities, outputs, and outcomes, thereby guiding program design and evaluative judgments (Chen, 2015; Weiss, 1998). Failure to examine assumptions may lead to misattributing outcomes, overlooking mechanisms, or producing incomplete assessments of program effectiveness.

Chen (2015) differentiates between descriptive and prescriptive assumptions, both of which are critical for understanding program functioning. Descriptive assumptions refer to beliefs about the causal processes underlying the targeted social problem, whereas prescriptive assumptions refer to beliefs about the actions, components, and activities necessary to achieve the desired change (pp. 66–69). A network-informed perspective reconceptualizes these assumptions as relational expectations embedded within networks of actors, organizations, and institutions, making the final analytical frame more explicit.

Why Assumptions Matter in Network-Informed Complex Evaluation

In complex networked programs, assumptions are critical because outcomes result from interactions among multiple actors rather than isolated interventions. Many assumptions lie beyond the direct control of program implementers and are shaped by broader social, organizational, and political contexts (Nkwake, 2012). Without explicit articulation and analysis, evaluators may misinterpret relational breakdowns, such as insufficient collaboration or weak information flow, as implementation failures instead of recognizing them as theoretically significant indicators of unarticulated assumptions.

Reconceptualizing assumptions from a network perspective enhances theory-driven evaluation by clarifying the conditions under which program mechanisms operate. This approach aligns with realist and complexity-informed evaluation methodologies, which emphasize interactions between context and mechanisms rather than linear causality (Pawson & Tilley, 1997; Rogers, 2008). Explicitly framing assumptions as relational allows evaluators to account for variations in outcomes across diverse settings and time periods. In practice, it helps evaluators identify which conditions support or hinder mechanisms in specific settings.

Conceptualizing Assumptions Through a Network Lens

SNA is particularly effective for examining descriptive and prescriptive assumptions because it translates these assumptions into observable relational patterns. This method allows evaluators to compare hypothesized and actual networks, assess whether assumed mechanisms were activated, and iteratively refine program theory. Through this process, network-informed evaluation transforms implicit assumptions into analytically tractable elements of program theory. This approach strengthens causal inference, supports learning-oriented evaluation, and provides a rigorous foundation for evaluating programs in complex, interdependent systems.

Table 5.5 incorporates Chen's (2015) distinction between descriptive and prescriptive assumptions by reframing them as relational conditions embedded within program networks, rather than as isolated beliefs held by individual actors. From a network perspective, the table clarifies how expectations regarding *causal processes* (descriptive assumptions) and *program actions* (prescriptive assumptions) manifest through patterns of interaction, influence, coordination, and authority within complex program environments. Instead of treating assumptions as abstract elements of program logic, the table presents them as analytically tractable components of program theory accessible via Social Network Analysis.

Table 5.5 serves as a conceptual bridge between theory-driven evaluation and network-informed methods by articulating theory-generating propositions that specify the relational conditions under which assumptions are expected to hold.

Table 5.5 Network-informed conceptualization of assumptions

Type of assumption	Role in program theory and evaluation	Network-informed conceptualization	Analytic proposition	Network concepts and measures
Descriptive assumptions (assumptions about causal processes)	Beliefs about how and why program activities are expected to address the underlying social problem; foundational to identifying program mechanisms	Expectations regarding the relational causal mechanisms through which change occurs, including information diffusion, social influence, collaboration, coordination, trust, and knowledge exchange	Program mechanisms are more likely to operate as theorized when observed relational configurations support the interaction patterns specified in program theory (e.g., adequate connectivity, effective brokerage, efficient pathways for information exchange, or cohesive subgroups)	Network density; average path length; diffusion reach; betweenness centrality; brokerage roles
Prescriptive assumptions (assumptions about actions and components)	Beliefs about the program components, activities, roles, and actions considered necessary for achieving desired outcomes	Normative expectations about relational behavior, roles, and coordination among actors within program networks	Prescriptive assumptions are more likely to be implemented consistently when expected relational behaviors are congruent with existing network norms and reinforced by structurally influential actors occupying central, brokerage, or governance positions	Degree and eigenvector centrality; multiplex ties (authority–collaboration); role equivalence; reputational or coordination networks

Note This table presents the author's network-informed reconceptualization of descriptive and prescriptive assumptions in program theory, drawing on Chen's framework (2015). It extends these assumption types by conceptualizing them as relational expectations examined through social network analysis. The analytical propositions are intended to support theory development and network-informed evaluation design rather than to represent empirically established causal relationships. The network concepts and measures are illustrative examples and should be selected and operationalized according to the theoretical framework, evaluation questions, and program context.
Source Author

This approach highlights the importance of examining both the content of program assumptions and the network structures necessary for these assumptions to function effectively. The following sections provide detailed elaboration on each type of assumption.

Descriptive Assumptions as Networked Causal Expectations

Descriptive assumptions are beliefs about the mechanisms by which an intervention is expected to operate. Chen (2015) emphasizes that assumptions "about the causal processes through which an intervention or a treatment is supposed to work are crucial for any program, because its effectiveness depends on their truthfulness" (p. 67). In complex social programs, these causal processes seldom follow linear or individualistic patterns; rather, they are mediated by interaction, influence, coordination, and collective behavior.

A network perspective reconceptualizes descriptive assumptions as expectations concerning relational mechanisms that SNA can help examine. For example, programs may propose that information diffuses through social ties, that peer influence shapes behavior, that collaboration among organizations enhances service coordination, or that trusted intermediaries legitimize new practices. These assumptions extend beyond technical causal claims and represent hypotheses about network functioning and the activation of change mechanisms via relationships.

SNA enables evaluators to assess whether the assumed relational mechanisms exist and operate as anticipated. By examining patterns of communication, collaboration, trust, and influence, evaluators can identify network structures essential for the assumed causal processes, such as sufficient connectivity, effective brokerage, or cohesive subgroups. Thus, descriptive assumptions become empirically testable network hypotheses through SNA rather than remaining abstract claims within logic models.

Prescriptive Assumptions as Normative Network Expectations

Prescriptive assumptions are beliefs regarding the actions, components, and activities considered essential to program success. Chen (2015) notes that these assumptions reflect what program designers and stakeholders "see as necessary to a program's success" (p. 68). Such assumptions often specify program components, including training, partnerships, participatory activities, roles, and implementation strategies.

From a network-informed perspective, prescriptive assumptions serve as normative expectations regarding relational behaviors within program networks. For example, programs may assume that organizations collaborate, frontline staff share information across boundaries, or community members actively participate in collective activities. These assumptions depend on expectations of trust, reciprocity, authority, and influence within networks.

Network analysis assesses whether prescriptive assumptions are supported or contradicted by actual relational patterns. For instance, a prescriptive assumption of collaboration may be undermined by fragmented networks, weak ties, or power imbalances that impede coordination. Conversely, these assumptions are strengthened when central actors broker relationships or when networks are characterized by dense, reciprocal ties that support collective action. Understanding these relational conditions is essential for interpreting implementation fidelity and for distinguishing whether challenges arise from program design failure or from contextual constraints.

Chapter Summary

This chapter reconceptualizes the input stage of evaluation by integrating principles from network analysis and complexity science within the NCE framework. This stage establishes the conceptual and analytical foundation for evaluation design through mapping relational mechanisms, clarifying program theory, and aligning governance structures with contextual constraints. The NCE framework offers a systematic method for defining program scope, articulating action plans, and specifying anticipated outcomes in complex, networked environments. By emphasizing relational dynamics and contextual interdependencies, the input stage ensures that interventions are guided by explicit, contextually grounded theories of change that address the interconnected nature of contemporary policy and social programs.

Incorporating network-informed concepts into the evaluation input stage advances evaluation theory by elucidating how relational mechanisms and contextual conditions influence program design and outcomes. The NCE framework is both theoretically rigorous and practically applicable for collaboratively developing program theory in multisector and networked interventions. Its structured approach facilitates interdisciplinary collaboration, clarifies assumptions regarding mechanisms and outcomes, and equips evaluators with analytic tools to examine governance structures, collaboration patterns, and resource flows. The network-informed conceptualizations presented in this chapter—including interpretations of program scope, action planning, program effects, contextual factors, and program assumptions—illustrate how evaluation components can be translated into measurable, empirically examinable relational and structural terms.

The NCE input stage presents a distinctive methodological perspective by integrating program theory evaluation with social network analysis and complexity-informed thinking. This integration enables evaluators to identify systemic constraints, analyze power and coordination dynamics, and explain variations in program outcomes within multi-actor environments. By emphasizing relational structures and evolving contextual conditions, the framework offers a practical, analytically robust approach to designing evaluations that capture real-world complexity. Appendix A, Network-Informed Complex Evaluation Program Theory Template, provides a structured tool to support the application of the NCE framework in developing network-informed, complexity-aware evaluations.

Reflection Questions

- How does reconstructing program theory through a network-informed lens change your assumptions about causality and change? When relational mechanisms, distributed governance, and contextual interdependence are treated as central rather than peripheral, how does this influence the understanding of outcome generation and the interpretation of causal claims?
- What methodological tensions emerge when designing evaluations within complex, multi-actor systems? How can evaluators balance the requirement for analytic clarity with the recognition of nonlinearity, feedback loops, and adaptive behavior? What trade-offs exist between simplifying theory for evaluation purposes and preserving system complexity?
- What ethical and political considerations arise when relational structures and power dynamics are explicitly integrated into program theory and evaluation design? How might the disclosure of patterns of influence, centrality, or exclusion impact stakeholder relationships? What responsibilities do evaluators hold when evaluation design uncovers structural inequities embedded within networks?

Applied Activities

Scenario: Select a program, partnership, initiative, or policy intervention that you are familiar with. The chosen case should involve multiple actors or sectors and operate within a context in which coordination, influence, or relational dynamics plausibly affect outcomes. This activity addresses the foundational question presented in this chapter: *How can a program's theory of change be reconstructed to explicitly incorporate relational mechanisms, governance structures, contextual constraints, and adaptive system dynamics?* Utilize Appendix A: Network-Informed Complex Evaluation (NCE) Program Theory Template to redesign the program's theory of change, reflecting the dynamics of operating within a complex, networked system rather than a linear intervention model. The goal is not to complete every element of the template, but to demonstrate conceptual alignment among program goals, organizational drivers, relational mechanisms, governance arrangements, contextual conditions, and anticipated system effects.

References

Borgatti, S. P., Mehra, A., Brass, D. J., & Labianca, G. (2009). Network analysis in the social sciences. *Science (American Association for the Advancement of Science), 323*(5916), 892–895. https://doi.org/10.1126/science.1165821

Chen, H. T. (1990). *Theory-driven evaluations*. Sage.

Chen, H. T. (2015). *Practical program evaluation: Theory-driven evaluation and the integrated evaluation perspective* (2nd ed.). Sage.

Coleman, J. S. (1988). Social capital in the creation of human capital. *The American Journal of Sociology, 94*(1988), S95–S120. https://doi.org/10.1086/228943

Fitzpatrick, J. L., Sanders, J. R., & Worthen, B. R. (2004). *Program evaluation: Alternative approaches and practical guidelines*. Pearson.

Funnell, S. C., & Rogers, P. J. (2011). *Purposeful program theory: Effective use of theories of change and logic models*. Jossey-Bass.

Laumann, E. O., Marsden, P. V., & Prensky, D. (1989). The boundary specification problem in network analysis. *Research Methods in Social Network Analysis, 61*(8), 176–179.

Mathison, S. (2005). *Encyclopedia of evaluation* (1st ed.). Sage.

Nkwake, A. M. (2012). *Working with assumptions in international development program evaluation*. Springer. https://doi.org/10.1007/978-1-4614-4797-9

Patton, M. Q. (2011). *Developmental evaluation: Applying complexity concepts to enhance innovation and use*. Guilford Press.

Pawson, R., & Tilley, N. (1997). *Realistic evaluation*. Sage.

Provan, K. G., & Kenis, P. (2008). Modes of network governance: Structure, management, and effectiveness. *Journal of Public Administration Research and Theory, 18*(2), 229–252. https://doi.org/10.1093/jopart/mum015

Provan, K. G., & Milward, H. B. (1995). A preliminary theory of interorganizational network effectiveness: A comparative study of four community mental health systems. *Administrative Science Quarterly, 40*(1), 1–33. https://doi.org/10.2307/2393698

Rogers, P. J. (2008). Using programme theory to evaluate complicated and complex aspects of interventions. *Evaluation, 14*(1), 29–48. https://doi.org/10.1177/1356389007084674

Stufflebeam, D. L. (2000). The CIPP model for evaluation. In D. L. Stufflebeam, G. F. Madaus, & T. Kellaghan (Eds.), *Evaluation models. evaluation in education and human services* (Vol. 49). Springer. https://doi.org/10.1007/0-306-47559-6_16

Stufflebeam, D. L., & Coryn, C. L. S. (2014). *Evaluation theory, models, and applications* (2nd ed.). Jossey-Bass.

Valente, T. W. (2010). *Social networks and health: Models, methods, and applications*. Oxford University Press.

Wasserman, S., & Faust, K. (1994). *Social network analysis: Methods and applications*. Cambridge University Press.

Weiss, C. H. (1998). *Evaluation: Methods for studying programs and policies* (2nd ed.). Prentice Hall.

Wholey, J. S., Hatry, H. P., & Newcomer, K. E. (2010). *Handbook of practical program evaluation* (3rd ed). Jossey-Bass.

Chapter 6
Evaluation Design and Knowledge Production in Networked Contexts

Introduction

The outcomes of complex interventions rarely follow linear cause-and-effect relationships; rather, they emerge from dynamic interactions among multiple actors, organizations, and contextual factors. This inherent complexity demands evaluation designs that uphold methodological integrity, credibility, and practical utility. Scholars emphasize that evaluators must explicitly address the multilevel, adaptive, and networked nature of interventions to generate findings that facilitate meaningful learning and informed decision-making (Mark et al., 2000; Patton, 2011). Mark et al. (2000) argue that the evaluation process itself shapes how stakeholders interpret and value program activities and outcomes. Therefore, evaluation design should be integrated with implementation realities and stakeholder perspectives. Collaborative engagement in developing evaluation purposes, questions, criteria, and communication strategies is essential in complex systems, where values, priorities, and interpretations are multiple, evolving, and often contested.

Stufflebeam's Context, Input, Process, and Product (CIPP) model provides a foundational framework that highlights the importance of the process stage in decision-oriented evaluation (Stufflebeam & Coryn, 2014). In this model, the process stage is intended to monitor implementation fidelity, identify deviations from planned activities, and deliver actionable feedback to facilitate ongoing program improvement. This stage serves several interconnected functions: it documents the relationship between intended and actual activities; uses various data-collection strategies—such as participant and independent observation, interviews, document analysis, and ongoing staff communication—to monitor progress and identify implementation challenges; and establishes feedback mechanisms that support process control, activity refinement, and timely midcourse corrections. Furthermore, the process stage produces a comprehensive record of implementation, which is critical for interpreting outcomes, assessing program quality, and informing decisions about replication or scaling.

L. Zhang, *Network-Informed Complex Evaluation*,
https://doi.org/10.1007/978-3-032-27495-3_6

The process stage is especially significant in network-informed complex evaluations (NCE), where program success depends on relational quality, communication structures, and patterns of resource exchange among participants, rather than solely on individual or organizational performance. A rigorous process stage enables evaluators to monitor and analyze evolving relational dynamics, ensuring responsiveness to the complex and adaptive nature of real-world networks. In this context, the process stage is both iterative and adaptive, functioning as a continuous evaluative cycle that compares real-time implementation with original plans, identifies emerging challenges, examines organizational and interpersonal responses, and systematically documents costs, effort, and quality (Stufflebeam & Coryn, 2014). These structured feedback loops facilitate ongoing refinement and adaptation, enabling evaluators and stakeholders to respond effectively to new information, changing contexts, or unforeseen circumstances (Patton, 2011).

The NCE process stage operationalizes the program theory developed during the input stage by translating abstract theoretical constructs into structured evaluative practices. During this phase, theoretical assumptions regarding mechanisms, relationships, and expected outcomes become empirically observable through clearly defined procedures and indicators. By incorporating network analysis methods, this stage establishes systematic procedures for collecting, analyzing, and interpreting relational data. These procedures facilitate the examination of interaction patterns, structural configurations, and relational dynamics that influence program implementation. Continuous stakeholder engagement informs and refines the evaluation design, thereby enhancing contextual responsiveness and methodological rigor. This integrated approach enables a systematic assessment of both implementation fidelity relative to core program activities and the quality and evolution of relationships within the intervention network. The following section outlines the sequential steps of this network-informed process stage, conceptually based on Carolan's (2014, pp. 266–267) network study steps, while introducing significant modifications to advance a network-informed evaluation design.

1. *Formulate Network-Informed Evaluation Objectives and Questions.* Articulate the evaluation's purpose to emphasize relational processes, interdependencies, and network dynamics, rather than focusing exclusively on isolated program components. In developing evaluation questions, consider how network variables, whether structural (such as patterns of connections) or relational (such as trust and collaboration), interact with other key program variables. This approach ensures that evaluation questions reflect the complexity and interconnectedness of networked interventions.
2. *Specify Network Scope and Boundary.* Delineate the network's scope and boundaries by specifying the network type, actors, relationships, levels of analysis, and time frames included. Careful boundary specification is essential for analytic validity, methodological feasibility, and transparency, supporting the credibility of network-informed evaluation findings.
3. *Align Evaluation Methods with Questions and Network Boundaries.* Select and justify evaluation methods, such as whole network analysis, ego network analysis,

qualitative network inquiry, or mixed-methods approaches, that are appropriate for the evaluation questions and consistent with the defined network boundaries. This alignment ensures methodological coherence and the generation of evidence relevant to both network structure and dynamics.
4. *Develop Data Collection and Analysis Plans.* Implement the evaluation design by specifying data sources, measurement instruments, data-collection timing, analytical strategies, and the integration of quantitative and qualitative network data. This phase translates the conceptual design into actionable procedures, supporting methodological rigor and nuanced interpretation.
5. *Design Reporting and Knowledge-Use Strategies.* Develop strategies for interpreting, visualizing, and disseminating network evaluation findings, with careful consideration of the needs and capacities of intended users. Network results are often complex, susceptible to misinterpretation, and may be politically sensitive. Thoughtful reporting and knowledge-use strategies are essential to maximize the utility, uptake, and responsible use of network-informed evaluation evidence.

Formulating Network-Informed Evaluation Objectives and Questions

Clarifying evaluation objectives and questions is essential in all evaluations, particularly in network-informed, complexity-aware contexts involving interdependent actors, multilevel processes, and nonlinear pathways of change. In these settings, vague or narrowly defined objectives may obscure the mechanisms through which programs produce effects, potentially resulting in incomplete or misleading conclusions (Patton, 2011; Rogers, 2008). Evaluation objectives link decisions to analytic focus by specifying what the evaluation seeks to understand, for whom, and for what purpose (Fitzpatrick et al., 2011). When clearly articulated in network contexts, these objectives support designs that reflect real-world complexity, rather than imposing linear models of causality. Additionally, network evaluations often entail sensitive relational data, complex boundary decisions, and political considerations. Well-defined objectives and questions provide critical justification for design choices, boundary specifications, and analytic strategies, enhancing the credibility and responsible use of evaluation findings (Carolan, 2014; Durland & Fredericks, 2005).

How Program Theory Shapes Evaluation Objectives and Questions

Program theory developed during the input stage plays a central role in shaping evaluation purposes and questions. This stage clarifies the program's scope by identifying the problem addressed, the affected population, key determinants, and program goals.

It also defines the action plan by specifying implementers, partners, resources, the ecological context, and activities at the individual, organizational, community, and policy levels.

In theory-driven evaluations, evaluation questions must derive from the program theory. For example, if the theory identifies community partnerships as central to implementation, evaluation questions should examine how these partnerships function, evolve, and influence program activities and outcomes. When the theory emphasizes multilevel actions, questions should address interactions across these levels rather than treating them as isolated domains (Funnell & Rogers, 2011). This alignment ensures that evaluation efforts reveal not only whether a program is effective but also the mechanisms and contextual factors that the program theory identifies as contributing to meaningful change.

Developing Network-Informed Objectives and Questions

Grounding evaluation objectives and questions in a collaboratively developed program theory during the input stage enables evaluators to design inquiries that are methodologically coherent, analytically rigorous, and practically relevant. This alignment ensures that evaluation findings not only address program effectiveness but also elucidate the mechanisms, target populations, and network conditions identified in the program theory as driving meaningful change.

- Evaluation objectives should explicitly reference the relational mechanisms identified in the program theory. For instance, objectives may examine coordination dynamics between implementers and community partners, resource flows within the network, or the influence of organizational roles on program delivery. This approach is consistent with network analysis, which emphasizes relational structures and mechanisms rather than purely descriptive accounts. Network-informed objectives must be linked to their intended use—whether formative, summative, developmental, or accountability-oriented. Establishing this connection ensures that evaluations inform decisions regarding refinement, scaling, sustainability, or policy influence, which is critical in complex systems where adaptation is as important as judgment (Patton, 2011, pp. 131–132).
- Evaluation questions should address the ecological aspects of program theory. Instead of focusing exclusively on outcome attainment, network-informed questions examine interactions among activities at the individual, organizational, community, and policy levels. For example, questions may explore how organizational collaboration supports community-level implementation or how policy alignment enables or constrains network functioning (Hawe et al., 2009; Provan & Kenis, 2008). Connecting network structural or relational variables to program outcomes yields a more causally informative understanding of how network structure or relationships influence programs.

Defining Network Scope and Boundaries

A central challenge in network-informed evaluation is specifying network boundaries, which requires precise identification of system actors and analytically relevant relationships among them (Knoke & Yang, 2008; Laumann et al., 1978). These boundary decisions are critical because they directly inform evaluation choices, such as the determination of intervention reach, stakeholder roles, and anticipated mechanisms of change. As noted by Laumann et al. (1989), boundary specification entails determining network membership and the types of relationships to be analyzed. It is used to "define the target population and construct a sampling frame that adequately provides access to that population of interest" (Carolan, 2014, p. 68). This foundational design decision shapes the system under evaluation, the operationalization of mechanisms of change, and the scope of claims that can be drawn from the findings.

Network research highlights two primary decisions in boundary specification: selecting the set of actors and establishing criteria for relevant ties (Marsden, 2014; Wasserman & Faust, 1994). Scholars such as Laumann et al. (1989) and Knoke and Yang (2008) identify three general approaches to identifying network boundaries: positional, relational, and event-based. Each approach offers distinct advantages. Positional strategies rely on formal attributes or roles, relational strategies emphasize actual connections and perceptions, and event-based strategies define boundaries through participation in specific activities. This section, together with Table 6.1, presents the boundary specification strategies employed in network-informed complex evaluation.

Boundary Specification Strategies

Positional Strategy

The *positional strategy* defines network boundaries based on actors' attributes, membership in formal organizations, or occupation of clearly defined institutional roles (Knoke & Yang, 2008, p. 16). Instead of identifying actors solely by observed relational ties, this approach emphasizes the positions they occupy within social and organizational structures. As a result, the network population consists of actors occupying comparable roles or structural positions within a broader institutional framework. Foundational research on network boundary specification highlights that such decisions require theoretical justification and transparent documentation, especially regarding the inclusion or exclusion of actors or positions within the network under study (Laumann et al., 1989; Wasserman & Faust, 1994).

Positional approaches direct analytical focus toward the structural logic that defines and differentiates roles and positions within institutional settings. By emphasizing shared attributes such as rank, functional responsibility, or organizational role, researchers identify network boundaries that may not be apparent from relational data

Table 6.1 Boundary specification strategies in network-informed complex evaluation across social-ecological levels

Social-ecological level	Primary unit of analysis	Boundary specification strategy	Boundary justification	Common network forms	Analytic purposes
Individual	Persons, actors, dyads	Relational boundary specification using ego network nomination procedures (e.g., name generators); positional strategies using role- or setting-based rosters (e.g., classroom, clinic, workgroup); explicit tie inclusion criteria (e.g., interaction type, time frame)	Boundary specification at the individual level should align with the interpersonal mechanisms articulated in the program theory (e.g., social influence, advice seeking support, information exchange). Relational nominations identify salient social ties, positional rosters define eligible actors, and explicit tie inclusion criteria strengthen conceptual clarity and construct validity.	Ego-centered networks; whole networks within bounded settings	Social influence; diffusion processes; peer effects; mobilization of social support
Organizational	Organizations; organizational subunits; formal representatives	Positional strategies based on institutional membership, mandate, or system participation; event-based strategies based on participation in initiatives, coalitions, or collaborative activities	Interorganizational networks are typically bounded through organizational membership, formal mandates, or participation within a defined system. Event-based strategies are appropriate when participation in collaborative initiatives constitutes the system of interest. Relational data are then used to assess coordination and governance within the defined boundary.	Interorganizational networks; governance networks	Coordination; resource exchange; implementation capacity; network governance and effectiveness

(continued)

Table 6.1 (continued)

Social-ecological level	Primary unit of analysis	Boundary specification strategy	Boundary justification	Common network forms	Analytic purposes
Community	Organizations, leaders, groups, and cross-sector actors	Positional strategies using place-based definitions (e.g., city, county, neighborhood); event-based strategies based on coalition or initiative participation; relational strategies using reputational nomination of locally relevant actors	Community networks frequently span multiple sectors and exhibit fluid or overlapping membership, making boundary specification an explicit theoretical and evaluative decision. Positional and event-based strategies provide nominalist anchors, while relational (reputational) strategies identify locally relevant actors when formal membership is diffuse, aligning the observed network with the community system specified in the evaluation's theory of change.	Multisector community networks; two-mode (actor–initiative) networks	Partnership functioning; collective capacity; coordination across sectors; systems integration
Policy	Government agencies, legislators, advocacy organizations, policy intermediaries	Positional strategies based on office, role, or jurisdiction; event-based strategies based on participation in formal decision processes (e.g., hearings, committees); relational strategies using reported influence, advice, or communication ties	Policy networks are most defensibly bounded through formal institutional authority, jurisdiction, and decision-making responsibility. Event-based strategies capture participation in policy processes, while relational strategies identify patterns of influence and coordination beyond formal roles, consistent with research on policy networks and advocacy coalitions.	Policy networks; governance networks; advocacy coalitions	Agenda-setting; policy diffusion; power and influence; regulatory coordination

Note This table presents the author's synthesis of established approaches to network boundary specification across social-ecological levels, drawing on foundational and applied literature in social network analysis and evaluation (e.g., Knoke & Yang, 2008; Marsden, 2014; Provan et al., 2007; Rhodes, 1997; Sabatier & Jenkins-Smith, 1993; Valente, 2010; Wasserman & Faust, 1994). It organizes positional, relational, and event-based boundary strategies into a multilevel framework for network-informed complex evaluation.
Source Author

alone (Borgatti et al., 2018). Thus, positional analysis offers a theoretically grounded basis for specifying the population of actors relevant to a given networked system. Membership criteria can be explicitly defined, enabling the construction of network datasets that reflect institutional arrangements rather than relying solely on reported interactions.

Within NCE, the positional strategy offers a valuable framework for identifying actors and structures that influence system functioning. By classifying actors according to their formal roles or positions, evaluators can map the institutional architecture that governs influence, authority, and resource allocation. This perspective is especially important in evaluations involving multiple organizations, sectors, or stakeholder groups, where formal positions frequently structure participation and accountability within collaborative arrangements (Provan et al., 2007).

Positional analysis facilitates the development of transparent sampling frames and analytically meaningful categories for network-based inquiry. By emphasizing formal roles and institutional positions, this approach enables evaluators to examine how governance structures, role differentiation, and organizational hierarchies influence the functioning of complex systems. These considerations are essential for understanding how networked interventions operate, adapt, and contribute to system-level change in multi-actor environments.

Relational Strategy

The *relational strategy* is a fundamental approach in social network analysis, particularly in ego-level networks, where data collection relies on knowledgeable informants or network actors to identify additional participants. This strategy encompasses several established methods, including the reputational approach, snowball sampling, fixed-list selection, expanding selection, and the k-core method (Knoke & Yang, 2008). For example, the *reputational method* solicits nominations from experts or well-informed insiders, enabling the identification of influential actors, brokers, or key leaders who may be overlooked by analyses confined to formal organizational boundaries (Knoke, 1990). These methods are especially significant in community and policy network research because they uncover the underlying dynamics of influence, coordination, and informal leadership that shape network functioning.

In evaluation research, relational strategies are crucial for capturing actual flows of information, resources, and influence, often revealing patterns that differ from those suggested by formal organizational charts. *Snowball sampling*, a widely used relational method, is particularly effective for accessing hard-to-reach or hidden populations (Knoke & Yang, 2008, p. 18). Starting with a small group of initial actors who nominate others within a specified relationship type enables evaluators to map network contours that might otherwise remain undetected. Variations of this method, including *fixed-list selection*, in which respondents report ties among a predefined roster, and expanding selection, in which respondents may nominate an unlimited number of contacts, provide flexibility to align data collection with evaluation objectives and network complexity (Knoke & Yang, 2008, p. 19).

To ensure methodological rigor, evaluators employing snowball sampling should establish clear stopping rules, such as terminating data collection after two consecutive waves yield no new nominations. This approach ensures that the resulting network remains manageable and empirically valid. The *k-core* method further strengthens relational analysis by identifying cohesive subgroups within large, sparse networks, highlighting clusters whose members are densely interconnected internally despite weak connections to the broader network (Knoke & Yang, 2008, p. 19; Seidman, 1983). These relational strategies provide a robust, evidence-based foundation for mapping, analyzing, and evaluating complex social systems, ensuring that both formal and informal influence structures are systematically and transparently incorporated into network-informed evaluation.

Event-Based Strategies

Event-based strategies draw network boundaries by "including actors who participate in a defined set of activities occurring at specific times and places" (Knoke & Yang, 2008, p. 20). This approach is particularly robust in studies of collaborative governance and community partnerships, where empirical inclusion criteria are grounded in formal membership rosters, attendance records, or documented participation in key events (Butterfoss, 2007; Nowell & Foster-Fishman, 2011). These strategies provide a transparent and replicable means of identifying network members, allowing evaluators to align network boundaries tightly with the intervention's logic of action and the mechanisms under investigation. The methodological strength of this approach lies in its ability to capture the dynamic and temporal aspects of network formation and participation, ensuring that the network reflects actors who are actively engaged in processes relevant to the evaluation's objectives.

A critical task for evaluators involves selecting events that are both theoretically and practically relevant to the mechanisms of change under investigation. Inclusion criteria must be justified by demonstrating that participation in these activities is logically or empirically linked to the outcomes or processes of interest (Knoke & Yang, 2008; Laumann et al., 1989). This approach improves construct validity and minimizes the risk of including peripheral or irrelevant actors whose involvement does not significantly influence the network dynamics under study. Furthermore, event-based strategies facilitate longitudinal analysis by enabling repeated measurement of participation across multiple events or time points, providing detailed insights into network evolution, actor engagement, and the development of collaborative patterns (Snijders, 2011). When applied rigorously, event-based strategies offer a methodologically robust framework for defining network boundaries in complex evaluations, integrating both structural and processual dimensions of network dynamics.

Network Boundaries at Social-Ecological Levels

NCE enhances the specification of network boundaries in complex evaluations by mapping strategies across individual, organizational, community, and policy levels. Table 6.1 presents a framework for defining network boundaries at each social-ecological level within complex programs.

Individual-Level Boundary Specification

At the individual and interpersonal levels, boundary specification is essential for ensuring construct validity in network-informed evaluation. Boundary decisions must define a social system that directly corresponds to the interpersonal mechanism under study, such as social support, social influence, or information diffusion. Consistent with established social network methodology, this process involves two analytically distinct but interrelated decisions: delineating the set of actors included in the network and establishing explicit criteria for what constitutes a relevant tie (Wasserman & Faust, 1994).

Boundary specification at this level employs both relational and positional strategies. Relational strategies typically use ego-centered designs with name-generator instruments that prompt respondents to nominate alters based on defined criteria. Conversely, positional strategies use role- or setting-based rosters to define a closed population that shares attributes or settings within bounded contexts such as classrooms, clinics, or workgroups (Marsden, 2014). In both approaches, evaluators must specify tie criteria carefully, including interaction type and relevant time window, to ensure alignment with the theoretical mechanism under investigation (Valente, 2010).

Organizational-Level Boundary Specification

At the organizational level, boundary specification is commonly achieved through positional strategies that define actors by institutional membership, formal mandates, or participation in designated systems such as service-delivery networks or governance arrangements. These strategies align with classic nominalist approaches and are widely regarded as defensible in evaluation research because they reflect formal structures that organize authority, accountability, and resources (Knoke & Yang, 2008). Event-based strategies are also appropriate at the organizational level, especially when the system of interest involves participation in defined collaborative activities such as coalitions, initiatives, or interagency working groups. In these cases, participation in specific events or activities serves as the inclusion criterion, enabling evaluators to delineate the network in alignment with program design and evaluation objectives.

After establishing organizational boundaries through positional or event-based strategies, relational data such as collaboration, coordination, or resource exchange are employed to assess network functioning, governance structures, and system effectiveness rather than to determine initial inclusion (Provan et al., 2007). Analyzing relational patterns enhances understanding of network dynamics; however, the defensibility of boundary specification depends on institutional or participation-based criteria. This distinction is critical in evaluation contexts, where clarity and transparency regarding system boundaries support credible interpretation and application of findings.

Community-Level Boundary Specification

Boundary specification at the community level presents distinct challenges due to the multisectoral and often informal nature of community systems. Unlike organizational or individual networks, community systems are seldom defined by a single institution or formal membership structure. As a result, boundary specification at this level represents a substantive, theory-driven decision rather than a purely technical process.

Evaluators define community network boundaries by integrating positional, event-based, and relational strategies. Positional strategies typically use place-based definitions such as city, county, or neighborhood, providing a nominalist anchor aligned with geographic conceptions of community. Event-based strategies determine inclusion based on participation in coalitions, initiatives, or partnerships that organize collective action around shared objectives. Relational strategies, often implemented through reputational nominations, apply realist boundary logic by identifying actors perceived as influential or relevant by others (Laumann et al., 1978). The theory of change guiding the evaluation should direct the selection and integration of these strategies to ensure that the observed network accurately represents the community system through which the intervention or policy operates.

Policy-Level Boundary Specification

At the policy level, boundary specification is most effectively justified through positional strategies that identify actors by institutional authority, formal roles, or jurisdictional authority within policy systems. Relevant actors comprise government agencies, legislative bodies, and advocacy organizations operating within clearly defined policy domains or decision venues. These strategies align with policy network and advocacy coalition frameworks, which conceptualize policy systems as structured by formal authority and institutionalized roles (Knoke, 1990; Rhodes, 1997; Sabatier & Jenkins-Smith, 1993).

Event-based strategies are also significant at the policy level, particularly when inclusion is determined by participation in formal policy processes such as hearings, committees, or task forces. These strategies enable evaluators to delineate networks focused on venues where policy decisions occur. Additionally, relational strategies, including nominations of influence, communication, or coordination, identify patterns of interaction and influence that extend beyond formal roles and hierarchies. Collectively, these approaches enable evaluators to define policy network boundaries that encompass both the formal structure of authority and the relational dynamics that shape policy influence and coordination.

Aligning Evaluation Methods with Questions and Network Boundaries

Methodological alignment is essential for maintaining rigor and credibility in network-informed complex evaluations. Unlike conventional approaches, which often select methods without fully accounting for system structure, network evaluations require the intentional integration of evaluation questions, network boundaries, and analytic strategies (Carolan, 2014; Prell, 2011). Such alignment strengthens analytic validity, ethical responsibility, and practical utility. Without this congruence, evaluations risk producing invalid inferences, misinterpreting network measures, or yielding findings irrelevant to decision-makers.

Assumptions regarding boundary completeness, relational mechanisms, and evaluation purposes shape network methods. For example, whole network analysis requires clearly defined boundaries and high participation rates to accurately capture structural properties. In contrast, ego network or two-mode approaches are better suited to exploratory contexts or situations in which boundaries are ambiguous (Laumann et al., 1989; Provan & Milward, 2001). Neglecting boundary considerations during method selection can lead to overinterpretation of partial data and reduce the explanatory power of network analysis. Furthermore, network evaluations frequently yield sensitive findings regarding centrality, exclusion, and power asymmetries, underscoring the importance of selecting methods that are analytically appropriate, interpretable, feasible, and ethically sound (Durland & Fredericks, 2005).

Program theory developed during the input stage provides the conceptual foundation for method selection by clarifying the pathways and mechanisms through which complex interventions are expected to produce change. When program theory emphasizes organizational coordination, structural network measures, such as density, centralization, and subgroup identification, become relevant because they align with that logic. Conversely, when theories highlight individual actors' access to resources or information, ego network methods or qualitative inquiry may be necessary to capture the range of experiences within the network (Carolan, 2014). The NCE context assessment further informs method selection by evaluating network relevance, intended use, stakeholder engagement, feasibility, technical capacity, and ethical risk, ensuring that the chosen methods are both contextually appropriate and decision-relevant (Fitzpatrick et al., 2011).

Effective methodological alignment consists of a series of interconnected processes. Network-informed evaluation generally begins with descriptive analyses to assess network properties, such as overall structure, group configurations, key positions, and relational patterns, establishing the basis for later interpretation. Subsequent phases may employ statistical inference to examine whether network structure affects individual attributes or organizational collaboration, depending on the evaluation questions (Carolan, 2014). Mixed-method integration is especially valuable in complex systems: quantitative measures identify structural patterns, whereas qualitative data elucidate underlying mechanisms, contextual factors, and stakeholder perspectives (Durland & Fredericks, 2005). Methodological alignment should be considered iterative and adaptive. As networks evolve and new evidence emerges, evaluators may need to refine analytic approaches, adjust boundaries, or conduct additional analyses. Systematic documentation of these adaptations enhances transparency and fosters a learning-oriented approach to evaluation (Patton, 2011; Rogers, 2008).

Developing Data Collection and Analysis Plans

Complex programs encompass multilevel action plans, multiple implementers and partners, and ongoing interaction with broader ecological and policy environments. These features create interdependencies that outcome measurement alone cannot fully capture. Therefore, data-collection strategies must address both program outcomes and the relational mechanisms linking activities to those outcomes. Within NCE, the evaluation design begins with the program theory developed during the input stage, which serves as the analytical foundation for identifying relevant data sources, specifying methodological approaches, and clarifying the mechanisms through which change is expected to occur. For instance, if the program theory posits that improved outcomes depend on enhanced collaboration among service providers, the evaluation design must generate evidence on both outcome indicators (e.g., service utilization, policy adoption, client well-being) and relational processes (e.g., referral patterns, information exchange, joint planning, shared decision-making). Relational mechanisms constitute central pathways through which complex interventions produce effects. Consequently, NCE requires data-collection strategies that explicitly align with the mechanisms articulated in the theory of change.

Findings from the NCE context assessment further inform the data collection and analysis plan by evaluating system readiness, governance capacity, resource availability, stakeholder alignment, and implementation risk. This contextual analysis guides decisions regarding feasibility, boundary specification, sampling strategies, and ethical considerations. Therefore, the data collection and analysis plan extends beyond technical instrumentation to represent the operational translation of theoretical assumptions within real-world constraints. Alignment among theory, context, and method strengthens internal validity, enhances interpretive credibility, and increases the likelihood that findings will be meaningful and actionable. Without such alignment, evaluations risk producing technically sound analyses that are theoretically disconnected or contextually misaligned.

Developing a coherent data collection and analysis plan within NCE requires attention to three interrelated considerations: theoretical clarity, contextual awareness, and practical feasibility. Evaluators must identify the relational processes hypothesized to drive change, assess whether the system can support specific data-collection methods (e.g., complete network surveys, longitudinal tracking, participatory mapping), and balance analytic rigor with resource constraints, respondent burden, and data accessibility. Aligning data-collection approaches with intended outcomes and contextual realities enhances both the credibility and utility of evaluation findings. By linking program theory, relational mechanisms, and empirical strategy, NCE advances a framework in which methodological rigor and contextual responsiveness reinforce each other within complex adaptive systems.

Network Data-Collection Procedures in Evaluation

Network-informed evaluation employs a diverse range of relational data-collection procedures. Before presenting these methods, it is essential to outline the criteria for selecting among them. The choice of data-collection procedures depends on factors such as the evaluation's purpose, network boundary definitions, system scale and complexity, available resources, and accessibility of relevant data sources. These procedures differ in how relational information is generated, how network boundaries are specified, and the types of inferences they permit. SNA literature demonstrates that no single data-collection method is universally optimal. Instead, method selection should be guided by the evaluation's theory of change, boundary specification approach, system scale and complexity, and practical considerations such as resource availability and data accessibility (Borgatti et al., 2024; Wasserman & Faust, 1994). The following categories summarize the primary network data-collection procedures commonly employed in evaluation and applied network research.

- *Survey-Based Network Data-Collection Methods.* Survey-based methods commonly collect network data through structured questionnaires in which respondents report their relationships with others. Techniques include name-generator surveys, roster-based sociometric surveys, and relational rating scales assessing tie strength, frequency, or quality (Marsden, 2005; Wasserman & Faust, 1994). These methods are useful when the evaluation seeks structured relational data from actors who can report on their ties, and they enable evaluators to identify collaboration patterns, highlight key connections, and detect gaps in communication or partnerships that can inform program improvements. Survey-based methods "are most useful when the actors are people, and the relation(s) that are being studied are ones that the respondent can report on" (Wasserman & Faust, 1994, p. 45). They may also be used when individuals report on behalf of organizations or collective entities. Survey designs facilitate formal structural analysis, such as examining centralization, cohesion, and brokerage. However, these methods require clearly defined network boundaries and are sensitive to missing data.

- *Egocentric Data-Collection Methods.* Egocentric network methods collect data from individuals (egos) regarding their personal networks without requiring participation from alters. These approaches, often implemented through name generators and ego–alter inventories, enable evaluators to examine network composition, diversity, and resource access at the individual level (Carolan, 2014; Perry et al., 2018). Egocentric methods are particularly valuable when network boundaries are ambiguous or when collecting complete network data is impractical. These methods are widely used in health, behavioral, and community-based evaluations to study processes of exposure, support, and influence. Although egocentric designs do not permit inference about the global network structure, they provide flexibility and feasibility in complex or hard-to-reach populations (Marsden, 2014).
- *Qualitative Network Data-Collection Methods.* Qualitative network methods generate relational data through interviews, observations, participatory mapping, and ethnographic engagement. These approaches are useful when the evaluation needs to understand meaning, context, and process. Examples include qualitative network interviews, participatory network mapping exercises, and observation of interactions among actors (Ryan et al., 2014). When survey methods are infeasible, interviews can generate egocentric relational data. Observing interactions among actors provides an additional means of collecting network data, particularly in small groups characterized by face-to-face engagement (Wasserman & Faust, 1994). In evaluation contexts, qualitative approaches are especially valuable for understanding how relationships function, how actors interpret their roles, and why network structures emerge or evolve. Although qualitative methods may not produce the standardized adjacency matrices required for formal network metrics, they enhance explanatory depth. They are often incorporated into mixed-method designs to support interpretation and stakeholder engagement (Creswell & Plano Clark, 2017).
- *Archival and Administrative Record Methods.* Archival and administrative methods infer network ties from existing records generated for operational or institutional purposes, such as administrative databases, public records, email logs, program participation records, organizational charts, or documented policy interactions (Carolan, 2014; Wasserman & Faust, 1994). These approaches are useful when the evaluation seeks nonreactive data or longitudinal evidence, and they may enable longitudinal analysis without imposing additional data collection burdens. They are frequently used in organizational, governance, and policy evaluations where formal records reflect coordination patterns. However, evaluators must carefully assess construct validity, as recorded interactions may not fully capture informal or emergent relational ties (Cross et al., 2002).
- *Longitudinal Network Data-Collection Methods.* Longitudinal network methods involve repeated measurements of network data over time, enabling analyses of network evolution, diffusion, and intervention effects (Wasserman & Faust,

1994). These designs are useful when the evaluation seeks to examine change processes within complex systems and may incorporate repeated surveys, egocentric interviews, or archival data extraction at multiple time points (Snijders et al., 2010). Such approaches are critical for evaluating change processes within complex systems. However, they demand substantial resources, sustained participant engagement, and careful management of boundary stability. These methods are most applicable in organizational or programmatic contexts characterized by relatively stable populations.
- *Census (Complete Network) Data-Collection Methods.* Census approaches aim to collect network data on all actors and relevant ties within a clearly bounded population. Typically, implemented through roster-based surveys or complete interorganizational data collection, census designs are useful when the evaluation requires a comprehensive structural analysis of a bounded system, including centralization, cohesion, and brokerage (Carolan, 2014; Wasserman & Faust, 1994). Census methods provide strong analytic power but are highly sensitive to missing data and require well-defined boundaries and high participation rates. Therefore, they are most appropriate in organizational or governance settings with clearly enumerated sets of actors.
- *Other and Hybrid Network Data-Collection Methods.* Hybrid approaches combine multiple procedures or generate relational data as part of intervention or experimental designs (Valente, 2012). These methods are increasingly common in implementation and systems evaluation, where methodological flexibility is necessary to capture dynamic change processes (Creswell & Plano Clark, 2017). For example, a team evaluating a multisector public health initiative combined roster-based surveys with participatory mapping workshops. While the survey revealed predictable service provider connections, the subsequent mapping identified an unexpected and influential partnership with a local housing advocacy group that had not been recognized in earlier planning stages. This insight enabled program leaders to engage new stakeholders and uncover additional pathways for impact. Such hybrid strategies can reveal hidden dynamics and foster more robust, actionable evaluations.

Table 6.2 synthesizes the primary categories of network data-collection procedures identified in social network analysis literature and maps their applications across social-ecological levels. It highlights differences in assumptions regarding boundary specification, scale, and actor accessibility, and how these differences affect the types of evaluative questions addressed. Organizing network data-collection methods by procedural category and ecological level offers a practical framework for selecting methods that align theoretically with program theories of change and are appropriate for studying complex, multilevel social systems.

Table 6.2 Common network data-collection methods by social-ecological level

Network data collection	Representative methods	Individual level	Organizational level	Community level	Policy level
Survey data	Name-generator surveys; roster-based sociometric surveys; relational rating scales	Well suited for measuring interpersonal relationships, social influence, information exchange, and diffusion processes within bounded populations	Widely used to assess collaboration, advice seeking, communication, and coordination among organizational actors	Applicable when community boundaries are reasonably defined, although feasibility decreases as systems become larger, more heterogeneous, and organizationally diffuse	Generally limited by challenges associated with boundary specification, respondent access, and participation among policy elites
Egocentric data	Ego-centered name generators; ego–alter inventories; network composition measures	Highly appropriate for examining individual relational environments, social capital, and mechanism-focused evaluation when complete network boundaries are impractical	Useful for studying leadership, professional relationships, and organizational subgroups without requiring complete network enumeration	Frequently employed with community leaders, key informants, or sampled residents to characterize local relational environments	Occasionally used to examine the personal networks of policymakers, advocates, or influential intermediaries
Qualitative data	Qualitative network interviews; participatory network mapping; ethnographic observation	Provides rich contextual understanding of relationship formation, interaction processes, and perceived network dynamics	Supports interpretation of collaboration, governance, organizational routines, and coordination mechanisms	Particularly valuable for understanding cross-sector partnerships, systems change, and locally embedded relational processes	Well suited for examining influence, negotiation, coalition formation, and governance processes among policy actors

(continued)

Table 6.2 (continued)

Network data collection	Representative methods	Individual level	Organizational level	Community level	Policy level
Archival/ administrative records	Attendance records; program participation logs; organizational records; communication logs	Limited applicability because routine administrative records seldom capture interpersonal relationships comprehensively	Highly appropriate for reconstructing formal coordination structures, communication patterns, workflow relationships, and administrative linkages	Moderately appropriate when records span multiple organizations, initiatives, or community sectors	Moderately to highly appropriate when legislative, regulatory, or administrative records document formal interactions among policy actors (e.g., legislative co-sponsorship or committee participation)
Longitudinal data	Panel network surveys; repeated egocentric interviews; longitudinal administrative data	Applicable when evaluating changes in interpersonal networks over time, although repeated data collection may increase respondent burden	Particularly well suited for examining network evolution, implementation processes, diffusion, organizational learning, and sustainability	Useful for longitudinal community evaluations but complicated by evolving system boundaries and participant turnover	Generally difficult due to substantial turnover, changing institutional arrangements, and unstable network boundaries
Census (Sociocentric design)	Whole network roster surveys; complete interorganizational network surveys	Most feasible in relatively small, bounded populations where complete network enumeration is possible	Highly appropriate when organizational membership and network boundaries are clearly specified	Often challenging because community systems are large, multi-sector, and characterized by porous boundaries	Rarely feasible because policy systems typically lack stable, fully bounded actor populations

(continued)

Table 6.2 (continued)

Network data collection	Representative methods	Individual level	Organizational level	Community level	Policy level
Other	Mixed-methods network designs; network intervention–generated data; experimental network interventions or agent-based simulation studies	Useful for evaluating interventions designed to modify interpersonal relationships or behavioral diffusion	Supports studies of organizational change, implementation strategies, and network interventions	Frequently used in systems-oriented and participatory evaluations	Emerging approaches for studying policy scenarios, governance interventions, and complex adaptive systems through simulation and experimental designs

Note This table presents the author's synthesis of common network data-collection procedures, drawing on social network analysis and evaluation literature (e.g., Borgatti et al., 2024; Carolan, 2014; Creswell & Plano Clark, 2017; Marsden, 2005, 2014; Perry et al., 2018; Snijders et al., 2010; Valente, 2010, 2012; Wasserman & Faust, 1994). It organizes these approaches across social-ecological levels to support method selection in network-informed complex evaluation.
Source Author

Analytic Strategies in Network-Informed Complex Evaluation

The selection of data-collection procedures determines the types of relational evidence available for evaluation; however, generating relational data alone does not yield evaluative insight. Relational evidence attains analytic significance only through methodologically rigorous, theoretically aligned, and explicitly justified analytic choices that correspond to the evaluation's objectives and research questions. Within NCE, analytic strategies are grounded in program theory and are designed to address distinct lines of inquiry related to structure, mechanism, process, and context. Consequently, network analysis extends beyond visualization or descriptive mapping to encompass multiple inferential logics aligned with evaluative aims (Borgatti et al., 2018; Wasserman & Faust, 1994).

Analytic approaches in NCE are selected according to the evaluation's primary purpose: diagnosing structural conditions, testing relational mechanisms, assessing temporal adaptation, or integrating structural evidence with contextual interpretation. Each strategy embodies a distinct inferential logic and produces a specific form of evaluative insight. Descriptive analysis characterizes observed relational architecture; statistical modeling evaluates structural tendencies under specified probabilistic assumptions; longitudinal analysis examines relational evolution over time; and mixed-method integration connects structural findings to lived experience and institutional context.

Table 6.3 provides an overview of the application of each analytic strategy across social–ecological levels in NCE. These approaches are cumulative and complementary rather than mutually exclusive. Descriptive analysis establishes structural baselines; statistical modeling evaluates hypothesized relational mechanisms; longitudinal analysis examines adaptive changes over time; and mixed-method integration contextualizes structural findings within lived and institutional settings. The following sections examine each strategy sequentially, beginning with descriptive network analysis as the foundational step for diagnosing structural conditions in complex systems.

Descriptive Network Analysis in Network-Informed Complex Evaluation

Descriptive network analysis represents a foundational analytic strategy for understanding the structural complexity of social systems. Rooted in classical social network theory, it emphasizes relational patterns, subgroup organization, and positional configurations rather than individual actor attributes (Wasserman & Faust, 1994, p. 23). Its purpose is to "represent the network's underlying social structure through data-reduction techniques or to characterize network properties through algebraic computations" (Carolan, 2014, p. 14). By focusing on structural properties, descriptive network analysis provides a systematic method for identifying how actors are embedded within relational systems and how those systems are organized.

Table 6.3 Network analytic approaches in network-informed complex evaluation (NCE)

Analytic approach	Purpose	Guiding question	Individual	Organizational	Community	Policy
Descriptive network analysis	Structural characterization and diagnostic assessment of network configurations	What structural patterns, positional arrangements, and subgroup structures are observable within the network?	Actor centrality, brokerage positions, role differentiation, and degree distribution	Network density, centralization, cohesion, and patterns of interorganizational connectivity	Whole network cohesion, segmentation, bridging structures, and inclusion patterns	Coalition structures, influence concentration, and cross-jurisdictional brokerage
Statistical network analysis	Model-based estimation and hypothesis testing of relational mechanisms under specified probabilistic assumptions	Which structural processes, actor attributes, or contextual conditions are associated with tie formation, network position, or diffusion of outcomes?	Relationships between positional embeddedness and behavioral or performance outcomes; peer exposure and influence effects	Structural drivers of collaboration, network determinants of organizational outcomes, and patterns of resource exchange	Predictors of participation and diffusion processes; structural constraints affecting integration or fragmentation	Modeling coalition formation, policy diffusion, resource dependence, and coordination among governing actors
Longitudinal network analysis	Examination of temporal dynamics in network structures and co-evolution of networks and behaviors	How do network structures evolve, and what mechanisms explain observed relational change?	Changes in centrality, brokerage, or exposure; co-evolution of relational ties and individual behaviors	Evolution of partnerships, tie formation and dissolution, and shifts in governance structure or coordination patterns	Structural integration, resilience, cross-group bridging, and diffusion processes over time	Changes in coalition alignment, redistribution of influence, and evolution of intergovernmental coordination
Mixed-methods social network analysis	Integration of quantitative network measures with qualitative evidence to strengthen contextual validity and explanatory depth	How are network structures enacted, experienced, and interpreted within institutional, cultural, and political contexts?	Lived experience of centrality, marginality, role strain, and perceived influence within networks	Interpretations of governance dynamics, trust relationships, and institutional constraints shaping collaboration	Community interpretations of cohesion, social capital, participation, and collective capacity	Interpretations of influence, negotiation processes, and power dynamics within governance networks

Note This table presents the author's synthesis of principal network analytic approaches, drawing on social network analysis and mixed-methods research (e.g., Borgatti et al., 2018; Creswell & Plano Clark, 2017; Edwards, 2010; Fetters et al., 2013; Hollstein, 2014; Knoke, 1990; Provan & Kenis, 2008). It organizes these approaches across social-ecological levels to support network-informed complex evaluation and integrates them into a multilevel evaluative framework. The analytic foci in each cell are illustrative rather than exhaustive.
Source Author

Descriptive analysis extends beyond visualization. Although sociograms illustrate relational patterns visually, rigorous descriptive approaches employ formal metrics to quantify structural features and enable systematic comparison across groups or time periods (Freeman, 1979). Measures such as degree, betweenness, and closeness centrality capture distinct dimensions of prominence and access; density and centralization clarify coordination and concentration of authority; clustering and cohesion illuminate subgroup formation and collective capacity. In NCE, descriptive analysis establishes a structural baseline against which relational change can be assessed. It also determines whether relational architecture aligns with the collaborative, diffusion, or coordination mechanisms specified in program theory.

Across levels of analysis, descriptive network analysis functions as both a diagnostic and interpretive tool. At the individual level, centrality measures reveal disparities in access and influence with equity implications (Freeman, 1979). At the organizational level, density and centralization clarify governance arrangements and coordination patterns (Provan & Kenis, 2008). At the community level, clustering and bridging structures illuminate social capital dynamics and collective efficacy (Putnam, 2000). At the policy level, brokerage and coalition clustering clarify the distribution of influence and agenda-setting processes (Knoke, 1990). Although descriptive measures do not establish causal relationships, they provide essential structural evidence that grounds subsequent statistical and longitudinal analyses in empirically observable relational conditions.

Statistical Inference in Network-Informed Complex Evaluation

While descriptive analysis characterizes relational structure, statistical network analysis advances evaluation by enabling model-based inference. This approach facilitates hypothesis testing regarding associations between network structures and program-relevant outcomes using probabilistic frameworks (Robins et al., 2007). By integrating network data with actor-, dyadic-, or contextual-level attributes, evaluators can assess whether centrality, brokerage, or exposure patterns are statistically associated with behavioral adoption, organizational performance, diffusion processes, or policy outcomes (Carolan, 2014, p. 276; Valente, 2010).

Exponential random graph models (ERGMs) examine whether tie formation reflects structural tendencies such as homophily, reciprocity, or triadic closure (Robins et al., 2007). In longitudinal contexts, stochastic actor-oriented models (SAOMs) assess the co-evolution of networks and behavior, distinguishing mechanisms of selection and influence under specified assumptions (Snijders et al., 2010). These modeling strategies enable evaluators to empirically examine relational mechanisms articulated in program theory while acknowledging the assumptions underlying statistical inference.

Applied across levels, statistical network modeling evaluates whether individual positions predict outcomes, whether partnership patterns reflect sector similarity or resource complementarity, whether diffusion pathways shape community participation, and whether policy coalitions reflect ideological alignment or resource dependence (Knoke, 1990; Provan & Kenis, 2008). Although statistical modeling enhances explanatory rigor, findings remain conditional on theoretical specification, model assumptions, and data quality. Within NCE, statistical network analysis functions as an iterative, theory-driven strategy that refines program assumptions and informs adaptive decision-making.

Longitudinal Network Analysis in Network-Informed Complex Evaluation

Complex interventions unfold within dynamic systems where relational structures evolve. Longitudinal network analysis captures this temporal dimension by examining changes in ties, positions, and structural configurations across repeated observations (Snijders et al., 2010; Wasserman & Faust, 1994). Rather than treating networks as static snapshots, this approach models processes of tie formation, persistence, and dissolution, enabling evaluators to assess whether hypothesized relational transformations occur during implementation. Longitudinal models further differentiate mechanisms such as selection (tie formation among similar actors), influence (behavioral convergence among connected actors), and structural opportunity effects (Snijders et al., 2010). These distinctions are critical when program theory posits that enhanced relational embeddedness precedes improved outcomes. Repeated measurement aligns relational evolution with intervention milestones and system adaptation, thereby increasing the plausibility of theorized change pathways.

Across levels, longitudinal analysis clarifies how governance structures stabilize or fragment (Provan & Kenis, 2008), how diffusion trajectories unfold within communities (Valente, 2010), and how coalition dynamics shift within policy domains (Knoke, 1990). Although temporal sequencing enhances causal plausibility, conclusions remain contingent on the rigor of design, the consistency of measurement, and theoretical coherence. Within NCE, longitudinal network analysis provides the temporal perspective necessary to evaluate adaptive change in complex systems.

Mixed-Method Social Network Analysis

Descriptive, statistical, and longitudinal network analyses progressively deepen structural and temporal understanding of relational systems. However, these approaches remain primarily structural: they identify patterns, associations, and trajectories but do not fully capture how actors interpret their positions, how trust and power shape relational processes, or how institutional contexts influence network formation and change. Mixed-method social network analysis addresses this limitation by integrating quantitative structural measurement with qualitative inquiry (Borgatti et al., 2018; Hollstein, 2014). Quantitative methods map and measure properties, such as centrality, brokerage, and cohesion, while qualitative approaches illuminate how relationships are experienced, negotiated, and embedded within organizational and cultural contexts (Edwards, 2010). The objective is the integration of inference rather than parallel reporting, combining structural evidence with interpretive insight into analytic dialogue (Fetters et al., 2013).

Within NCE, mixed-method social network analysis functions as an interpretive bridge connecting structure, process, and context. It clarifies whether structural prominence translates into influence or burden, whether collaboration reflects genuine trust or strategic dependency, and whether policy centrality corresponds to agenda-setting authority (Knoke, 1990; Provan & Kenis, 2008). By situating structural findings within lived experience and institutional environments, mixed-method integration strengthens explanatory coherence and enhances causal plausibility within complex adaptive systems (Creswell & Clark, 2017; Fetters et al., 2013).

Data Collection and Analysis Planning in Network-Informed Complex Evaluation

Careful planning of data collection and analysis is essential for translating conceptual designs into credible and actionable evidence in network-informed, complex evaluations. Grounding methodological decisions in program theory and findings from context assessment ensures that data are both theoretically justified and contextually relevant. Such alignment strengthens construct validity and enhances the interpretability of relational findings within dynamic systems. In addition, comprehensive documentation, ethical safeguards, and sustained methodological rigor increase the trustworthiness, transparency, and practical utility of evaluation results (Durland & Fredericks, 2005; Patton, 2011). The development of a data collection and analysis plan for network-informed evaluation, therefore, requires systematic consideration of several interrelated decisions, outlined below.

- Data sources and instruments must align with network boundaries and evaluation questions. Potential sources include network surveys, administrative data, digital trace data, and qualitative interviews or observations. Instruments should define ties, recall periods, and units of analysis to ensure consistency and validity (Carolan, 2014; Prell, 2011). Table 6.2 summarizes the types of network data used within NCE.
- The timing and frequency of data collection must correspond to program cycles and decision timelines. In this respect, cross-sectional designs are appropriate for diagnostic or formative purposes, whereas longitudinal or panel designs are necessary to assess network change or adaptation over time. Design choices should be guided by program theory assumptions concerning the pace of relational change (Hawe et al., 2009).

- Data quality assurance requires plans for entity resolution, monitoring response rates and handling missing data, and documenting protocols for managing incomplete or asymmetric ties. Implementing explicit error-control strategies improves transparency and reproducibility in complex relational datasets (Durland & Fredericks, 2005).
- Analytic strategies require theoretical justification and accessibility for intended users. As detailed in Table 6.3, these strategies include descriptive network measures such as density and centrality; comparative or longitudinal analyses; statistical inference about relationships between network variables and individual attributes; and equity-focused metrics such as participation inequality. Integrating mixed methods connects quantitative network findings with qualitative insights, revealing mechanisms and contextual factors that structural metrics alone cannot capture. This integration enables nuanced interpretation and supports equitable sense-making (Funnell & Rogers, 2011).
- Documentation and governance are essential components. Version-controlled data dictionaries, analytic decision logs, and protocols for data storage, access, and long-term learning plan.

Designing Reporting and Knowledge Use Strategies

Russ-Eft and Preskill (2001) emphasize that "communicating and reporting about an evaluation's activities and findings can easily be seen as one of the most critical aspects of an evaluation" (p. 348). Effective communication and reporting should address several key dimensions, including the identification of relevant audiences, the clarification of purpose, the determination of optimal timing, and the selection of appropriate formats (Russ-Eft & Preskill, 2001). In network-informed complex evaluation, robust reporting and knowledge utilization are essential for informed decision-making. Network analyses generate relational, multilevel, and often visual findings that provide valuable insights but are susceptible to misinterpretation without sufficient contextualization. Unlike traditional evaluation outputs, network findings may disclose sensitive information, thereby increasing ethical, political, and interpretive risk (Durland & Fredericks, 2005). Comprehensive reporting strategies are necessary to ensure accurate interpretation, responsible application, and effective communication of network evidence. Inadequate reporting can lead to oversimplification, such as equating centrality with effectiveness, reinforcing existing structural patterns, or unintentionally causing harm to individuals or organizations (Borgatti et al., 2009). From a utilization-focused perspective, the value of network-informed evaluation lies in translating findings into actionable learning while maintaining analytic rigor.

The NCE context assessment checklist informs product-stage strategies by clarifying readiness, feasibility, and risk across multiple domains. Identifying intended users and decision pathways guides the selection of the most suitable type, format, and timing for evaluation products. Technical reports are generally designed for analysts or system leaders, whereas executive briefs, dashboards, or community summaries are more appropriate for policymakers or frontline partners (Russ-Eft & Preskill, 2001, see Chapter 13). The degree of stakeholder engagement and buy-in affects the feasibility and effectiveness of collaborative interpretation methods, such as facilitated sense-making workshops. Ethical and equity considerations influence decisions regarding disclosure, visualization, and dissemination. When relational data are politically sensitive or significant power asymmetries are present, NCE recommends anonymization, phased disclosure, and structured interpretation to reduce the risk of harm or stigmatization. For example, node labels in network data presentations may be anonymized by replacing real names with numeric codes or generic identifiers (e.g., Individual A, Group 1), thereby preserving confidentiality while enabling meaningful analysis. Consequently, network-informed evaluation products are deliberately tailored to context, ensuring alignment with both decision-making needs and ethical responsibilities.

Developing Effective Evaluation Reports

Evaluation reporting is a foundational component of evaluation practice, shaping the credibility, utility, and ethical application of findings (Fitzpatrick et al., 2011; Patton, 2008). High-quality reports clearly state their purpose, offer methodological transparency, ensure accessibility for diverse audiences, and align with intended use. Reporting that is contextually responsive and well-designed not only disseminates results but also facilitates organizational learning, reinforces accountability, and informs evidence-based decision-making (Mark et al., 2000).

Stakeholder engagement is essential for effective evaluation reporting. Russ-Eft and Preskill (2001) argue that involving stakeholders throughout the evaluation process enhances both relevance and utility. NCE approaches build on this principle by engaging stakeholders in co-constructing the program theory of change, clarifying evaluation purposes, selecting appropriate designs and methods, organizing logistics, and planning communication and reporting strategies. This collaborative approach situates evaluation activities within context, ensures ethical responsiveness, and aligns with stakeholder priorities, thereby increasing the likelihood that findings will be interpreted and applied meaningfully.

Reporting products should be explicitly aligned with the evaluation's purpose and intended use. Formative and developmental evaluations benefit from interim products such as learning memos, briefings, and rapid-feedback reports that support ongoing adaptation. In contrast, summative or accountability-oriented evaluations require comprehensive, formal reporting structures and clear interpretive guidance. Deliberate alignment among evaluation purpose, reporting format, and anticipated use helps prevent misinterpretation or misuse of network evidence and promotes responsible, timely decision-making (Fitzpatrick et al., 2011; Patton, 2008).

Given their abstract nature, network visualizations and summaries require careful attention to interpretability and accessibility. Best practices include transparent documentation of layout and analytic decisions, clear legends, explanatory primers, color-blind-accessible palettes, and limited technical complexity. Network maps should be presented as analytic tools rather than as definitive representations of reality. They should be accompanied by narrative interpretations that clarify underlying assumptions, analytic limitations, and appropriate uses of network metrics (Carolan, 2014). Detailed methodological notes or technical appendices further enhance transparency and credibility, particularly for technical audiences, and help prevent overinterpretation or inappropriate application of findings.

The evaluation findings must be communicated in formats that are accessible and meaningful to diverse stakeholder groups. Consistent with the NCE framework, layered communication strategies such as executive summaries, interactive dashboards, visual network representations, and plain-language community briefs facilitate differentiated access to evaluation evidence. Policymakers, program administrators, and community partners may prioritize different aspects of network findings, including coordination, representation, or relational equity. Adapting reporting formats to stakeholder needs and capacities enhances both the perceived legitimacy and practical utility of evaluation results, thereby increasing the likelihood that findings will inform action and decision-making (Mark et al., 2000; Russ-Eft & Preskill, 2001).

Table 6.4 presents example reporting strategies. Consistent with utilization-focused and developmental evaluation scholarship, the table highlights that network evidence is inherently contextual and interpretive, and is designed to complement other evaluative data. Network visualizations and findings function as tools to demonstrate how network structures or relationships may influence program outcomes, rather than as performance rankings or objective representations of relational structures. By explicitly stating assumptions, analytic decisions, ethical considerations, and audience-specific applications, these reporting strategies comply with established evaluation standards and address concerns about overinterpretation of network measures and the potential for inequitable or unintended consequences in reporting.

Facilitating Sense-Making and Action Translation

The NCE framework emphasizes the significance of sense-making and action translation, acknowledging that evaluation use is fundamentally a social and interpretive process (Weiss, 1998). In network-informed evaluation, findings often reveal complex patterns of coordination, influence, or exclusion that require contextualized, collective interpretation for meaningful understanding. NCE operationalizes sense-making through structured processes, such as facilitated workshops and guided reflection sessions, in which stakeholders and intended users collaboratively examine findings, challenge interpretations, and elicit tacit and experiential knowledge.

Table 6.4 Network-informed complex evaluation reporting products by audience, purpose, timing, and format

Primary audience	Evaluation purpose	Timing in evaluation lifecycle	Reporting product	Typical formats and features	Primary methodological and ethical considerations
Policymakers and funders	Accountability; summative judgment; policy and funding decisions	End of evaluation cycle; key decision milestones	Summative evaluation report with integrated network findings	Formal written report; executive summary; static, clearly annotated network visualizations; summary tables	Requires interpretation, transparency, and explicit limitations. Network metrics (e.g., density, centralization) are presented as contextual evidence rather than direct indicators of performance to prevent misuse or oversimplification
Senior system leaders (e.g., executives)	Strategic learning; system alignment; resource prioritization	Midpoint and end of evaluation; strategic planning cycles	Strategic network briefing	Concise briefing document; annotated network maps; comparative visuals across time points	Emphasizes system-level patterns (e.g., coordination, fragmentation, hubs) supported by narrative interpretation. Visuals are paired with facilitated or written sense-making to reduce overreliance on graphical representations

(continued)

Table 6.4 (continued)

Primary audience	Evaluation purpose	Timing in evaluation lifecycle	Reporting product	Typical formats and features	Primary methodological and ethical considerations
Program managers and implementers	Formative learning; adaptive management; implementation improvement	Ongoing; iterative feedback cycles	Learning memos or rapid-feedback briefs	Short written memos; dashboards; preliminary network snapshots	Prioritizes timeliness and actionability. Findings are explicitly framed as provisional and hypothesis generating, supporting reflection and adaptation rather than summative judgment
Evaluation and research teams	Methodological rigor; analytic transparency; replication and knowledge building	Throughout the evaluation; finalized at the reporting stage	Technical or methodological report	Detailed technical appendix; analytic codebooks; methodological tables; reproducible procedures	Documents boundary specification, tie definitions, missing data treatment, metric selection, and visualization algorithms. Supports peer review, reproducibility, and methodological credibility

(continued)

Table 6.4 (continued)

Primary audience	Evaluation purpose	Timing in evaluation lifecycle	Reporting product	Typical formats and features	Primary methodological and ethical considerations
Community partners and network participants	sense-making; relational learning; inclusion	Midpoint and end; facilitated reflection or dissemination sessions	Community-facing network brief or workshop materials	Plain-language briefs; simplified network maps	Emphasizes accessibility, ethical interpretation, and relational sensitivity. Visuals are contextualized to avoid stigmatization, labeling, or unintended consequences for individuals or groups
Cross-Sector collaboratives or coalitions	Coordination improvement; shared learning; collective accountability	Periodic checkpoints; coalition or partnership meetings	Interactive network products for shared reflection	Interactive dashboards; participatory network maps	Designed for facilitated use to support constructive dialogue. Careful framing prevents competitive comparison and reinforces a learning-oriented interpretation of network patterns

(continued)

Table 6.4 (continued)

Primary audience	Evaluation purpose	Timing in evaluation lifecycle	Reporting product	Typical formats and features	Primary methodological and ethical considerations
Academic and scholarly audiences	Theory development; methodological contribution; generalizable knowledge	Post evaluation dissemination	Peer-reviewed journal articles or academic book chapters	Theory-driven figures; analytic tables; formal narrative interpretation	Emphasizes conceptual clarity, methodological justification, and theoretical contribution. Network findings are situated within broader evaluation and systems literature and integrated with complementary sources of evidence

Note This table presents the author's synthesis of network-informed evaluation reporting strategies, drawing on established evaluation scholarship on reporting, utilization, and stakeholder engagement (e.g., Fitzpatrick et al., 2011; Mark et al., 2000; Patton, 2008; Russ-Eft & Preskill, 2001). It organizes reporting products by audience, purpose, timing, and format within a network-informed complex evaluation framework. The strategies emphasize the contextual, interpretive, and ethical use of network evidence and are intended to be illustrative rather than prescriptive.
Source Author

Collaborative sense-making democratizes the evaluation process by integrating technical expertise with lived experience, fostering the shared ownership of results, and increasing the likelihood of meaningful application (Cousins & Whitmore, 1998; Patton, 2008). In network contexts, where findings may reveal inequities or politically sensitive dynamics, these sessions function as essential forums for ethical reflection and contextualization. Facilitation techniques prompt stakeholders to discuss power dynamics, question the beneficiaries of existing patterns, and consider implications for marginalized or peripheral actors. For example, facilitators may ask, "Whose perspectives are missing in the current analysis, and how might their inclusion change our understanding?" or "In what ways do existing power structures influence the actions or decisions made within this network?" Addressing these questions directly advances the equity and learning objectives central to the NCE approach.

The NCE framework links sense-making to the translation of insights into structured action. Rather than viewing interpretation as a final step, the framework prioritizes converting findings into actionable plans with defined responsibilities, timelines, and progress indicators (Patton, 2008). For instance, evidence of over-centralization may prompt strategies to strengthen connections among less connected actors, whereas findings of homophily can inform initiatives that promote cross-sector or cross-group collaboration. Decision logs and monitoring mechanisms institutionalize accountability by documenting how evaluation findings inform subsequent policy, program, or governance decisions. This approach transforms evaluation products from static reports into dynamic blueprints for improvement and system change, ensuring that network evidence is both understood and implemented.

Integrating Feedback and Adaptive Learning Loops

The NCE framework highlights the importance of feedback and adaptive learning loops, positioning evaluation products as catalysts for ongoing cycles of reflection, adjustment, and organizational learning rather than as static, one-time outputs. This perspective is especially relevant in network-informed complex evaluations, where networks are dynamic and evolve in response to internal interactions, external pressures, and changes in policy or funding environments (Byrne & Callaghan, 2014).

Drawing on developmental evaluation principles, the NCE framework conceptualizes learning in complex systems as iterative and path-dependent, with knowledge, action, and adaptation continuously informing one another (Patton, 2011). Interim evaluation products, structured reflection sessions, and explicit documentation of adaptation rules, such as those in Table 6.4, enable findings to guide mid-course corrections, refine network boundaries, and support ongoing adjustments to data-collection strategies. When contextual readiness is high, feedback loops can be integrated into governance or planning processes, facilitating real-time learning and adaptation. In contexts with lower readiness, learning may be supported through phased dissemination, targeted capacity building, or incremental feedback mechanisms.

By integrating feedback and adaptive learning loops into the reporting and use of evaluation findings, the NCE framework transforms evaluation products into "learning infrastructures" that enhance system responsiveness, flexibility, and resilience (Patton, 2011; Preskill & Torres, 1999). Living repositories, which are dynamic archives capturing findings, adaptations, and decisions across evaluation cycles, build institutional memory and support both cumulative learning and the capacity to respond effectively to emerging challenges and opportunities. This approach fosters continuous, adaptive system improvement rather than episodic or reactive change and develops the adaptive coordination capacity required for success in complex, networked environments.

Prioritizing Equity-Centered Communication and Use

Equity considerations are fundamental to NCE reporting and knowledge-use strategies. Without intentional safeguards, network evaluations may overlook power dynamics or underrepresent marginalized actors through metrics or visualizations that lack adequate context (Borgatti & Molina, 2005). NCE addresses these risks by providing contextualized insights into structural measures, emphasizing strengths rather than deficiencies, and intentionally incorporating diverse perspectives in interpretation and planning. The use of terms such as "emerging connectors" instead of "less-connected actors" demonstrates a commitment to asset-based language, highlighting potential and opportunities within the network.

Network-Informed Complex Evaluation Design and Reporting Checklist

Table 6.5 presents the five steps of the network-informed process within a quality assurance framework. While the previous section described these steps in theory, this table outlines methods essential to ensuring rigor, transparency, and responsible application in complex network interventions. These methods are grounded in established evaluation theories and network science. Explaining why and how processes function aligns with theory-driven, contribution-focused evaluation (Chen, 1990; Weiss, 1998). Emphasizing adaptive learning and stakeholder engagement corresponds to utilization-focused and developmental evaluation approaches (Patton, 2008, 2011). Consideration of relationships, boundaries, and structure derives from social network analysis, which recognizes that relational data require specialized methods and a clearly defined network scope (Borgatti et al., 2018, 2024; Wasserman & Faust, 1994).

Table 6.5 Network-informed complex evaluation design and reporting checklist

Domain and stage	Focus and rationale	Quality assurance considerations
A. Conceptualization and design		
Network-informed objectives, questions, and mechanisms	Establish theoretical coherence and articulate explicit causal reasoning linking network processes to program outcomes	• Articulation of evaluation purpose in relational or structural terms • Identification of intended users and alignment with decision timelines • Development of theory-informed structural and relational evaluation questions • Specification of hypothesized mechanisms linking network processes (e.g., diffusion, brokerage, coordination) to outcomes • Clarification of assumed temporal ordering and causal sequencing • Definition of relational equity objectives (e.g., inclusion, influence, access to resources) • Alignment between unit of analysis and level of inference
Network scope, boundaries, and levels of analysis	Promote analytic validity and transparency through explicit boundary specification and attention to levels of analysis	• Clear specification of network type (e.g., whole network, ego network, two-mode, multiplex, multilevel) and analytic scale • Definition of actors, tie constructs, nomination rules, and temporal scope • Clarification of multilevel structures and cross-level relationships where applicable • Theoretical and practical justification of inclusion and exclusion criteria • Assessment of potential bias arising from boundary specification • Articulation of ecological, theoretical, and contextual scope conditions • Distinction among analytic, statistical, and theoretical forms of generalization

(continued)

Table 6.5 (continued)

Domain and stage	Focus and rationale	Quality assurance considerations
Methodological alignment, causal logic, and comparative design	Ensure coherence between evaluative questions, causal ambition, and analytic strategy	• Selection of analytic approaches consistent with evaluation questions and boundary decisions • Clarification of whether the design supports descriptive analysis, contribution analysis, quasi-experimental inference, or causal attribution • Alignment between the strength of causal claims and the rigor of the evaluation design • Distinction between structural change and compositional change in longitudinal designs • Identification of implementation fidelity indicators in network interventions • Explicit specification of the explanatory and causal claims supported by the evaluation design
B. Data collection and implementation		
Data collection, measurement validity, and integration	Support rigorous operationalization and defensible measurement of relational constructs	• Theory-consistent operational definitions of tie constructs • Explicit nomination rules and boundary constraints • Justification of measurement scales (binary, ordinal, weighted) and coding decisions • Instrument piloting and assessment of recall bias, nomination error, and ceiling effects • Pre-specified strategies for addressing missing data and non-response • Assessment of the validity and reliability of relational measures • Cross-validation of data sources where feasible • Alignment of data-collection timing with hypothesized mechanisms • Explicit mixed-method integration strategy where applicable

(continued)

Table 6.5 (continued)

Domain and stage	Focus and rationale	Quality assurance considerations
Ethics, governance, and reflexivity	Address relational risk, structural power asymmetries, and evaluator positionality	• Informed consent procedures acknowledging relational inference risks • Disclosure thresholds and anonymization standards for network visualization • Assessment of differential reputational or participation risks for actors with limited network visibility or influence • Analysis of structural power concentration, brokerage, and exclusion patterns • Consideration of the normative implications of observed structural configurations • Documentation of evaluator positionality and reflexive practice • Specification of data governance and long-term stewardship arrangements
Fieldwork quality, fidelity, and monitoring	Protect data integrity and implementation credibility during collection	• Reporting of response-rate benchmarks overall and by subgroup • Monitoring of intervention fidelity in network-building initiatives • Maintenance of comprehensive audit trails documenting data-collection processes • Comparison of participation patterns with design assumptions and readiness indicators

(continued)

Table 6.5 (continued)

Domain and stage	Focus and rationale	Quality assurance considerations
C. Analysis, inference, and interpretation		
Data processing, missingness, and reproducibility	Promote transparency, robustness, and reproducibility of analytic procedures	• Entity reconciliation and validation of relational ties • Assessment of missingness patterns and potential subgroup bias • Sensitivity analyses addressing boundary effects and non-response bias • Archiving analytic scripts and reproducible workflows • Documentation of data transformations and analytic assumptions
Theory-driven metrics and inference analysis	Support theoretically grounded interpretation and methodologically defensible inference	• Selection of network metrics aligned with program theory and hypothesized mechanisms • Use of inferential approaches that account for relational interdependence • Reporting of model diagnostics and fit indices where modeling is applied • Presentation of uncertainty estimates where appropriate • Clear distinction between descriptive patterns and inferential conclusions • Separation of structural and compositional change in longitudinal analyses • Examination of centralization, brokerage, variation in participation, and access to influence • Interpret findings in relation to the evaluation theory, consider plausible alternative explanations, and clarify the contexts in which conclusions are expected to hold

(continued)

Table 6.5 (continued)

Domain and stage	Focus and rationale	Quality assurance considerations
Visualization, interpretation, and responsible communication	Promote clarity and prevent misinterpretation of complex network findings	• Documentation of layout algorithms and visual encoding decisions • Provision of legends, metric explanations, and interpretive guidance • Application of anonymization and disclosure controls • Explicit statement of uncertainty and analytic limits • Avoid unsupported normative interpretations (e.g., assuming higher density implies effectiveness) without explicit theoretical justification
D. Reporting, use, and institutional learning		
Knowledge translation and decision integration	Promote responsible and context-sensitive application of findings	• Adaptation of reporting formats to user capacity and decision cycles • Facilitation of structured sense-making processes among stakeholders • Maintenance of decision logs linking evidence to action • Documentation of intended and unintended structural consequences

(continued)

Table 6.5 (continued)

Domain and stage	Focus and rationale	Quality assurance considerations
Feedback, adaptation, and comparative learning	Encourage adaptive rigor and cross-cycle reflection	• Dissemination of findings aligned with decision timelines • Documentation of boundary and instrument revisions across evaluation waves • Comparison of findings across networks or time periods where appropriate • Reflection on the ethical implications and potential consequences of disclosure • Planning of subsequent evaluation cycles informed by accumulated evidence
Documentation, stewardship, generalizability, and capacity	Institutionalize methodological memory and clarify limits of transferability	• Maintenance of version-controlled repositories of instruments, metrics, and analytic scripts • Archiving sufficient documentation to support replication • Clarification of long-term data stewardship responsibilities • Explicit articulation of transferability conditions and analytic limits • Development of organizational capacity in network literacy, governance, and relational analysis

Note Drawing on established principles from social network analysis, theory-based evaluation, and mixed-methods evaluation research (e.g., Borgatti et al., 2018; Creswell & Clark, 2017; Rogers, 2008; Wasserman & Faust, 1994), this checklist presents an integrated framework for designing, analyzing, and reporting network-informed evaluations in which relational processes are conceptualized as central mechanisms of change.

The domains of Conceptualization and Design correspond to Steps 1 through 3 of the proposed framework. The section on Network-Informed Objectives, Questions, and Mechanisms formalizes Step 1 by ensuring that evaluation purposes are relational, theoretically grounded, and attentive to mechanisms within interdependent systems. Network Scope, Boundaries, and Levels of Analysis operationalize Step 2 by requiring defensible boundary specification, consideration of multilevel structures, and clarity regarding generalization. Methodological Alignment, Causal Logic, and Comparative Design advance Step 3 by aligning analytic strategies with evaluation questions, network boundaries, and the causal aims supported by the design. These elements ensure coherence among program theory, network theory, and empirical strategy.

The second domain, Data Collection and Implementation, corresponds to Step 4, which translates conceptual design decisions into structured procedures. Sections on measurement validity, relational constructs, missing-data strategies, and mixed-methods integration ensure that abstract theoretical assumptions become empirically observable and methodologically defensible. This translation is critical in network-informed evaluations because relational constructs such as trust, collaboration, and brokerage require precise operationalization to prevent construct drift. The inclusion of ethics, governance, and reflexivity safeguards acknowledges that network data are inherently relational and thus socially and politically significant. Monitoring response rates, fidelity, and structural anomalies during fieldwork further strengthens this stage by linking implementation realities to analytic interpretation.

The third domain, Analysis, Inference, and Interpretation, elaborates Step 4 by specifying standards for interdependence-aware inference, transparency, and reproducibility. Because network data violate conventional independence assumptions, analytic procedures must account for relational dependence. The checklist requires sensitivity analyses, documentation of analytic transformations, reporting of uncertainty, and a clear distinction between descriptive and inferential claims to prevent overinterpretation and support proportional causal reasoning. Additionally, the explicit examination of power concentration, participation inequality, and access to influence acknowledges that networks distribute resources and authority in patterned ways that affect program implementation and outcomes.

The domain of Reporting, Use, and Institutional Learning operationalizes Step 5. Network findings are often complex, visually compelling, and potentially sensitive, requiring structured communication strategies. The checklist emphasizes interpretive guidance, disclosure safeguards, structured sense-making, and documentation of both intended and unintended structural consequences. By integrating feedback loops, boundary revisions, and longitudinal comparisons, the framework reinforces the iterative process described by Stufflebeam and Coryn (2014) and the adaptive learning principles outlined by Patton (2011). Network-informed evaluation extends beyond reporting to inform subsequent evaluation cycles, thereby enhancing institutional memory and evaluative capacity.

The inclusion of Table 6.5 in this volume reflects both a conceptual commitment and practice-informed judgment. Conceptually, the table aims to align network science and evaluation theory more closely at the methodological level. Whereas much of the network analysis literature emphasizes structural description, evaluation theory focuses on purpose, use, and judgment. In complex systems, these domains must remain connected. The table articulates standards integrating attention to interdependence, mechanisms of change, boundary conditions, proportional causal reasoning, and responsible knowledge-use within a unified evaluative framework.

The inclusion of this table is grounded in accumulated experience. Across numerous network applications in evaluation, I have observed recurring patterns: boundaries are sometimes defined too broadly or too narrowly; mechanisms are often implied rather than explicitly theorized; power structures may be mapped but not critically interpreted; and causal claims are occasionally extended beyond what the research design can legitimately support. These observations highlight the necessity of a structured framework that fosters methodological discipline without constraining adaptive inquiry. The checklist emerged at the intersection of scholarship and practice. It is not intended as a prescriptive template but rather as a set of guardrails designed to protect the credibility of analytics, ethical integrity, and the relevance of decisions in relational evaluation. By rendering implicit assumptions explicit and insisting on alignment among theory, design, analysis, and use, the table articulates the view that rigor in complex systems evaluation is achieved not solely through technical precision but through sustained attention to coherence, proportionality, and reflexivity.

Chapter Summary

Chapter 6 presents evaluation approaches to designing and implementing network-informed evaluations in complex, networked systems. The NCE approach enables evaluators to address adaptive, multilevel, and relational dynamics in these contexts. The chapter offers structured guidance on formulating evaluation objectives and questions, defining network scope and boundaries, aligning methodological approaches with evaluation aims and contextual conditions, and developing data collection, analysis, and reporting strategies that accommodate system complexity and ethical considerations. It highlights the iterative and participatory nature of evaluation, incorporating stakeholder engagement and equity as essential components.

A central contribution of the chapter is the systematic articulation of network boundary specification and knowledge-use strategies in network-informed evaluation. It explains how positional, relational, and event-based boundary strategies enhance analytic validity, transparency, and interpretability of network data when aligned with program theory, evaluation objectives, and stakeholder input. By emphasizing explicit decision rules and transparent methodological choices, the chapter strengthens rigor and replicability in evaluation design. It also advances reporting and knowledge-use practices that support interpretability, collaborative sense-making, and equitable dissemination through layered communication strategies tailored to diverse audiences. Within the NCE framework, continuous feedback loops, adaptive learning processes, and stakeholder collaboration facilitate the translation of evaluation findings into actionable knowledge and system improvements. Appendix B: Network-Informed Complex Evaluation Design and Planning Template provides a practical tool for evaluation design and planning.

Reflection Questions

- How do the specification and justification of network boundaries affect the validity, utility, and ethical rigor of network-informed evaluations? Based on your experience, how have decisions regarding network boundaries, including inclusion criteria and boundary definitions, influenced the results, ethical considerations (such as representation, consent, and power dynamics), or broader implications of your work?
- What challenges and opportunities have you encountered when integrating network analysis? Describe a specific instance in which a methodological challenge or decision influenced the intended use of your evaluation findings. How can methodological decisions be optimized to ensure rigor and practical relevance within complex systems, particularly regarding how findings will be used and by whom?
- How can evaluation reporting be designed to maximize knowledge utilization and knowledge translation? Which strategies from Chapter 6, including accessible reporting formats, participatory dissemination, and equity-focused metrics, should be prioritized to ensure findings are actionable and accessible to diverse stakeholders? What types of misinterpretations or misunderstandings might arise among varied audiences, and how can intentional report design anticipate and mitigate these issues?

Applied Activities

Scenario: The City Health Department is evaluating its vaccination response network, which coordinates immunization delivery and outreach during both routine campaigns and emergency response efforts. The current network includes hospitals, public health clinics, pharmacies, schools, and established community organizations. However, there is ongoing debate about whether to formally include private mobile vaccination providers and neighborhood associations, both of which have contributed informally to previous vaccination campaigns but are not officially recognized as network members.

Recent community engagement sessions identified several key behavioral drivers, including:

- Thinking and feeling factors, such as trust in vaccines and confidence in health authorities.
- Social processes, including the influence of community leaders, peer networks, and local norms.
- Motivation, reflected by the willingness to seek vaccination or encourage others to do so.
- Practical issues, including transportation barriers, language access, clinic hours, and cost.

These findings suggest that trust, social influence, motivation, and practical access shape both participation in the vaccination response network and the reach of vaccination services within the community. The task is to design a network-informed evaluation that combines network analysis with community perspectives to determine which organizations and community groups should be included in the vaccination response network, using the chapter's boundary and knowledge-use approaches.

Activity:

- List the formal and informal actors involved in vaccination delivery, outreach, and coordination and briefly describe their roles in the vaccination response network.
- Develop at least two boundary definitions (e.g., an inclusive boundary that includes community groups and mobile providers, and a more restrictive boundary limited to formal health organizations). Provide a short rationale for each.
- Discuss how including or excluding certain actors may affect network structure (e.g., connectivity, brokerage, or reach) and behavioral drivers of vaccination, such as trust, social influence, motivation, and practical access.
- Select the boundary definition you consider most appropriate and explain your reasoning. Briefly outline how this decision and its rationale should be communicated to stakeholders, and how stakeholder feedback should be collected.

References

Borgatti, S. P., Everett, M. G., & Johnson, J. C. (2018). *Analyzing social networks* (2nd ed.). SAGE Publications.

Borgatti, S. P., Everett, M. G., Johnson, J. C., & Agneessens, F. (2024). *Analyzing social networks* (3rd ed.). Sage Publications Ltd

Borgatti, S. P., & Molina, J.-L. (2005). Toward ethical guidelines for network research in organizations. *Social Networks, 27*(2), 107–117. https://doi.org/10.1016/j.socnet.2005.01.004

Borgatti, S. P., Mehra, A., Brass, D. J., & Labianca, G. (2009). Network Analysis in the Social Sciences. *Science (American Association for the Advancement of Science), 323*(5916), 892–895. https://doi.org/10.1126/science.1165821

Butterfoss, F. D. (2007). *Coalitions and partnerships in community health.* Jossey-Bass.

Byrne, D., & Callaghan, G. (2014). *Complexity theory and the social sciences: The state of the art* (1st ed.). Routledge. https://doi.org/10.4324/9780203519585

Carolan, B. V. (2014). *Social network analysis and education: Theory, methods & applications.* SAGE.

Chen, H. T. (1990). *Theory-driven evaluations.* Sage.

Cousins, J. B., & Whitmore, E. (1998). Framing participatory evaluation. *New Directions for Evaluation, 1998*(80), 5–23. https://doi.org/10.1002/ev.1114
Creswell, J. W., & Clark, V. L. P. (2017). *Designing and conducting mixed methods research*. Sage Publications.
Cross, R., Borgatti, S. P., & Parker, A. (2002). Making invisible work visible: Using social network analysis to support strategic collaboration. *California Management Review, 44*(2), 25–46. https://doi.org/10.2307/41166121
Durland, M. M., & Fredericks, K. A. (2005). An introduction to social network analysis. *New Directions for Evaluation, 2005*(107), 5–13. https://doi.org/10.1002/ev.157
Edwards, G. (2010). *Mixed-method approaches to social network analysis*.
Fetters, M. D., Curry, L. A., & Creswell, J. W. (2013). Achieving integration in mixed methods designs-principles and practices. *Health Services Research, 48*(6pt2), 2134–2156. https://doi.org/10.1111/1475-6773.12117
Fitzpatrick, J. L., Sanders, J. R., & Worthen, B. R. (2011). *Program evaluation: Alternative approaches and practical guidelines* (4th ed.). Pearson.
Freeman, L. C. (1979). Centrality in social networks conceptual clarification. *Social Networks, 1*(3), 215–239.
Funnell, S. C., & Rogers, P. J. (2011). *Purposeful program theory: Effective use of theories of change and logic models*. Jossey-Bass.
Hawe, P., Shiell, A., & Riley, T. (2009). Theorising interventions as events in systems. *American Journal of Community Psychology, 43*(3–4), 267–276. https://doi.org/10.1007/s10464-009-9229-9
Hollstein, B. (2014). Mixed methods social networks research: An introduction. In *Mixed methods social networks research* (pp. 3–34). Cambridge University Press. https://doi.org/10.1017/CBO9781139227193.003
Knoke, D. (1990). *Political networks: The structural perspective*. Cambridge University Press.
Knoke, D., & Yang, S. (2008). *Social network analysis* (2nd ed.). SAGE.
Laumann, E. O., Galaskiewicz, J., & Marsden, P. V. (1978). Community structure as interorganizational linkages. *Annual Review of Sociology, 4*(1), 455–484. https://doi.org/10.1146/annurev.so.04.080178.002323
Laumann, E. O., Marsden, P. V., & Prensky, D. (1989). The boundary specification problem in network analysis. *Research Methods in Social Network Analysis, 61*(8), 176–179.
Mark, M. M., Henry, G. T., & Julnes, G. (2000). *Evaluation: An integrated framework for understanding, guiding, and improving public and nonprofit policies and programs*. Jossey-Bass.
Marsden, P. V. (2005). Recent developments in network measurement. In P. J. Carrington, J. Scott, & S. Wasserman (Eds.), *Models and methods in social network analysis* (pp. 8–30). Cambridge University Press.
Marsden, P. V. (2014). Survey methods for network data. In J. Scott & P. J. Carrington (Eds.), *The SAGE handbook of social network analysis* (pp. 370–388). SAGE Publications Ltd. https://doi.org/10.4135/9781446294413.n25
Nowell, B., & Foster-Fishman, P. (2011). Examining multi-sector community collaboratives as vehicles for building organizational capacity. *American Journal of Community Psychology, 48*(3–4), 193–207. https://doi.org/10.1007/s10464-010-9364-3
Patton, M. Q. (2008). *Utilization-focused evaluation* (4th ed.). Sage Publications.
Patton, M. Q. (2011). *Developmental evaluation: Applying complexity concepts to enhance innovation and use*. Guilford Press.
Perry, B. L., Pescosolido, B. A., & Borgatti, S. P. (2018). *Egocentric network analysis: Foundations, methods, and models* (Vol. 44). Cambridge University Press. https://doi.org/10.1017/9781316443255
Prell, C. (2011). *Social network analysis: History, theory and methodology*. SAGE.
Preskill, H. S., & Torres, R. T. (1999). *Evaluative inquiry for learning in organizations* (1st ed.). Sage Publications.

Provan, K. G., Fish, A., & Sydow, J. (2007). Interorganizational networks at the network level: A review of the empirical literature on whole networks. *Journal of Management, 33*(3), 479–516. https://doi.org/10.1177/0149206307302554

Provan, K. G., & Kenis, P. (2008). Modes of network governance: Structure, management, and effectiveness. *Journal of Public Administration Research and Theory, 18*(2), 229–252. https://doi.org/10.1093/jopart/mum015

Provan, K. G., & Milward, H. B. (2001). Do networks really work? A framework for evaluating public-sector organizational networks. *Public Administration Review, 61*(4), 414–423. https://doi.org/10.1111/0033-3352.00045

Putnam, R. D. (2000). *Bowling alone: The collapse and revival of American community*. Simon & Schuster.

Rhodes, R. A. W. (1997). *Understanding governance: Policy networks, governance, reflexivity and accountability*. Open University Press.

Robins, G., Pattison, P., Kalish, Y., & Lusher, D. (2007). An introduction to exponential random graph (p) models for social networks. *Social Networks, 29*(2), 173–191. https://doi.org/10.1016/j.socnet.2006.08.002

Rogers, P. J. (2008). Using programme theory to evaluate complicated and complex aspects of interventions. *Evaluation, 14*(1), 29–48.

Russ-Eft, D. F., & Preskill, H. S. (2001). *Evaluation in organizations: A systematic approach to enhancing learning, performance, and change*. Perseus Pub.

Ryan, L., Mulholland, J., & Agoston, A. (2014). Talking ties: Reflecting on network visualisation and qualitative interviewing. *Sociological Research Online, 19*(2), 1–12. https://doi.org/10.5153/sro.3404

Sabatier, P. A., & Jenkins-Smith, H. C. (1993). *Policy change and learning: An advocacy coalition approach*. Westview Press.

Seidman, S. B. (1983). Network structure and minimum degree. *Social Networks, 5*(3), 269–287. https://doi.org/10.1016/0378-8733(83)90028-X

Snijders, T. A. B., van de Bunt, G. G., & Steglich, C. E. G. (2010). Introduction to stochastic actor-based models for network dynamics. *Social Networks, 32*(1), 44–60. https://doi.org/10.1016/j.socnet.2009.02.004

Snijders, T. A. B. (2011). Network dynamics. In J. Scott & P. J. Carrington (Eds.), *The handbook of social network analysis* (pp. 501–513). SAGE Publications.

Stufflebeam, D. L., & Coryn, C. L. S. (2014). *Evaluation theory, models, and applications* (2nd ed.). Jossey-Bass.

Valente, T. W. (2010). *Social networks and health: Models, methods, and applications*. Oxford University Press.

Valente, T. W. (2012). Network interventions. *Science, 337*(6090), 49–53. https://doi.org/10.1126/science.1217330

Wasserman, S., & Faust, K. (1994). *Social network analysis: Methods and applications*. Cambridge University Press.

Weiss, C. H. (1998). Have we learned anything new about the use of evaluation? *The American Journal of Evaluation, 19*(1), 21–33. https://doi.org/10.1016/S1098-2140(99)80178-7

Chapter 7
Making Network-Informed Complex Evaluation Work for You

What Network-Informed Complex Evaluation Offers

Alkin and Christie's (2004) "evaluation theory tree" offers a foundational schema for understanding the primary theoretical orientations in the evaluation field, including accountability and control, social inquiry, methods, value, and use. Network-informed complex evaluation (NCE) addresses these criteria and provides a comprehensive framework for evaluating the complexity, dynamism, and relationality inherent in complex social programs.

Accountability and Control

Accountability is a central principle of traditional evaluation, ensuring that programs are held responsible for their outcomes through compliance, performance monitoring, and summative assessment (Alkin & Christie, 2004, p. 14). Alkin and Klein (1972) identify three types of accountability in evaluation: goal accountability, program accountability, and outcome accountability. From a network-informed and complexity-oriented perspective, NCE strengthens each of these dimensions by making them more explicit and actionable.

- *Goal accountability* evaluates whether a program's goals and objectives are appropriate, well-formulated, and responsive to stakeholder needs. This process supports formative evaluation by clarifying how a program is designed to achieve its goals (Alkin & Klein, 1972). NCE enables evaluators to determine whether program goals reflect the distributed resources, interests, and capacities of network members, ensuring that objectives remain relevant and attainable within a collaborative system.
- *Program accountability* examines whether a program is implemented as intended, emphasizing the fidelity and quality of processes and procedures. This focus is

L. Zhang, *Network-Informed Complex Evaluation*,
https://doi.org/10.1007/978-3-032-27495-3_7

central to process evaluation, which examines the pathways and mechanisms linking program activities to outcomes (Alkin & Klein, 1972). From a network-informed perspective, NCE enables evaluators to analyze both formal action plans and informal relational structures within the program, including communication patterns, resource flows, and collaboration across multiple levels. By making these relational elements explicit, NCE allows evaluators to identify implementation strengths and gaps that traditional process evaluation may overlook.
- *Outcome accountability* assesses the extent to which a program's goals and objectives have been achieved, typically through summative evaluation that measures impacts over short, medium, and long terms (Alkin & Klein, 1972). NCE enables evaluators and stakeholders to move beyond isolated assessments of individual or organizational outputs by facilitating the evaluation of collective, system-wide impacts and the equity of collaborative achievements. By examining how network functioning influences outcomes, NCE provides a comprehensive understanding of success in complex, multi-actor environments. This approach is particularly valuable in contexts of networked governance and cross-sectoral collaboration, where assessing the effectiveness of the entire system is essential for meaningful accountability (Provan & Milward, 2001).

Social Inquiry

Social inquiry is defined as "the systemic study of the behavior of groups of individuals in various kinds of social settings by a variety of methods" (Alkin & Christie, 2004, p. 15). NCE addresses the need for evaluation approaches that capture the complexity, contextual factors, and relational dynamics present in complex programs while sharpening attention to outcomes. Through network analysis, NCE equips evaluators with tools to measure structural relationships within program networks and to explain how these relationships cause and shape program outcomes. This approach enables the identification of underlying social mechanisms, such as structural holes, key influencers, and pathways of trust or information diffusion, that shape program outcomes. These network-based inquiries are essential for understanding not only what works but also how and why programs succeed or encounter challenges within complex social systems.

Method

Effective evaluation in complex systems requires the intentional selection and ongoing adaptation of methods tailored to the specific context, ensuring the production of rigorous, credible evidence. Leading scholars emphasize that evaluators must customize their methodological approaches to reflect the unique characteristics, dynamics, and evolving conditions of each evaluation setting (Bamberger et al.,

2016; Patton, 2011). NCE supports these principles by providing evaluators with a suite of methodological options designed to address the dynamic, interconnected, and often unpredictable realities of complex interventions. Rather than promoting a uniform methodology, NCE encourages evaluators to select and adapt methods (e.g., qualitative network mapping, quantitative network analysis, mixed-methods network analysis, and statistical inference) that best align with the evaluation's evolving context and needs. This methodological flexibility ensures that evaluations remain relevant and responsive within dynamic environments, fostering continuous learning and innovation as programs develop (Bamberger et al., 2016; Patton, 2011; Rogers, 2008). Ultimately, such context-sensitive approaches increase the robustness and practical utility of evaluation findings, providing stakeholders with actionable insights for decision-making in complex, rapidly changing settings.

Value

NCE emphasizes the role of values in evaluation by beginning with careful consideration of how programs should be judged and which outcomes are most meaningful, ensuring that these decisions are firmly rooted in the program's specific context and needs (Alkin & Christie, 2004, p. 32). Recognizing that stakeholders bring diverse and legitimate perspectives on what constitutes value, NCE employs participatory network mapping and inclusive engagement strategies to systematically identify whose voices are represented or marginalized in decision-making and resource allocation. By making these relational dynamics visible, NCE facilitates the transparent negotiation of value claims, democratizes the evaluative process, and cultivates more equitable judgments (Greene, 2006).

This approach aligns with Patton's (2011) emphasis on stakeholder engagement and utilization-focused evaluation, which supports inclusive processes that surface and negotiate diverse interests and priorities. Funnell and Rogers (2011) underscore the importance of participatory approaches and collaborative program theory development to ensure that evaluative judgments reflect multiple stakeholder perspectives. Bammer (2013) further highlights the value of interdisciplinarity and integrative methods for addressing the complexity of real-world problems, arguing that equitable participation is foundational to producing just and actionable evaluation outcomes.

Use

Alkin and Christie (2004) define use as the intention to conduct evaluations designed to assist key stakeholders in making informed program decisions (p. 44). Consistent with this principle, NCE is oriented toward practical use, addressing both instrumental (direct decision-making) and conceptual (shaping understanding) applications (Christie, 2007; Weiss, 1998). NCE operationalizes this commitment by systematically identifying key stakeholders who can meaningfully contribute to the evaluation process (context assessment) and by ensuring their continuous involvement throughout the evaluation's design (input stage), implementation (process stage), and reporting (product stage).

Participatory processes such as network mapping and iterative feedback foster stakeholder ownership and build evaluation capacity, while increasing the likelihood that evaluation findings will inform evidence-based decision-making (Patton, 2011; Preskill & Torres, 1999). The visual outputs generated by network analysis, including accessible diagrams and relational narratives, make complex program dynamics visible and actionable to a wide range of audiences. By identifying leverage points and systemic bottlenecks within program networks, NCE enables stakeholders to translate evaluation findings into concrete actions, ensuring that evaluation serves as a catalyst for ongoing improvement and transformative impact rather than a procedural exercise.

Foundational Questions in Network-Informed Complex Evaluation

Is Network-Informed Complex Evaluation a Theoretically Coherent Framework?

This question is central to advancing evaluation as a scholarly discipline. Alkin and Christie (2004) caution that superficial borrowing of theory leads to fragmented, conceptually weak frameworks, underscoring the importance of theory accumulation grounded in logical coherence and integrative synthesis. Rogers (2008) contends that credible evaluation must extend beyond description to provide robust causal explanations, particularly for complex interventions in which linear models are inadequate. Furthermore, Hopson (2009) asserts that evaluation theory should explicitly address power, context, and equity to ensure social relevance and credibility. In response, the NCE framework is purposefully constructed to address these critiques. Rather than merely aggregating contemporary ideas, NCE offers a theoretically integrative and methodologically rigorous approach that aligns ontological assumptions, conceptual models, and analytic strategies, as described in Chapters 1–3.

Figure 7.1 demonstrates that NCE is rooted in health equity programs designed to reduce systematic, avoidable, and unjust disparities in health outcomes. These programs are influenced by the social determinants of health (SDOH) and function across the nested levels of the socio-ecological model (SEM), encompassing individual, organizational, community, and policy domains. Determinants interact across these levels, shaping health opportunities through interconnected pathways and forming complex adaptive systems characterized by cross-level interactions, feedback loops, and adaptation. These processes generate nonlinear, dynamic, and emergent patterns of health inequity. Complex adaptive systems (CAS) theory provides the foundation for understanding these dynamics, redirecting the evaluative focus from isolated variables and discrete interventions to systems defined by interdependence. Conventional models are inadequate for capturing system dynamics, relational processes, and cross-level effects, leading to partial or misleading explanations of program effectiveness within complex social systems. NCE addresses this gap through methodological innovation. By representing actors, programs, policies, and determinants as nodes and their relationships as ties, social network analysis (SNA) offers a mathematical representation of the system's structure. This methodology enables evaluators to examine relational causality, identify leverage points, and reveal the structural configurations through which inequities are produced, sustained, or transformed.

By integrating complexity theory, the socio-ecological model, and network analysis, NCE advances evaluation practices from linear attribution to a focus on structural and relational contributions. This shift emphasizes system structure, feedback mechanisms, and power relations within evaluative inquiry. It directly responds to longstanding calls in evaluation theory to strengthen causal explanations while explicitly considering context and equity, thereby offering a coherent and practically relevant framework for evaluating health equity initiatives within complex adaptive systems.

Is Network-Informed Complex Evaluation a Good Evaluation Theory?

Shadish et al. (1991) state that "the fundamental purpose of program evaluation theory is to specify feasible practices that evaluators can use to construct knowledge of the value of social programs that can be used to ameliorate the social problems to which programs are relevant" (p. 36). Their framework posits that a robust evaluation theory must articulate (1) a theory of social programming, (2) a theory of knowledge construction, (3) a theory of valuing, (4) a theory of use, and (5) a theory of practice. The following section examines how NCE addresses these criteria, highlighting its relevance and rigor within contemporary evaluation scholarship.

- *Social Programming.* Shadish et al. (1991) argue that a robust evaluation theory must be grounded in a nuanced and realistic conceptualization of social programming that accounts for how programs are structured, enacted, and evolve within their specific social contexts (pp. 37–40). They further emphasize that "better theories should be more comprehensive, more accurate in their content, and should prioritize more acutely those things worth attending to" (p. 39). NCE addresses this requirement by challenging the limitations of conventional evaluation approaches,

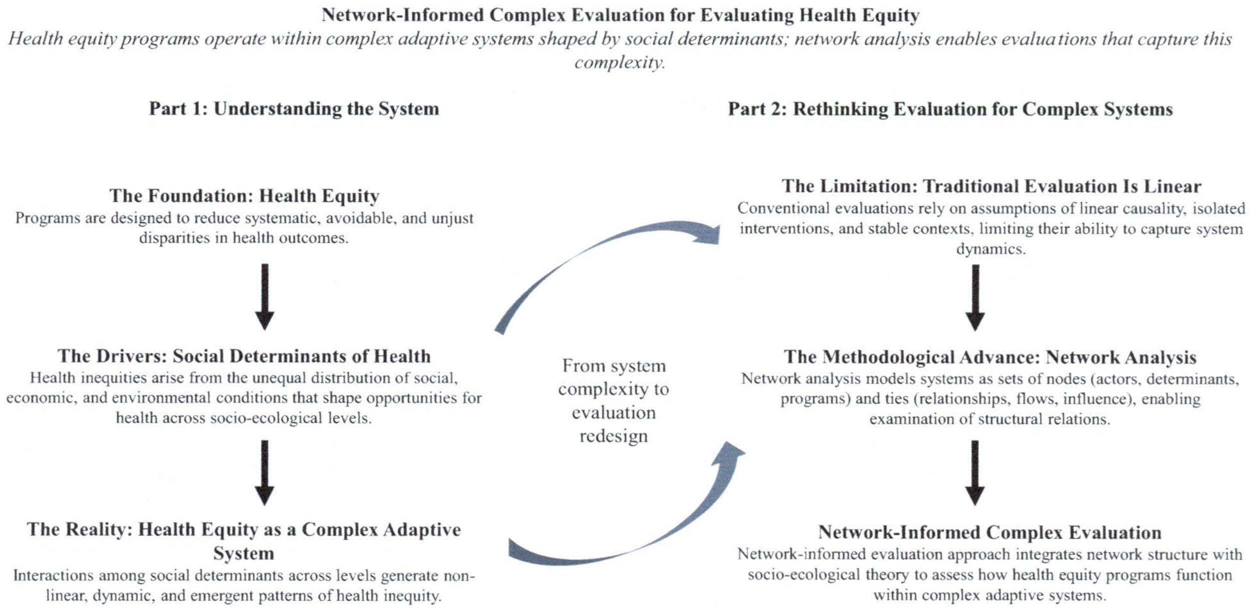

Fig. 7.1 Network-informed complex evaluation of health equity programs. The figure presents the author's conceptual synthesis integrating complex adaptive systems theory, social determinants of health, and network-informed evaluation. Health equity programs operate within complex adaptive systems shaped by social determinants across socio-ecological levels. Network analysis models these systems as relational structures, enabling evaluation approaches that capture multilevel interactions, feedback, and adaptive dynamics

which frequently overlook the complexity and dynamism inherent in contemporary programs. Instead of treating programs as static or linear, NCE conceptualizes them as embedded within dynamic, adaptive networks of diverse actors, relationships, and contextual influences. This network-informed, complexity-oriented perspective yields an authentic understanding of how complex programs operate. Through systematic mapping and analysis of these networks, NCE enables evaluators to identify leverage points, detect bottlenecks, and reveal the often-invisible social structures that ultimately shape program outcomes.

- *Knowledge Construction.* A central requirement of evaluation theory, as outlined by Shadish et al. (1991), is the explicit specification of ontology (the nature of reality), epistemology (the characteristics and standards of evaluation knowledge), and methodology (the techniques for constructing evaluation knowledge) (pp. 42–44). NCE addresses these dimensions comprehensively. Drawing on CAS, SEM, and SNA, NCE enables evaluators to detect, represent, and analyze nonlinear and emergent patterns in real-world programs. This approach is both a methodological advancement and a distinct epistemological stance, emphasizing relational, adaptive, and network-informed knowledge generation. NCE operationalizes these principles through guiding evaluation principles, network concepts, and an evaluation approach adaptable across individual, organizational, community, and policy levels. Furthermore, NCE supports iterative, adaptive learning cycles, aligning with developmental and systems-oriented evaluation paradigms that are increasingly vital in rapidly evolving contexts (Patton, 2011; Williams & Hummelbrunner, 2010).
- *Valuing.* Shadish et al. (1991) argue that evaluation theory must explicitly address how values are identified, negotiated, and integrated into evaluation (pp. 46–52). They emphasize that explicit attention to values "helps evaluators understand what steps to undertake to make value statements about programs, to see what value judgments implicit in their work…to make decisions about implementing those recommendations in their work" (p. 52). NCE addresses this challenge through a value-attentive and participatory approach. It employs descriptive valuing to elicit and clarify stakeholders' values, collaboratively determines evaluation criteria, and systematically investigates whether stakeholders perceive the program as worthwhile and what improvements they recommend based on evaluation findings. By engaging a diverse range of stakeholders in network mapping and analysis, NCE reveals not only formal program objectives but also the underlying values, power dynamics, and perspectives that shape program meaning and interpretation. Visual and analytical tools, such as network diagrams that distinguish central, peripheral, and excluded actors, make these dynamics explicit and foster reflective, transparent dialogue about what is valued, by whom, and with what consequences. NCE thus provides a practical and ethical framework for inclusive, context-sensitive assessment of values, ensuring that multiple perspectives are meaningfully and transparently integrated into evaluation practice.
- *Use.* Shadish et al. (1991) emphasize that "evaluators need a theory to tell how, when, where, and why they can produce useful results" (p. 52). In alignment with

this perspective, Chapters 1 and 2 establish foundational ontological assumptions regarding evaluation and provide epistemological justifications for the development of NCE, with a focus on the complexities inherent in health equity programs. Chapter 3 extends this foundation by specifying the core components of NCE, including guiding principles, network terms, and evaluation methodologies. Chapters 4 through 6 elaborate on the context, input, process, and product stages of the NCE evaluation cycle, presenting a stage-based approach. NCE is purposefully designed for maximum utility and sustained relevance. Its participatory processes, such as stakeholder mapping, joint sense-making, and visual feedback, foster stakeholder ownership and trust while enhancing evaluation capacity and collective learning. Network analysis within NCE generates actionable insights for diverse audiences and directly informs program improvement, adaptation, and strategic decision-making. Furthermore, the framework's iterative and adaptive orientation ensures that evaluative knowledge remains timely and responsive as program contexts evolve.

- *Practice.* Shadish et al. (1991) emphasize that evaluation theory must be operationalizable, providing concrete methods, tools, and guidance to inform real-world evaluation practice (pp. 57–64). They specify that theories of practice should address critical questions, such as whether an evaluation should be conducted, the intended purpose of the evaluation, and the evaluator's role. NCE addresses these requirements with a robust, adaptable approach grounded in established practices. Its network-informed context assessment enables evaluators to determine the appropriateness and readiness of programs for NCE, guiding decisions about whether to proceed with network analysis and at what level of complexity. During the input stage, NCE assists stakeholders in clarifying program plans and articulating theories of change from a network perspective, thereby informing subsequent evaluation design and implementation. This alignment of context, input, and process ensures that evaluation designs are both methodologically rigorous and contextually relevant. NCE employs a collaborative, participatory, and iterative approach to maximize utility and stakeholder engagement from the outset of evaluation design.

How Does Network-Informed Complex Evaluation Advance and Operationalize Complexity-Oriented Evaluation Frameworks?

A central challenge in contemporary evaluation scholarship is translating complexity-oriented frameworks into analytically rigorous and practically coherent approaches. Over the past two decades, several traditions have advanced evaluation beyond linear, reductionist causal models. Developmental Evaluation emphasizes adaptive learning within innovative and emergent initiatives (Patton, 2011). Realist Evaluation explains what works, for whom, and under what conditions through context–mechanism–outcome configurations (Pawson & Tilley, 1997). Systems Thinking in evaluation highlights feedback loops, interdependence, and nonlinear dynamics that influence program effects (Williams & Hummelbrunner, 2010). Collectively, these approaches have expanded evaluators' conceptualization of complexity. However, as Rogers (2008) notes, complexity-informed approaches are often conceptually persuasive but offer limited procedural guidance. Evaluators frequently face challenges in defining appropriate system boundaries, specifying mechanisms in empirically tractable terms, and translating abstract interdependencies into analytic strategies that support decision-making. Although equity has gained prominence in evaluation discourse, the relational structures that produce and sustain disparities remain insufficiently examined.

NCE addresses this gap by positioning relational configuration as a central analytic focus. Instead of treating networks merely as metaphors for connectedness, NCE conceptualizes them as observable and measurable structures that shape collaboration, power dynamics, and resource exchange. Outcomes emerge from patterned interdependence among actors, organizations, and institutional arrangements. Mechanisms extend beyond individual responses or program components to include structural positioning and connectivity. Consequently, NCE extends existing complexity-oriented traditions without replacing them.

NCE builds upon these contributions by emphasizing the empirical examination of relational configurations as structures that condition mechanisms, allocate opportunities, and contribute to inequities. By making network positioning and connectivity analytically visible, NCE enables evaluators to investigate how structural relations within systems shape outcomes. This relational perspective integrates adaptive learning, causal reasoning, and systemic analysis into a coherent framework that enhances both explanation and strategic action. Table 7.1 situates NCE alongside developmental evaluation, realist evaluation, and systems thinking to clarify areas of convergence and theoretical extension.

How Can Network-Informed Complex Evaluation Be Operationalized in Real-World Evaluation Settings?

A central challenge in evaluation is translating conceptually rich, complexity-informed frameworks into practical approaches suitable for real-world application. Rogers (2008) notes that although these frameworks are intellectually stimulating, they often lack operational clarity, leaving evaluators without concrete guidance for implementation. Williams and Hummelbrunner (2010) contend that effective systems-based frameworks must balance adaptability with sufficient structure to support evaluators' decision-making amid uncertainty and change. Patton (2011) emphasizes that iterative and adaptive processes are essential for evaluations to remain practical, credible, and sustainable, particularly under resource, time, or data constraints. This body of scholarship highlights a persistent tension: complexity-informed evaluation must be both theoretically rigorous and operationally applicable.

Table 7.1 Comparison of network-informed complex evaluation (NCE), developmental evaluation, realist evaluation, and systems thinking in evaluation

Dimension	NCE	Developmental evaluation	Realist evaluation	Systems thinking in evaluation
Primary purpose	Examine how patterned relationships and network structures shape outcomes and inequities in complex systems	Support adaptation and innovation through real-time learning	Explain what works, for whom, in which contexts, and through which mechanisms	Understand dynamic system behavior, feedback processes, and interdependencies that influence system performance and change
Unit of analysis/scope	Relational networks that connect individuals, organizations, sectors, and multilevel systems to facilitate collaboration, knowledge exchange, and resource sharing	Programs or initiatives operating in emergent or adaptive contexts	Interventions or programs guided by explicit program theories and context–mechanism–outcome (CMO) configurations	Systems, subsystems, interacting actors, and structural relationships within complex systems
View of context	Context is constituted through evolving configurations of relationships; outcomes and context are mutually co-produced through network interactions	Context emergent and continually interpreted through iterative learning processes	Context shapes whether and how underlying generative mechanisms are activated to produce outcomes	Context emerges from interactions among system elements, structures, feedback processes, and environmental conditions
Conceptualization of mechanisms	Mechanisms are understood as relational processes embedded in network structures and patterns of interaction	Change is understood through adaptive learning, experimentation, and developmental feedback rather than explicitly theorized mechanisms	Mechanisms are conceptualized as generative causal processes triggered in specific contexts	Mechanisms are represented as dynamic feedback interactions, reinforcing and balancing loops, and emerging system behaviours over time

(continued)

Table 7.1 (continued)

Dimension	NCE	Developmental evaluation	Realist evaluation	Systems thinking in evaluation
Core methods	Social network analysis, relational mapping, influence and resource-flow tracing, network visualization	Iterative feedback cycles, rapid-cycle learning, adaptive learning	Realist interviews, context–mechanism–outcome configurations, theory refinement, mixed-method inquiry	Systems mapping, causal loop diagrams, system dynamics modeling, participatory systems methods
Equity orientation	Examines how differential network positioning and structural connectivity shape disparities in access, influence, and outcomes	May incorporate equity through inclusive stakeholder engagement and adaptive design, depending on evaluation purpose	Explores variation in outcomes across groups and contexts; equity emphasis varies	Equity considerations may be incorporated through system analysis but are not intrinsic to the framework itself

Note This table presents the author's interpretive synthesis of network-informed complex evaluation (NCE) relative to established complexity-oriented evaluation frameworks, including developmental evaluation, realist evaluation, and systems thinking in evaluation (e.g., Patton, 2011; Pawson & Tilley, 1997; Williams & Hummelbrunner, 2010). It integrates key theoretical dimensions to clarify areas of convergence and conceptual extension. The descriptions are interpretive and intended to highlight analytic distinctions rather than to provide exhaustive representations of each framework.
Source Author

In response to these critiques, Fig. 7.2 presents a structured decision framework for determining when to apply network-informed complex evaluation. Rather than assuming that complexity or collaboration automatically justifies network analysis, the framework establishes a sequenced set of criteria to guide methodological decisions. It begins by assessing whether relational mechanisms are central to the program's theory of change, a necessary condition, followed by an examination of relationally relevant properties of complex adaptive systems. Only when these conditions are satisfied does the framework proceed to determine the appropriate scope of relational analysis and assess feasibility and epistemic value. By integrating theoretical rigor with explicit screening steps, the framework translates abstract complexity principles into a transparent decision process. This approach provides the operational clarity emphasized in the evaluation literature and supports the responsible, context-sensitive application of NCE.

Building on this decision logic, NCE is operationalized through a structured, phase-based process adaptable to diverse contexts. The process begins with a network-informed assessment of the evaluation context and program readiness, as detailed in Chapter 4. This initial phase enables evaluators to determine whether NCE is appropriate within the specific program environment and to guide decisions regarding timing, boundaries, and the identification of key actors and system-level

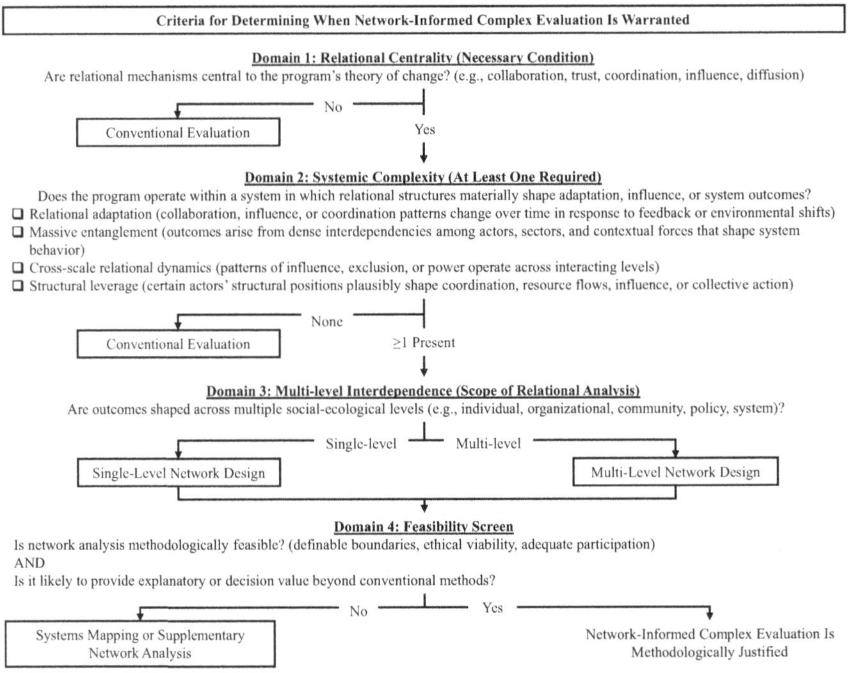

Fig. 7.2 Criteria framework for determining when network-informed complex evaluation is methodologically warranted. *Source* Author

influences. By clarifying the system's relational architecture early, evaluators align methodological choices with contextual realities.

NCE supports the development of a network-informed program theory by articulating how relational mechanisms are expected to influence outcomes within a complex adaptive system, as described in Chapter 5. Clarifying the scope of relational analysis, as outlined in Fig. 7.2, enables evaluators to differentiate between single-level and multilevel dynamics and to design evaluations accordingly. This stage also facilitates the creation of a contextually grounded action plan and the articulation of anticipated results from a network perspective, thereby fostering a shared understanding among stakeholders.

Building on this foundation, NCE delivers tailored evaluation designs and products responsive to the specific context and inputs defined in earlier phases. By embedding feasibility and value-added criteria within its decision framework, NCE guides evaluators toward methods that are both rigorous and practically sustainable. This approach remains theoretically grounded while producing actionable, context-sensitive insights. Through this structured and adaptive process, NCE addresses longstanding critiques of complexity-informed evaluation by providing both conceptual rigor and operational clarity. It enables evaluators to apply network-informed methods systematically, transparently, and responsibly in real-world settings.

Does Network-Informed Complex Evaluation Provide Sufficient Methodological Rigor to Ensure Credible and Valid Evaluation?

Maintaining methodological rigor is a foundational concern in advancing evaluation practice. Greene (2007) argues that methodological innovation should not compromise the credibility or validity of evaluation findings. Crossley et al. (2015) and Borgatti et al. (2024) warn that the superficial application of network methods reduces their utility and explanatory power. These scholars underscore the importance of theory-driven, context-sensitive metric selection and the thoughtful integration of qualitative and quantitative evidence.

NCE addresses these concerns by embedding methodological rigor throughout the evaluation process. It prioritizes selecting network metrics (such as centrality, density, and brokerage) based on program theory and evaluation questions. This theory-driven approach ensures that measurement strategies are tailored to the specific mechanisms and contextual factors identified during the NCE input stage. NCE also employs mixed-method triangulation to systematically integrate findings from social network analysis with qualitative data from interviews, focus groups, and document analysis. This methodological pluralism, as advocated by Greene (2007), enhances explanatory value and ensures that diverse perspectives inform interpretation. Additionally, NCE supports iterative and longitudinal analysis, allowing evaluators to monitor changes in network structure and program context over time and to adapt their approaches as new insights arise. By aligning measurement strategies with theoretical frameworks and equity considerations, NCE maintains analytic rigor across diverse evaluation environments, ensuring that findings are both credible and contextually meaningful.

How Does Network-Informed Complex Evaluation Ensure that Network Mapping and Analysis Do not Perpetuate Inequity?

The ethical and equity implications of network-informed and data-driven evaluation approaches are increasingly recognized as critical concerns for the field. As numerous scholars have argued, data and network analysis methods are not neutral and may reproduce or amplify social inequities unless guided by explicit ethical frameworks (Borgatti & Molina, 2005; Molina et al., 2014). Mertens (2019) and Hopson (2009) further emphasize the importance of transformative, culturally responsive evaluation practices that foreground issues of power, justice, and consent throughout the evaluation process. These scholars argue that evaluators must move beyond procedural ethics to actively address structural inequities, ensure meaningful participation, and protect the rights and interests of marginalized communities.

NCE is purposefully structured to embed ethics and equity throughout the evaluation lifecycle. It requires participatory boundary definition during the process stage, ensuring that stakeholders, particularly those from underrepresented groups, are substantively involved in decisions regarding what is mapped, whose networks are visualized, and how data are interpreted and utilized. NCE emphasizes shared ownership and governance of network data, thereby supporting collective control over the visualization, dissemination, and application of findings. This strategy mitigates the risk of data misuse and builds community trust. Ethical reflexivity is integral to NCE, requiring evaluators to assess the potential risks and unintended consequences of network analysis. Power analysis is systematically embedded, employing social network analysis to identify both visible structures of influence and hidden patterns of exclusion and marginalization (Valente, 2010). By adopting these practices, NCE transforms potential ethical risks into opportunities to advance social justice, aligning with the standards of contemporary evaluation.

How Can Evaluators Build Capacity for Network-Informed Complex Evaluation?

Capacity building for network-informed, complexity-aware evaluation requires intentional, multidimensional strategies that integrate individual skill development, organizational learning, and the cultivation of a supportive, adaptive culture. More specifically, the evaluation literature emphasizes that capacity building should address not only technical training but also relational, cultural, and systemic components, thereby fostering environments where evaluation is valued and routinely practiced (Labin et al., 2012; Preskill & Boyle, 2008). Williams and Hummelbrunner (2010) argue that sustainable systems change depends on an organization's ability to learn from feedback and embed evaluation as an ongoing, adaptive process. In complex contexts, participatory approaches and stakeholder engagement are essential, as they promote inclusivity and responsiveness to diverse stakeholder needs (Cousins et al., 2014; King & Volkov, 2005). Accordingly, the NCE framework operationalizes capacity building across three interrelated domains: technical, relational, and cultural, making it a practical tool for advancing complexity-aware evaluation.

- *Technical Capacity*: Developing technical expertise is essential for evaluators applying the NCE framework. This requires acquiring knowledge of network concepts and understanding their practical applications in evaluation contexts. Foundational works by Borgatti et al. (2024), Carolan (2014), Knoke and Yang (2008), and Prell (2011) provide comprehensive guidance on social network analysis. For complexity and systems thinking in evaluation, Patton (2011), Renger (2022), and Williams and Hummelbrunner (2010) present key frameworks that support evaluators in applying complexity- and system-oriented approaches in practical settings.
- *Relational Capacity*: The NCE framework emphasizes the cultivation of trust, collaboration, and shared sense-making among stakeholders. Relational capacity is developed through participatory evaluation strategies and the co-creation of evaluation plans. Practical approaches include organizing network-weaving sessions to foster relationship building and conducting co-interpretation workshops to facilitate joint data analysis. These practices enhance stakeholder engagement and increase credibility, relevance, and utilization of evaluation findings.
- *Cultural Capacity*: Embedding evaluation within organizational culture is essential for sustainability. To support this, the NCE framework encourages organizations to integrate evaluation into daily routines, strategic planning, and feedback mechanisms, transforming evaluation from a compliance-driven activity into a dynamic system of inquiry and improvement. Common strategies to develop cultural capacity include establishing regular evaluation and review forums, initiating participatory evaluation approaches, incorporating evaluation feedback into program design, and providing routine staff training sessions. These initiatives cultivate a culture where evaluation informs strategic decision-making and facilitates adaptation to emerging challenges.

What Are Other Common Applications of Network-Informed Complex Evaluation?

Previous chapters established the significance of NCE in evaluating complex programs addressing health equity. The theoretical foundations and core methodologies of NCE have been synthesized and described. Beyond program evaluation, NCE is relevant across multiple stages of program planning and implementation. Specifically, NCE contributes to strategic planning, clarifies program plans, supports implementation, and monitors program processes.

- *Strategic Planning.* Strategic planning in complex systems can be daunting, but the NCE framework helps evaluators and organizations feel capable by embedding relational and network mapping within planning processes. This approach aligns with Patton's (2011) call for complexity-informed evaluation, which emphasizes understanding and adapting to system dynamics rather than relying on linear models, and with Williams and Hummelbrunner's (2010) advocacy for mapping real-world interconnections to inform decision-making. Systematic analysis of both formal and informal relationships among stakeholders, organizations, and community actors enables planners to visualize, assess, and manage the network dynamics that drive adaptive decision-making (Provan & Kenis, 2008). Furthermore, NCE conceptualizes strategic planning as a participatory process. Facilitated network mapping exercises engage evaluators and stakeholders in co-constructing evaluation plans, supporting the identification of key actors, leverage points, and vulnerabilities. This collaborative approach fosters a shared understanding and commitment to strategic action, empowering evaluators to lead adaptive changes with confidence.
- *Clarifying Program Plans.* The quality of program planning is widely recognized as a foundational determinant of implementation and outcomes. Chen (2015) emphasizes the importance of evaluators supporting stakeholders in program planning and development, particularly for complex programs characterized by nonlinearity, emergence, adaptation, and dynamic interdependencies (Byrne & Callaghan, 2014; Patton, 2011; Rogers, 2008). The NCE framework provides a structured, network-informed approach for refining program plans in such environments. As detailed in Chapter 5, NCE offers stakeholders a systematic process to clarify "what the problem is; why it is important to address; what needs to be done to address it; and what and who will do what, when, and where" (Chen, 2015, p. 97). Such clarity is essential for developing actionable, responsive program plans that reflect the realities of dynamic, real-world contexts.
- *Supporting Program Implementation.* Programs frequently encounter persistent challenges, including mission drift, siloed workgroups, and shifting stakeholder dynamics, all of which can undermine effectiveness, sustainability, and equity in collaborative efforts (Provan & Kenis, 2008; Provan & Milward, 2001). Chen (2015) asserts that "an implementation must be a success before a program can be considered effective" (p. 151). Without mechanisms for ongoing assessment and adaptation, evolving relationships and changes in power structures

may erode performance and collaboration over time. NCE addresses these issues by providing opportunities for continuous diagnostic and adaptive management. Regular network diagnostics, conducted at defined intervals such as quarterly or biannually, allow organizations to monitor changes in collaboration and engagement, facilitating early detection of emerging silos or overburdened nodes before they lead to critical failures (Provan & Kenis, 2008). Integrating these network findings into ongoing stakeholder learning cycles fosters adaptive learning and supports real-time program adjustments.

Can Network-Informed Complex Evaluation Be Applied in Other Contexts?

Although initially developed to evaluate complex health equity programs, the NCE framework's theoretical basis and methods are adaptable to various sectors. Its flexible approach enables scholars and practitioners to understand, assess, and improve outcomes in diverse contexts, including education, community development, and environmental programs. The following examples demonstrate how NCE's principles can be applied across multiple sectors, highlighting its broad utility in complexity and network analysis.

- *Education.* Educational systems operate as CASs, consisting of interacting agents such as students, teachers, administrators, and policymakers embedded within multilevel institutional and community contexts (Mason, 2008; Moolenaar et al., 2010). Educational outcomes emerge from dynamic interactions, feedback mechanisms, and ongoing adaptation, rather than from linear processes (Mason, 2008). Additionally, variables such as sex, age, and socioeconomic status are social determinants that influence educational opportunities and outcomes (Carolan, 2014, p. 4). Building on this, the NCE framework synthesizes CAS and SEM by mapping flows of information, influence, and collaboration among educational stakeholders. It specifies key roles, such as opinion leaders and knowledge brokers, and identifies bottlenecks or silos that may hinder reform. By tracing the effects of policy changes and peer dynamics within educational networks, the NCE framework supports accountability, continuous improvement, and targeted interventions at the micro-, meso-, and macro-levels.
- *Health Services.* Health systems exemplify CAS characteristics, in which outcomes are shaped by nonlinear, interdependent relationships among clinicians, administrators, patients, and external actors (Braithwaite et al., 2018; Plsek & Greenhalgh, 2001). These relationships are further influenced by social-ecological factors, including team dynamics, governance, and policy environments (Provan & Milward, 2001). Network analysis has been employed to examine referral patterns, care coordination, and professional collaboration, revealing how network gaps or hubs can affect quality and the diffusion of innovation (Cunningham et al., 2012; Valente, 2010). NCE can visualize and analyze

these networks, enabling evaluators to identify strengths, weaknesses, and opportunities for adaptive improvement. By embedding quality-of-care metrics within broader social networks, NCE supports organizational learning, adaptation, and more resilient responses to challenges such as care transitions and chronic disease management across multiple levels of the healthcare system.

- *Community Development.* The NCE framework is useful in community development because initiatives function as CASs shaped by intricate interdependencies among individuals, families, organizations, and policy actors, in which social capital, trust, and collective agency drive emergent outcomes (Christens & Inzeo, 2015; Woolcock & Narayan, 2000). Peer-reviewed studies have utilized social network analysis to map resource flows, social support, and collaboration in community initiatives, underscoring the significance of network structure for program success and sustainability (Prell et al., 2009; Varda et al., 2008). NCE employs network analysis by engaging communities to map their assets and needs, clarify pathways of support or exclusion, and identify opportunities for empowerment and participation. This approach aligns with empowerment and participatory evaluation traditions, fostering local ownership and systemic change across multiple social-ecological levels.
- *Environment and Sustainability.* The NCE framework is applicable to environmental and sustainability programs because they operate within multi-scale socio-ecological systems, where feedback loops and cross-sector collaborations among social and ecological actors are essential for adaptive management and resilience (Bammer, 2013; Ostrom, 2009). Social network analysis has been widely applied in natural resource management to examine stakeholder networks, identify collaboration bottlenecks, and map knowledge diffusion (Bodin & Crona, 2009; Prell et al., 2009). NCE utilizes network analysis to visualize partnerships and information flows, enabling evaluators to identify leverage points for intervention and monitor the development of resilient, sustainable systems. By integrating network perspectives, NCE supports adaptive management, learning, and long-term impact across ecosystem, community, and policy levels.
- *International Development and Humanitarian Response.* International development and humanitarian efforts function within unpredictable, multi-actor systems characterized by shifting political, cultural, and resource landscapes (Bamberger et al., 2016; Ramalingam et al., 2008). Bamberger et al. (2016) describe development interventions as embedded in complex systems, characterized by multiple interacting actors, feedback loops, emergent properties, and unpredictable outcomes. Network analysis has demonstrated value in mapping partnerships, resource flows, and influence in development and humanitarian contexts, facilitating more effective coordination and adaptive response. NCE adds distinct value by integrating network analysis with complexity awareness, enabling evaluators to map flows of knowledge, resources, and influence in ways that support interventions aligned with local realities and global standards, such as the Sustainable Development Goals. Participatory network mapping, as emphasized in complexity-aware evaluation, enhances legitimacy, ownership, and adaptability, which are essential for effective humanitarian response (Bamberger

et al., 2016). By combining network and complexity perspectives, NCE advances accountability, innovation, and equitable outcomes.

Conclusion

This book addresses a central challenge in contemporary evaluation: the persistent misalignment between traditional evaluation approaches and the realities of programs operating within complex social systems. Interventions targeting structural inequities in public health, education, community development, and cross-sector governance operate within environments characterized by multiple actors, evolving relationships, and shifting contextual conditions. These initiatives rarely follow simple causal chains or bounded interventions; rather, they emerge through interactions among individuals, organizations, institutions, and communities shaped by networks of influence, collaboration, and resource exchange.

Conventional evaluation approaches often fail to capture these dynamics. Rooted in assumptions of linear causality, stable contexts, and clearly defined program boundaries, many traditional evaluation models prioritize measuring discrete program components and short-term outputs. While these approaches offer valuable tools for accountability and performance monitoring, they frequently overlook relational and systemic processes through which meaningful social change occurs. In programs designed to advance equity, such limitations obscure the mechanisms shaping outcomes, including flows of information and resources among actors, the distribution of influence and authority across networks, and adaptive system responses to evolving conditions.

This volume addresses these challenges by introducing NCE as a conceptual and methodological framework for evaluating programs operating within complex, networked environments. By integrating insights from CAS theory, SEM, and SNA, NCE reconceptualizes programs not as isolated interventions but as configurations of relationships embedded within broader systems of interaction. Within this perspective, program outcomes are understood as emergent properties arising from patterns of relationships, interactions, and feedback processes unfolding across multiple levels of social organization.

Throughout this book, the NCE framework is developed through a sequence of conceptual and methodological steps. The initial chapters establish theoretical foundations by integrating perspectives from complexity science, social-ecological theory, and network analysis. Subsequent chapters translate these foundations into methodological guidance for designing and implementing network-informed evaluations. Collectively, these contributions demonstrate how relational structures, interaction patterns, and contextual conditions influence program implementation and outcomes.

A key contribution of this work is reframing relationships as the primary unit of analysis for evaluating complex systems. Instead of focusing solely on individual actors or isolated program components, NCE emphasizes relational structures through which information, resources, and influence circulate. Network structures shape opportunities for collaboration, determine access to resources, and influence the diffusion of innovations and practices across systems. Analyzing these relational dynamics enables evaluators to gain deeper insight into how programs function within complex environments and the causes of outcome variation across contexts.

Although the framework was developed with particular attention to health equity initiatives, its relevance extends beyond the public health sectors. Many contemporary policy challenges, including educational reform, climate governance, community development, and cross-sector collaboration, share similar characteristics. These challenges involve multiple actors operating across institutional boundaries, require sustained collaboration among diverse stakeholders, and unfold within adaptive, nonlinear systems deeply embedded in social and political contexts. In such environments, evaluation approaches that account for relational dynamics and system-level interactions are essential.

NCE offers a framework that supports evaluation across diverse contexts in which programs operate within complex, interconnected systems. Its flexibility enables adaptation to diverse program environments and stakeholder configurations, while its theoretical grounding ensures that the evaluation design remains conceptually coherent and methodologically rigorous. By linking theory, analytical methods, and practical evaluation strategies, the framework equips evaluators with tools to navigate complexity while maintaining analytical clarity.

A Call to Action for Evaluation Scholars and Practitioners

The growing complexity of social challenges requires parallel advancements in evaluation theory and practice. Issues such as health inequities, educational disparities, climate adaptation, and governance failures are systemic phenomena influenced by patterned relationships, power dynamics, and adaptive interactions over time. Persisting with methods that overlook complexity risks generating insufficient understanding and ineffective interventions. Oversimplifying change pathways may result in significant losses at both the human and societal levels.

This work advocates for ongoing theoretical development and empirical investigation of network-informed evaluation approaches within the field of evaluation. The NCE framework offers multiple avenues for scholarly inquiry, including comparative analyses of network structures across policy domains, examinations of relational mechanisms that influence program outcomes, and theoretical refinement of the interactions between network dynamics and broader social systems. Such research can strengthen the explanatory power and theoretical coherence of evaluation scholarship.

For evaluation practitioners, the NCE framework presents both challenges and opportunities. The primary challenge involves redesigning evaluations to emphasize relationships, interactions, and system dynamics rather than focusing on isolated program components. The opportunity is to produce evaluations that are more credible to stakeholders within complex systems and more effective in supporting adaptive decision-making. Practitioners should integrate network-informed approaches as fundamental elements of complexity-aware evaluation design, particularly in initiatives that aim to foster collective action and structural change.

Emerging scholars and doctoral students play a critical role in advancing this work. The convergence of network science, complexity theory, and evaluation offers fertile ground for methodological innovation and interdisciplinary scholarship. Early engagement with these perspectives prepares emerging evaluators to contribute to a field better equipped to address system-level change and equity-driven transformation.

The NCE framework is introduced as a generative model rather than a definitive theory, which encourages critique, adaptation, and empirical investigation. The evolution of evaluation theory has historically depended on scholars and practitioners who challenge established assumptions and broaden the field's scope. NCE exemplifies this expansion. Its future relevance and impact rely on the collective efforts of the evaluation community to refine, test, and apply network-informed complex evaluation to contemporary challenges.

Final Reflection

Throughout my work as an evaluator, I have frequently encountered a persistent tension: the realities of the programs assessed rarely align with the simplified diagrams of traditional evaluation models. Many initiatives I have evaluated—such as public health collaborations, cross-sector partnerships, community coalitions, and family violence response networks—do not operate within clear organizational boundaries or linear action chains. Instead, they function through complex webs of relationships among diverse actors whose influence, resources, and decisions shape program trajectories in ways that conventional frameworks fail to capture. Over time, I recognized that what is often termed a "program" is, in practice, a dynamic network of relationships. However, evaluation methods have largely continued to treat programs as isolated interventions rather than relational systems. This insight became the foundation for developing the NCE framework presented in this book.

At the core of this work is a powerful insight: many mechanisms driving change in complex interventions are inherently relational. Information disseminates through connection patterns; collaboration arises from evolving organizational ties; leadership often reflects structural network positions; and access to resources depends on actors' embeddedness within exchange systems. Evaluations focusing solely on activities or outputs risk neglecting the deeper relational structures that enable or constrain collective action. Consequently, NCE centers these dynamics in evaluation design by translating program theory into network structures, relational mechanisms, and measurable indicators. Rather than merely assessing whether a program succeeded, the framework encourages evaluators to analyze how relationships evolved, how influence traversed networks, and how these changing patterns shaped outcomes across interconnected systems.

This book begins with a central question: *how can evaluation effectively assess programs addressing complex and systemic inequities when conventional methods fail to capture the relational and adaptive dynamics driving change?* NCE was developed to address this challenge. Unlike traditional logic-model approaches that emphasize linear cause-and-effect relationships between inputs and outcomes, NCE examines the web of interactions through which programs operate within complex systems. By integrating principles from social network analysis and complexity science, the framework explores how relational structures, system dynamics, and contextual forces influence program implementation and outcomes across multiple social–ecological levels. Importantly, NCE is not simply the application of network analysis as a standalone method; it provides a systematic approach that embeds relational analysis throughout the evaluation lifecycle—from contextual assessment and program theory development to evaluation design, implementation, and knowledge generation.

Through network-informed methods, NCE enables evaluators to assess program readiness, refine program theory, and analyze the relational mechanisms driving program processes and outcomes. This approach reveals how context, power, and interdependence influence implementation, uncovering patterns that sustain inequities while identifying opportunities for transformation. In this way, evaluation moves beyond retrospective assessment. Rather than merely documenting whether programs achieve predetermined targets, evaluators using the NCE framework map relationships among partners, facilitate knowledge and resource exchange, and help stakeholders identify structural barriers or leverage key connections that enable change. Through sustained engagement, evaluation becomes a process of collective learning that supports adaptive decision-making, strengthens trust among actors, and enables collaborative responses to persistent social challenges.

As evaluation evolves in response to increasingly interconnected and dynamic problems, approaches integrating complexity, relationality, and systems thinking become essential. NCE contributes to this progression by reorienting evaluation toward the networks through which change unfolds. By recognizing relationships as central drivers of system dynamics, NCE equips evaluators with conceptual and methodological tools to generate more meaningful evidence, support adaptive action, and promote equity within complex social systems. It also prompts evaluators to ask a critical question: whose relationships are most influential within a system, and whose remain invisible? By revealing hidden power dynamics and identifying marginalized actors whose connections are often overlooked, NCE opens new possibilities for more inclusive evaluation practice and transformative change within the systems we seek to improve. Ultimately, if programs operate through networks of relationships, evaluation must learn to identify, understand, and engage these relationships so that meaningful and lasting change can unfold within them.

References

Alkin, M. C., & Christie, C. A. (2004). An evaluation theory tree. *Evaluation Roots: Tracing Theorists' Views and Influences, 2*(19), 12–65.

Alkin, M. C., & Klein, S. P. (1972). Accountability defined. Evaluating teachers for outcome accountability. *UCLA Evaluation Comment, 3*(3), 1–11.

Bamberger, M., Vaessen, J., & Raimondo, E. (Eds.). (2016). *Dealing with complexity in development evaluation: A practical approach.* SAGE Publications, Inc.

Bammer, G. (2013). *Disciplining interdisciplinarity: Integration and implementation sciences for researching complex real-world problems.* ANU Press.

Bodin, Ö., & Crona, B. I. (2009). The role of social networks in natural resource governance: What relational patterns make a difference? *Global Environmental Change, 19*(3), 366–374. https://doi.org/10.1016/j.gloenvcha.2009.05.002

Borgatti, S. P., Everett, M. G., Johnson, J. C., & Agneessens, F. (2024). *Analyzing social networks* (3rd ed.). Sage Publications Ltd.

Borgatti, S. P., & Molina, J. L. (2005). Toward ethical guidelines for network research in organizations. *Social Networks, 27*(2), 107–117. https://doi.org/10.1016/j.socnet.2005.01.004

Braithwaite, J., Churruca, K., Long, J. C., Ellis, L. A., & Herkes, J. (2018). When complexity science meets implementation science: A theoretical and empirical analysis of systems change. *BMC Medicine, 16*(1), Article 63. https://doi.org/10.1186/s12916-018-1057-z

Byrne, D., & Callaghan, G. (2014). *Complexity theory and the social sciences: The state of the art.* Routledge.

Carolan, B. V. (2014). *Social network analysis and education: Theory, methods & applications.* SAGE.

Chen, H. (2015). *Practical program evaluation: Theory-driven evaluation and the integrated evaluation perspective* (2nd ed.). SAGE Publications, Inc.

Christens, B. D., & Inzeo, P. T. (2015). Widening the view: Situating collective impact among frameworks for community-led change. *Community Development (Columbus, Ohio), 46*(4), 420–435. https://doi.org/10.1080/15575330.2015.1061680

Christie, C. A. (2007). Reported influence of evaluation data on decision makers' actions: An empirical examination. *The American Journal of Evaluation, 28*(1), 8–25. https://doi.org/10.1177/1098214006298065

Cousins, J. B., Goh, S. C., Elliott, C. J., & Bourgeois, I. (2014). Framing the capacity to do and use evaluation. *New Directions for Evaluation, 2014*(141), 7–23. https://doi.org/10.1002/ev.20076

Crossley, N., Bellotti, E., Edwards, G., Everett, M. G., Koskinen, J. H., & Tranmer, M. (2015). *Social network analysis for ego-nets: Social network analysis for actor-centred networks* (1st ed.). SAGE Publications.

Cunningham, F. C., Ranmuthugala, G., Plumb, J., Georgiou, A., Westbrook, J. I., & Braithwaite, J. (2012). Health professional networks as a vector for improving healthcare quality and safety: A systematic review. *BMJ Quality & Safety, 21*(3), 239–249.

Funnell, S. C., & Rogers, P. J. (2011). *Purposeful program theory: Effective use of theories of change and logic models.* Wiley.

Greene, J. C. (2006). Evaluation, democracy, and social change. In J. C. Greene, M. M. Mark, & I. F. Shaw (Eds.), *Handbook of evaluation: Policies, programs and practices.* SAGE Publications Ltd. https://doi.org/10.4135/9781848608078.n5

Greene, J. C. (2007). *Mixed methods in social inquiry.* Wiley.

Hopson, R. (2009). Chapter 24. reclaiming knowledge at the margins: Culturally responsive evaluation in the current evaluation moment. In K. E. Ryan & J. B. Cousins (Eds.), *Chapter 24. Reclaiming knowledge at the margins: Culturally responsive evaluation in the current evaluation moment* (pp. 429–446). SAGE Publications, Inc. https://doi.org/10.4135/9781452226606.n24

King, J. A., & Volkov, B. (2005). A framework for building evaluation capacity based on the experiences of three organizations. *CURA Reporter*, 10–16.

Knoke, D., & Yang, S. (2008). *Social network analysis*. SAGE Publications.
Labin, S. N., Duffy, J. L., Meyers, D. C., Wandersman, A., & Lesesne, C. A. (2012). A research synthesis of the evaluation capacity building literature. *American Journal of Evaluation, 33*(3), 307–338. https://doi.org/10.1177/1098214011434608
Mason, M. (2008). Complexity theory and the philosophy of education. *Educational Philosophy and Theory, 40*(1), 4–18. https://doi.org/10.1111/j.1469-5812.2007.00412.x
Mertens, D. M. (2019). *Research and evaluation in education and psychology: Integrating diversity with quantitative, qualitative, and mixed methods*. Sage Publications.
Molina, J. L., Maya-Jariego, I., & McCarty, C. (2014). giving meaning to social networks: Methodology for conducting and analyzing interviews based on personal network visualizations. In *Mixed methods social networks research* (pp. 305–335). Cambridge University Press. https://doi.org/10.1017/CBO9781139227193.015
Moolenaar, N. M., Daly, A. J., & Sleegers, P. J. C. (2010). Occupying the principal position: Examining relationships between transformational leadership, social network position, and schools' innovative climate. *Educational Administration Quarterly, 46*(5), 623–670. https://doi.org/10.1177/0013161X10378689
Ostrom, E. (2009). General framework for analyzing sustainability of social-ecological systems. *Science (American Association for the Advancement of Science), 325*(5939), 419–422. https://doi.org/10.1126/science.1172133
Patton, M. Q. (2011). *Developmental evaluation: Applying complexity concepts to enhance innovation and use*. Guilford Press.
Pawson, R., & Tilley, N. (1997). *Realistic evaluation*. Sage.
Plsek, P. E., & Greenhalgh, T. (2001). Complexity science: The challenge of complexity in health care. *BMJ, 323*(7313), 625–628. https://doi.org/10.1136/bmj.323.7313.625
Prell, C. (2011). *Social network analysis: History, theory and methodology*.
Prell, C., Hubacek, K., & Reed, M. (2009). Stakeholder analysis and social network analysis in natural resource management. *Society & Natural Resources, 22*(6), 501–518. https://doi.org/10.1080/08941920802199202
Preskill, H., & Boyle, S. (2008). A multidisciplinary model of evaluation capacity building. *American Journal of Evaluation, 29*(4), 443–459. https://doi.org/10.1177/1098214008324182
Preskill, H. S., & Torres, R. T. (1999). *Evaluative inquiry for learning in organizations* (1st ed.). Sage Publications.
Provan, K. G., & Kenis, P. (2008). Modes of network governance: Structure, management, and effectiveness. *Journal of Public Administration Research and Theory, 18*(2), 229–252. https://doi.org/10.1093/jopart/mum015
Provan, K. G., & Milward, H. B. (2001). Do networks really work? A framework for evaluating public-sector organizational networks. *Public Administration Review, 61*(4), 414–423. https://doi.org/10.1111/0033-3352.00045
Ramalingam, B., Jones, H., Reba, T., & Young, J. (2008). *Exploring the science of complexity: Ideas and implications for development and humanitarian efforts* (Vol. 285, pp. 1–89). Overseas Development Institute.
Renger, R. (2022). *System evaluation theory: A blueprint for practitioners evaluating complex interventions operating and functioning as systems*. IAP.
Rogers, P. J. (2008). Using programme theory to evaluate complicated and complex aspects of interventions. *Evaluation, 14*(1), 29–48. https://doi.org/10.1177/1356389007084674
Shadish, W. R., Cook, T. D., & Leviton, L. C. (1991). *Foundations of program evaluation: Theories of practice*. Sage Publications.
Valente, T. W. (2010). *Social networks and health: Models, methods, and applications*. Oxford University Press.
Varda, D. M., Chandra, A., Stern, S. A., & Lurie, N. (2008). Core dimensions of connectivity in public health collaboratives. *Journal of Public Health Management and Practice, 14*(5), E1–E7. https://doi.org/10.1097/01.PHH.0000333889.60517.46
Weiss, C. H. (1998). *Methods for studying programs and policies* (2nd ed.). Prentice Hall.

Williams, B., & Hummelbrunner, R. (2010). *Systems concepts in action: A practitioner's toolkit* (1st ed.). Stanford University Press. https://doi.org/10.1515/9780804776554

Woolcock, M., & Narayan, D. (2000). Social capital: Implications for development theory, research, and policy. *The World Bank Research Observer, 15*(2), 225–249. https://doi.org/10.1093/wbro/15.2.225

Appendix A
Network-Informed Complex Evaluation Program Theory Template

This appendix presents a structured template for articulating and evaluating network-informed program theory within interorganizational and complex systems. The template serves as an analytic guide to support disciplined causal reasoning and implementation alignment rather than as a prescriptive checklist. Evaluators should tailor the depth and scope of its application to contextual constraints, governance arrangements, and available resources, recognizing that network configurations function as mediating mechanisms rather than as intrinsic objectives.

The template distinguishes three interrelated components:

- the Change Section, specifying determinants and causal mechanisms linking intervention to outcomes;
- the Action Section, defining the organizational and relational structures required to activate those mechanisms; and
- the Effects Section, outlining the progression from outputs to outcomes and ultimately to long-term impacts.

Structural indicators included in the template are intended as empirically observable expressions of hypothesized relational mechanisms and should be interpreted in light of contextual conditions rather than as universally optimal benchmarks.

Section I: Program Scope

Program Scope specifies the causal logic of change by defining the problem, identifying a limited number of influenceable determinants, articulating the intervention strategy, and distinguishing practical and ultimate goals (Table A.1). In network-informed evaluation, observed network structures (e.g., density, modularity, centrality, and reciprocity) are interpreted as indicators of structural conditions and hypothesized mediators rather than as outcomes in themselves.

L. Zhang, *Network-Informed Complex Evaluation*,
https://doi.org/10.1007/978-3-032-27495-3

Table A.1 Network-informed program scope with examples

Component	Evaluator task	Network-informed clarification	Illustrative example (BeSD context)
Problem Definition	Define the systemic performance gap requiring intervention	Identify network structures and relational conditions that may contribute to the problem. Distinguish observed structural patterns from the mechanisms through which they may influence outcomes	Vaccination uptake remains below target levels. Network analysis suggests segmentation between health professionals and community clusters (high modularity), strong homophily among vaccine-skeptical households, and limited bridging ties to trusted opinion leaders. These structural conditions may reduce exposure to credible information, constrain trust formation, and reinforce normative isolation.
Target Population & Boundaries	Specify beneficiaries and participating actors; define analytic boundaries	Define relevant actors and relational domains (e.g., trust, advice, referral). Clarify network boundaries and assess positional inequities affecting access to information, influence, and resources. Consider whether multiple networks should be analyzed separately or as multiplex systems	Actors include caregivers, community health workers (CHWs), clinic staff, religious leaders, and local media representatives. Trust, advice, and referral relationships are analyzed as distinct but related networks. Peripheral rural households occupy sparsely connected positions that may limit access to provider networks and trusted information sources.

(continued)

Table A.1 (continued)

Component	Evaluator task	Network-informed clarification	Illustrative example (BeSD context)
Determinants (Structural Drivers)	Identify structural conditions that may constrain or enable outcomes	Describe network structures that are plausibly relevant to outcomes while distinguishing them from the mechanisms through which effects occur	Determinants include insufficient bridging ties between clinicians and community leaders, high homophily reinforcing skepticism, and low reciprocity between clinics and community groups. These mechanisms plausibly reduce credible exposure and inhibit normative diffusion supporting vaccination.
Program Description	Describe the intervention strategy and theory of action	Specify how intervention activities are expected to influence relational opportunities, interaction patterns, or network structures that support desired mechanisms	The intervention establishes cross-sector working groups, formalizes CHW referral pathways, and trains peer ambassadors among mothers. These activities aim to create new cross-group connections, strengthen reciprocity, and improve access to trusted information pathways.
Program Goals	Distinguish practical outcomes, structural mediators, and ultimate goals	Specify outcome goals separately from hypothesized network mediators. Treat network indicators as evidence of mechanism activation rather than ends in themselves	Practical goal: Increase vaccination coverage by 15% within 12 months. Structural mediator hypotheses: Increased cross-cluster connectivity, stronger CHW brokerage, and reduced fragmentation between health and community networks. Ultimate goal: Sustained community trust and equitable participation in vaccination systems.

Section II: Action Plan

The Action Plan specifies how implementation activities are expected to influence identified determinants through the implementation design. Governance arrangements and relational infrastructure are treated as integral components of program theory (Table A.2).

Table A.2 Network-informed program action plan with examples

Component	Evaluator task	Network-informed clarification	Illustrative example (BeSD context)
Resources	Specify financial, technical, and human capacity required for implementation fidelity	Ensure capacity for relational mapping, facilitation, longitudinal monitoring, and ethical data management	Budget supports baseline and follow-up network surveys, network analysis software, facilitator training, and community engagement workshops. Safeguards protect relational confidentiality and prevent stigmatization based on positional status.
Implementing Organizations & Governance	Clarify implementing authority and accountability structure	Identify governance mode (lead organization, shared governance, network-administrative form) and its implications for coordination, information flow, and diffusion	The District Health Office functions as the lead organization; a cross-sector advisory council provides shared governance. CHWs are positioned as brokers linking clinics and households. Governance structure is hypothesized to influence coordination efficiency and information flow.
Partnering Organizations	Map collaborations and formal coordination routines	Assess opportunities for cross-sector bridging and the potential closure of structural holes across sectors	Partnerships formalized between clinics, religious councils, women's cooperatives, and local media outlets. These ties aim to close structural gaps between formal health institutions and informal community opinion networks.

(continued)

Table A.2 (continued)

Component	Evaluator task	Network-informed clarification	Illustrative example (BeSD context)
Ecological Context	Identify contextual supports and constraints influencing feasibility and sustainability	Examine macro-conditions shaping network evolution and moderating expected relational and structural effects	Historical distrust of government health campaigns, decentralized governance structures, and competitive NGO funding patterns may moderate reciprocity, authority distribution, and integration processes.
Program Activities	Specify determinant-activating activities and expected proximal effects	Define anticipated structural indicators and relational processes consistent with the program theory while recognizing contingency	Monthly cross-sector meetings are expected to increase inter-cluster density; peer ambassador outreach is expected to increase exposure among peripheral mothers; a coordinated referral system is expected to reduce average path length between households and clinics. These structural shifts are hypothesized to enhance credible exposure and normative reinforcement supporting vaccination uptake.

Section III: Program Effects

Program effects are conceptualized as a layered transformation in which relational activation may contribute to structural reconfiguration and, over time, institutionalized relational capacity:

- Outputs: relational activation
- Outcomes: structural reconfiguration consistent with theory
- Impacts: institutionalized and resilient relational capacity

Structural change increases the probability of substantive outcomes but does not guarantee them. Behavioral and social effects remain contingent on contextual, cultural, and institutional dynamics operating alongside relational mechanisms (Table A.3).

Table A.3 Network-informed program effects with examples

Level	Evaluator focus	Network-informed clarification	Illustrative example (BeSD context)
Outputs	Did implementation activate hypothesized relational mechanisms?	Formation or strengthening of ties, coordination routines, and relational processes supporting hypothesized mechanisms	Twelve cross-sector meetings convened; 45 new ties formed between clinicians and faith leaders; referral agreements signed between clinics and CHWs. These outputs indicate relational activation consistent with the action model.
Outcomes	Did structural reconfiguration occur consistent with program theory?	Measurable change in network structure aligned with hypothesized mediating mechanisms	Greater connectivity between health and community actors is reflected in a 20% reduction in modularity, a 15% increase in cross-cluster density, increased reciprocity between clinics and women's groups, and shorter pathways to trusted providers.
Impacts	Has relational transformation become institutionalized and resilient?	Stabilized relational infrastructure demonstrating durability, adaptive capacity, and governance embedding	The cross-sector advisory council continues beyond the funding cycle; the CHW brokerage role is formalized in district policy; the network remains connected despite leadership turnover; vaccination rates stabilize at higher levels across previously peripheral villages. Institutionalization indicates embedded collaborative capacity rather than temporary activation.

Appendix B
Network-Informed Complex Evaluation Design and Planning Template

A five-step, theory-aligned template for rigorous and ethically responsible network-informed evaluation design

Purpose

This appendix details the five sequential design steps of Network-Informed Complex Evaluation (NCE) as outlined in Chapter 6. The template supports evaluators in producing decision-relevant relational evidence by ensuring explicit alignment among program theory, relational mechanisms, network scope and boundary decisions, methodological and analytic choices, and reporting and knowledge-use pathways. Given that network evidence is relational, multilevel, and potentially sensitive, the template emphasizes inferential transparency, equity-aware interpretation, and ethical stewardship throughout the process. Evaluators are advised to complete the steps sequentially and maintain a concise decision log that documents major choices, assumptions, trade-offs, and adaptations made during design and implementation.

Step 1. Formulate Network-Informed Evaluation Objectives and Questions

Goal: Articulate evaluation purposes that foreground relational processes, interdependencies, and network dynamics, and translate program theory into network-informed inquiry.

L. Zhang, *Network-Informed Complex Evaluation*,
https://doi.org/10.1007/978-3-032-27495-3

1.1 Program theory anchor

Provide a concise summary of the theory of change, specifying:

☐ Core intervention mechanisms (what the program does and how change is expected to occur)
☐ Relational mechanisms central to implementation or outcomes (e.g., collaboration, coordination, trust, influence, brokerage, diffusion, feedback loops)
☐ Expected direction of relational influence (e.g., strengthened coordination is expected to increase implementation consistency; increased bridging ties are expected to support diffusion)
☐ Pace and sequencing assumptions (when and how relational change is expected to precede, accompany, or follow outcome change)

1.2 Relational constructs to be examined

For each relational construct, specify:

- Construct name
- Conceptual definition (theoretical meaning)
- Operational definition (how the construct will be observed/measured)
- Unit of analysis (actor, dyad, subgroup, whole network; including directed vs. undirected ties if relevant)
- Level(s) of analysis (individual, organizational, community, policy/governance)
- Expected mechanism of influence (how the construct functions within the theory of change)
- Theoretical justification (why this construct is central to the evaluation)

1.3 Evaluation objectives

State objectives that explicitly reference relational structure or dynamics and intended use. Example formats:

- "To diagnose whether the network exhibits [structural condition] relevant to [mechanism] within [level/system]."
- "To assess whether [relational mechanism] is associated with [outcome] within [level/system]."
- "To examine how [network structure/relationship] evolves across [time period] during implementation."

List Objectives 1–3 (as needed):

- Objective 1:
- Objective 2:
- Objective 3:

1.4 Evaluation questions by inferential logic

Organize questions by the inferential logic they require. (Selecting a question type commits the evaluation to the corresponding design and data requirements.)

A. Descriptive network analysis

- What structural configurations, positions, and subgroup patterns are observable?
- Are there patterns of centralization, fragmentation, clustering, brokerage concentration, or marginalization?

B. Statistical inference

- Which structural tendencies, actor attributes, or contextual factors are statistically associated with tie formation, network position, or program-relevant outcomes?
- Are exposure, embeddedness, or brokerage positions associated with adoption, performance, or implementation outcomes under specified modeling assumptions?

C. Longitudinal network analysis

- How does network structure change over time (formation, persistence, dissolution of ties)?
- Do changes in relational configuration align with implementation milestones or theorized mechanisms of change?

D. Mixed-method social network analysis

- How are network structures experienced, interpreted, and enacted by participants?
- How do trust, power dynamics, institutional rules, and history shape observed patterns and change?

1.5 Equity and power considerations

Specify how equity-relevant network conditions will be examined and communicated:

- How participation inequalities or exclusion will be identified (e.g., peripheralization, segmentation, unequal access to central actors)
- How power asymmetries and influence concentration will be interpreted responsibly
- Safeguards against stigmatizing individuals/organizations (e.g., avoid treating centrality as "performance")
- How equity implications will be incorporated into interpretation and use

Step 2. Specify Network Scope and Boundary

Goal: Delineate the system under evaluation by defining actors, ties, levels, and timeframes. Boundary choices directly shape feasibility, analytic validity, and the scope of defensible claims.

2.1 Network type(s) and representation

Specify:

- Network domain/type (e.g., advice, collaboration, referral, trust, information exchange, governance coordination)
- Directed or undirected (is the relation directional?)
- Binary or weighted (presence/absence vs. strength/frequency/quality)
- Multiplexity (single relation vs. multiple relation types measured separately)
- Justification (why this network representation best fits the program theory and evaluation questions)

2.2 Actors (nodes) and inclusion criteria

Specify:

- Primary unit of analysis (persons, organizations, coalitions, agencies, etc.)
- Boundary specification approach (positional, relational, event-based, or a justified combination)
- Inclusion criteria and exclusion criteria
- Network data-collection method (roster, name generator, administrative list, participation records)
- Anticipated turnover (entry/exit) and design implications (e.g., boundary stability rules for longitudinal work)

2.3 Tie definition and measurement integrity

Tie specification must align with the relational construct and evaluation purpose. Specify:

- Exact tie wording (survey item or extraction rule)
- Recall period (time window referenced)
- Strength/frequency/quality scale (if weighted)
- Context qualifiers (e.g., "regarding implementation decisions," "in the past 3 months")
- Justification linking tie definition to construct (why this item captures the intended mechanism)

Instrument alignment and measurement integrity

Document:

- Instrument type (roster-based survey, name generator, administrative/archival extraction, digital trace, interview-based elicitation)
- Why this instrument fits the boundary and construct
- Pilot testing or cognitive testing plans (if new or adapted items)
- Known limitations (e.g., recall bias; incomplete records; interpretive ambiguity) and how these will be handled

2.4 Temporal scope

Specify:

- Baseline timing and follow-up timing (if applicable)
- Alignment with program cycles, decision timelines, and implementation milestones
- Assumptions about the pace of relational change (why the chosen interval is defensible)
- Constraints (access, burden, organizational calendars)

2.5 Boundary decision log (recommended)

For each major boundary decision:

- Decision made
- Alternative(s) considered
- Rationale
- Risks introduced
- Mitigation strategies

Step 3. Align Evaluation Methods with Questions and Network Boundaries

Goal: Select methods that are appropriate for the questions and consistent with the boundary choices. Method selection should be theory-driven, feasible, interpretable, and ethically responsible.

3.1 Evaluation design type

Select and justify one or more designs:

- Whole network (census) design (appropriate when boundaries are clear and participation is feasible)
- Ego network design (appropriate when boundaries are diffuse or focus is individual access/exposure)
- Two-mode (bipartite) design (e.g., actors–events, organizations–initiatives)
- Longitudinal panel or repeated cross-section (when assessing change over time)
- Mixed-method network design (when interpretation, mechanism explanation, or contextualization is central)

Justification should explicitly reference: program theory, evaluation questions, boundary feasibility, and intended inferential scope.

3.2 Analytic strategy selection aligned to inferential logic

Utilize the table to document analytic decision-making processes. The provided entries serve as illustrative examples; evaluators are expected to adapt selections according to program theory, contextual conditions, and intended inference.

Evaluation questions	Theoretical rational	Analytical approach	Key measures	Network data	Level(s) of analysis (I/O/C/P)	Temporal design	Intended inference	Key assumptions/ risks
Specify relational structures, mechanisms, or dynamics to be examined	Identify hypothesized relational mechanisms and expected direction of influence	☐ Descriptive ☐ Statistical ☐ Longitudinal ☐ Mixed-Method	Specify measures aligned with the identified mechanism	Specify network boundary, actors, ties, and data sources	Individual/ Organizational/ Community/ Policy	Cross-sectional/ Longitudinal	Structural; Associational; Temporally Ordered; Developmental	Boundary instability; missing data; measurement inconsistency; model misspecification; confounding

Notes

1. **Evaluation Question** should be explicitly derived from program theory and specify a relational structure, mechanism, or dynamic rather than an isolated program outcome.
2. **Theoretical Rationale** must identify the relational mechanism (e.g., coordination, brokerage, diffusion, trust, influence) and the expected direction of influence, ensuring that analytic choices are theory-driven.
3. **Analytic Approach** reflects the inferential logic required: *descriptive* (structural characterization and pattern identification), *statistical* (model-based association under stated assumptions), *longitudinal* (analysis of relational change over time), or *mixed-method* (integration of structural and qualitative evidence).
4. **Key Measures** should correspond directly to the relational mechanism identified and be appropriate to the selected analytic approach.
5. **Network Data Required** should align with the network boundary specification, tie operationalization, measurement procedures, and construct operationalization.
6. **Level(s) of Analysis** should be consistent with the multilevel orientation of NCE (individual, organizational, community, policy) and should not conflate actor-level, subgroup-level, and whole network conclusions.
7. **Temporal Design** (cross-sectional or longitudinal) should reflect assumptions about the pace and sequencing of relational change. Designs may be cross-sectional or longitudinal.
8. **Intended Inference** should not exceed what the design supports. Descriptive and statistical analyses do not automatically justify causal claims; longitudinal designs strengthen temporal plausibility but require explicit disclosure of assumptions.
9. **Key Assumptions/Risks** should document critical threats to validity, including boundary instability, missing data, measurement inconsistency, model misspecification, selection effects, and potential confounding.

3.3 Mixed-method integration plan (if applicable)

If mixed methods are used, specify the integration strategy:

- Stage of integration: design, data collection, analysis, interpretation
- Integration type: convergent, explanatory sequential, exploratory sequential, embedded
- Linkage mechanism: how qualitative cases/participants will be selected using network evidence (e.g., central actors, brokers, peripheral actors, bridging ties, subgroup members)
- Handling divergence: procedures for reconciling or reporting conflicting findings
- Rationale: why this integration approach strengthens interpretation and use relative to program theory

Step 4. Develop Data Collection and Analysis Plan

Goal: Translate the conceptual design into actionable procedures: data sources, instruments, timing, analysis workflow, quality assurance, and explicit inferential assumptions.

4.1 Data sources and instruments

Specify all planned sources, with justification for each:

- Network surveys
- Administrative/archival records
- Digital trace data (if ethically permissible and construct-valid)
- Qualitative interviews/observations/participatory mapping
- Outcome measures (individual, organizational, community, policy indicators)

For each instrument/source: define what it measures, who provides it, how often, and how it aligns with constructs and boundaries.

4.2 Timing and frequency

Document:

- Data-collection schedule (waves, intervals)
- Alignment with program cycles and decision points
- Rationale based on theory (expected pace of relational change)
- Plans to manage respondent burden and organizational feasibility

4.3 Data quality assurance and error control

Specify protocols for:

- Entity resolution (deduplication, naming conventions, organization matching)
- Response rate monitoring (targets and follow-up plan)
- Missing data (diagnosis and handling; implications for network measures)

- Asymmetric ties (rules for handling discrepancies in directed relations)
- Documentation (version-controlled data dictionary; cleaning scripts; decision log)

4.4 Analytic workflow and reproducibility

Document:

- Data preparation steps (coding, matrix construction, attribute integration)
- Planned analytic sequence
- Software and analytic environments (as appropriate)
- Decision rules for reporting (which measures/models will be prioritized and why)

Step 5. Design Reporting and Knowledge-Use Strategies

Goal: Ensure network evidence is interpreted, visualized, and communicated in ways that maximize utility while minimizing misinterpretation and harm.

5.1 Reporting products aligned with intended users

Specify audiences and products, aligned with the evaluation purpose:

- Technical or methodological report (for analysts/research teams)
- Strategic synthesis brief (for system leaders)
- Learning memos/rapid feedback (for implementers; developmental use)
- Community-facing briefs/workshops (for partners/participants)
- Policy briefs (for decision-makers/funders)

For each product: purpose, timing, and how network evidence will be contextualized.

5.2 Visualization and interpretation guidance

Because network visuals and metrics can be misused, specify guardrails:

- Provide interpretive guidance (what the metric does and does not imply)
- Communicate uncertainty and limitations (missing data, boundary assumptions)
- Use anonymization or aggregation when politically/ethically warranted
- Provide equity-aware framing to avoid stigmatizing peripheral actors or groups

5.3 Ethical stewardship and governance (embedded in reporting and use)

Document:

- Informed consent procedures appropriate to relational data
- Confidentiality safeguards and anonymization rules for outputs
- Data storage, access control, and sharing protocols
- Harm mitigation strategies (e.g., phased disclosure; facilitated sense-making; restrictions on identifiable maps)

5.4 Knowledge-use pathway and adaptive learning

Specify:

- Decisions the evaluation is intended to inform
- Responsible parties for acting on findings
- Feedback loops (how findings will be used to adapt implementation)
- Plans for stakeholder sense-making (e.g., facilitated interpretation sessions)

Final coherence check (recommended quality assurance overlay)

Before implementation, confirm:

☐ Objectives and questions are derived from program theory to specify relational mechanisms
☐ Boundaries and tie definitions align with constructs and intended inference
☐ Methods and analytic strategies fit the questions and feasibility constraints
☐ Data collection timing matches program cycles and expected pace of relational change
☐ Assumptions, validity risks, and limits of conclusion are explicitly documented
☐ Equity and power implications are addressed in interpretation and reporting plans
☐ Ethical safeguards and governance protocols are adequate for relational data
☐ Reporting products and knowledge-use pathways are clear and decision-relevant

Provide a brief narrative summary ($\leq$300 words) explaining how design coherence has been achieved across Steps 1–5.

Index

A
Accountability
  community, 5, 7, 57, 164
  outcome, 8, 138, 207, 208, 225
  program, 2, 5–7, 138, 141, 143, 153, 164, 170, 186, 192, 207, 225
  See also Outcome accountability; Program accountability
Accountability-oriented evaluation, 186
Action plan
  policy implementation plan, 69
  program action plan, 155
  See also Program plan
Adaptation (systems), 47–49, 60, 95
Adaptive evaluation, 87, 95
Adaptive learning
  adaptive learning loops, 192, 193
  institutional learning, 200
Advocacy coalition framework (ACF), 49–51, 171
Agenda-setting positions, 76
Analytic validity, 162, 172, 194, 201
Assortativity
  attribute-based clustering, 91
  sectoral alignment, 85
Assumptions
  descriptive, 154–157, 180
  network-informed, 8, 94, 132, 154–159
  ontological, 210, 214
  prescriptive, 154–158
Average path length. *See* Distance (network)

B
Betweenness centrality
  brokerage across sectors, 52, 83, 89, 151, 156
  See also Brokerage roles
Bonding social capital, 46
Boundary specification
  institutional boundaries, 9, 226
  network boundary specification, 74, 165, 167, 201
  system boundaries, 102, 103, 129, 171, 215
Bridging social capital, 46
Brokerage roles
  boundary spanning, 51, 139
  gatekeeping, 83, 89, 90

C
Capacity building
  evaluation capacity, 94, 214
  evaluation capacity building, 72, 117, 210
  institutional capacity, 83, 94, 193, 200
Causal explanation, 210, 211
Causality, 13, 25, 155, 159, 163, 211, 225
Causal loop diagram, 217
Causal mechanisms, 20, 68, 94, 131, 156
Central actors. *See* Centrality
Centrality
  betweenness, 7, 38, 42, 44, 51, 52, 54, 73, 76, 81–83, 89, 150, 151, 182
  closeness, 76, 79, 80, 88, 182
  degree, 37, 38, 42, 54, 73, 76, 81–83, 150, 156
  eigenvector, 37, 38, 51, 76, 81–83, 89, 151, 156

L. Zhang, *Network-Informed Complex Evaluation*,
https://doi.org/10.1007/978-3-032-27495-3

network centralization, 42, 43, 81, 82, 89, 150
power concentration, 13
structural position, 14, 52
CIPP evaluation framework, 123, 127
Clique formation, 77
Closeness centrality, 79, 80
Clustering (network science)
policy subgroups, 90
transitivity, 83, 84, 90, 151
Coalitions, 17, 18, 32, 35, 50, 51, 52, 68, 79, 81, 82, 84, 85. *See also* Advocacy coalition framework (ACF)
Collaboration
collaboration networks, 17, 45, 48, 75
cross-sector collaboration, 10, 45, 46, 48, 87, 112, 136, 137, 192, 208, 224, 226
interorganizational collaboration, 77, 102, 104
Collective impact, 44, 47–49, 105
Community accountability circle, 5, 7, 57
Community health, 26, 58, 68
Complex adaptive systems (CAS)
adaptive capacity, 13
cross-scale interactions, 14
dynamic systems, 13, 15
emergence, 13–15, 18, 25, 34, 49
emergent outcomes, 14, 31, 36
interdependence, 13, 15, 19, 45
leverage points, 14, 15, 213
longitudinal network analysis, 13, 16
massive entanglement, 13
multilevel dynamics, 13, 32
power concentration (cross-level), 13
resource flow reconfiguration, 13, 14, 19
scale independence, 13, 16
sensemaking (ongoing), 13
system transformation, 19
Complexity
complexity theory, 8, 14, 19, 33, 67, 211, 227
nonlinearity, 15, 25, 159, 222
system complexity, 105, 159, 201
Complexity-aware evaluation, 158, 220, 221, 224, 227
Complex systems, 8, 13, 17–19, 25, 56, 57, 67, 73, 75, 78, 87, 94, 95, 104, 111, 114, 116, 161, 164, 168, 173, 176, 180, 183, 192, 201, 202, 208, 216, 222, 224, 225, 227, 228
Components (network)
fragmentation, 80, 89, 135, 137
isolates, 80, 89
policy silos, 89
Confidentiality, 71, 96, 97, 103, 113, 115, 118, 127, 128, 141, 186
Constraint (network)
limits on brokerage, 90
redundancy, 38, 76, 83
Context assessment
institutional context, 2, 38, 87, 180, 183
political context, 57, 155, 226
Context (contextual factors), 43, 70, 93, 94, 120, 135, 143, 149, 151, 158, 161, 164, 185, 208, 219
contextual support, 143, 144, 148
Contribution analysis, 195
Coordination, 10, 12, 14, 16–18, 21, 27, 42–44, 47, 48, 50, 52, 55, 57, 58, 68, 75, 77–84, 86–88, 90, 92, 98, 104, 106, 124, 125, 129, 135, 137, 139, 140, 142–144, 147, 149, 150, 153, 156, 157, 159, 166, 167, 171, 175, 181, 182, 187, 194, 224
Core–periphery structure
governance resilience, 86

D

Data availability, 101, 104, 127
Data collection, 73, 94, 97, 101, 107, 109, 113, 116, 118, 122, 123, 138, 141, 161, 163, 168, 169, 173–177, 179, 184, 192, 195, 196, 201
Data governance, 108, 109, 118, 140, 141, 196
Data quality assurance, 185
Data sources, 69, 70, 108, 114, 126, 163, 173, 174, 184, 195
Degree centrality, 38, 73, 81, 89
Density (network), 31, 37, 38, 48, 51, 52, 73, 75–77, 83, 96, 138, 147, 152, 156, 181, 219
cohesion, 46, 48, 83
Determinants, 1, 8, 10, 31, 38, 49, 58, 59, 128, 129, 134, 135, 137, 163, 181, 210–212, 223
Developmental evaluation, 22, 24, 71, 186, 187, 192, 193, 214, 215, 217
Diameter (network)
global span, 79, 80, 88
maximum geodesic distance, 79, 88
structural reach, 79
Diffusion
global health diffusion, 9, 36, 47

policy diffusion, 88, 167, 181
Distance (network)
average path length, 56, 79, 80, 88
coordination speed, 88
Dynamic systems, 13, 15, 20, 67, 102, 183, 184
structural dynamics, 18, 24

E

Ego-network analysis, 162
Eigenvector centrality, 38, 81–83, 156
institutional influence, 51, 82
Emergence, 14, 18–20, 27, 32, 36, 47, 53, 67, 82, 95, 146, 147, 222
emergent properties, 8, 57, 58, 67, 131, 224, 225
Empowerment evaluation, 72
Equity
equity-focused evaluation, 22, 23
health equity, 1, 4, 8–10, 13, 14, 25, 31–33, 36, 40, 49, 65, 210–212, 214, 222, 223, 226
inclusion, 68, 85, 98, 110, 115, 119, 127, 190, 194
marginalization, 3, 5, 84, 121, 128, 192
marginalized stakeholders, 3, 121, 128, 220
Ethical considerations, 66, 71, 96, 173, 187, 201, 202
Ethical evaluation, 23, 25, 66, 96, 118–120
Evaluability assessment, 94, 101, 104
Evaluation
capacity, 5, 20, 25, 38, 65, 72, 78–80, 86, 87, 103, 113, 117, 128, 147, 172, 200, 214, 220, 221
criteria, 6, 7, 26, 27, 114, 120–123, 127, 136, 138, 161, 169–171, 174, 202, 207, 211, 213, 218, 219
design, 1, 3, 13, 20, 23, 66, 70, 72, 87, 93–97, 101, 103, 110, 112, 113, 119, 123, 125, 126, 131, 132, 137, 156, 158, 159, 161–163, 170, 173, 186, 194, 195, 199, 201–203, 210, 214, 219, 221, 226–228
frameworks, 8, 10, 39, 103, 214, 215, 217, 220, 221
indicators, 1, 6, 8, 14, 40, 44, 78, 84, 117, 126, 146
methods, 2, 8, 13, 19, 65, 104, 111, 117, 155, 162, 227
objectives, 4, 74, 75, 79, 94, 101, 129, 162–164, 169, 170, 180, 201, 207, 208
planning, 87, 96, 104, 107, 126, 134, 148, 199, 202, 221
practice, 1, 2, 4, 6, 8, 10, 23, 25, 58, 67, 68, 78, 93, 95, 111, 139, 145, 186, 211, 213, 219, 220, 228
questions, 6, 25–27, 31, 59, 69–71, 74, 75, 78, 88–91, 96, 103, 112, 120, 122, 126, 129, 161–164, 172, 173, 176, 184, 200, 201, 210, 219, 228
readiness, 41, 96, 102, 104, 114, 117, 119, 127, 129, 218
reporting, 70, 95, 163, 185–187, 191, 193, 199–202, 210
standards, 65, 66, 69, 213, 220
theory, 21, 32, 38, 87, 104, 119, 131, 132, 148, 158, 167, 200, 201, 210, 211, 213, 214, 226, 227
use, 10, 23, 71, 72, 107, 111, 117, 119, 120, 122, 123, 125, 126, 151, 153, 163, 186, 187, 193, 201, 202, 209
Evaluation approaches
developmental, 22, 67, 71, 72, 193, 215
empowerment, 21, 44, 224
equity-focused, 2, 22
formative, 22, 95, 186
outcome, 1, 2, 8, 14, 18, 21, 22, 32, 72, 94, 104, 111, 112, 121, 131, 132, 208, 228
participatory, 21, 71, 72, 95, 96, 133, 175, 209, 213, 214, 221, 222, 224
process, 71, 112, 120, 127, 149, 186, 219
realist, 21, 22, 211, 214
summative, 164, 208
theory-driven, 22, 68, 131, 155, 157, 193, 197, 219
utilization-focused, 22, 69, 193, 209
value-based, 213
Evidence-based decision-making, 108, 210

F

Feedback loops, 1, 2, 22, 32, 36, 40, 56–58, 60, 67, 71, 97, 98, 131, 133, 159, 162, 192, 200, 201, 211, 215, 224
feedback mechanisms, 15, 18, 50, 59, 95, 161, 192, 211, 221, 223
Formative evaluation, 207

G

Governance structures
multilevel governance, 14
transnational governance, 34, 88

Groups (network), 7, 38, 45, 52, 73, 74, 79, 85, 152, 170

H
Health disparities, 8, 32
Health equity. *See* Equity
Health outcomes, 1, 3, 8–12, 17, 25, 31, 32, 44, 45, 57, 67, 210
Hierarchical partitioning, 76, 78
Homophily
  ideological alignment, 85
  sectoral clustering, 85

I
Implementation science, 225, 228
Implementation strategy, 133, 195
Information exchange, 16, 18, 19, 52, 74, 78, 79, 101, 125, 128, 133, 166, 173
Interconnectedness, 2, 65, 162
Interdependence, 16, 17, 20, 21, 34, 48, 95, 111, 132, 139, 159, 197, 200, 201, 211, 215, 228
Intergovernmental networks, 76
Interorganizational networks, 41–43, 46, 48, 52, 135, 166, 178
Isolates (network). *See* Components (network)

K
K-core analysis, 83, 84
  institutional cores, 84
Knowledge production, 6, 96, 117
Knowledge utilization, 185, 202

L
Leverage points, 2, 8, 14–16, 18, 20, 21, 25, 47, 50, 56, 137, 142, 210, 211, 222, 224
Logic model, 1–3, 25, 67, 96, 102, 112, 133, 157

M
Marginalization. *See* Equity
Methodological alignment, 102, 172, 173, 195, 200
Methodological rigor, 25, 26, 69, 102, 103, 117, 127, 162, 163, 169, 174, 184, 189, 219
Mixed-methods approaches, 163
Modularity
  polarization, 91
  sectoral segmentation, 91
Multilevel analysis, 14, 185
Multiplexity, 75, 76, 86, 92, 150
  cross-domain ties, 86, 150

N
Network boundaries, 74, 94, 103, 114, 127, 135, 136, 162, 163, 165, 169–172, 174, 175, 178, 184, 192, 200, 202
Network centralization, 16, 42, 43, 46, 51, 76, 78, 81, 82
Network complexity
  adaptive capacity, 86
  robustness, 86
Network density. *See* Density (network)
Network dynamics, 32, 98, 111, 162, 169, 171, 222, 226
Network efficiency, 149
  reachability, 76, 79, 80
Network-informed complex evaluation (NCE), 1–3, 6–8, 10, 14–23, 25, 26, 32, 33, 36, 38–41, 43, 44, 47–49, 51, 52, 56–58, 65–75, 78, 87, 88, 93–97, 101, 102, 104, 105, 111, 115, 116, 119, 123, 127, 131, 133, 144, 145, 152, 154, 158, 159, 162, 165–168, 172–174, 179–188, 191–194, 201, 202, 207–228
Network mapping, 3, 16, 23, 45, 50, 58, 94, 122, 175, 209, 210, 213, 222, 224
Network mechanisms, 7, 10, 53
  relational mechanisms, 17, 19
Network methods, 102, 141, 172, 175, 219
Network metrics, 43, 52, 78, 122, 138, 175, 187, 197, 219
Network position, 24, 38, 59, 118, 123, 125, 142, 152, 227
  positional variables, 75, 76
Network properties, 138, 145, 173, 180
  structural properties, 86, 134, 172, 180
Network readiness, 19, 40, 41, 53, 87, 111, 114
Network scope, 79, 162, 165, 193, 194, 200, 201
Network size, 43, 46, 52, 75, 76, 79–81, 88, 150, 152
Network structure
  relational variables, 75, 76, 164
  structural control, 81, 82, 89
  structural differentiation, 85, 91

structural span, 79, 88
Nonlinear dynamics, 1, 2, 22, 215

O
Outcome accountability, 207, 208
Outcome evaluation, 141
Outcome relevance, 93
Outcomes, 1–4, 6–8, 13–20, 22–24, 26, 27, 31, 32, 34, 36, 43, 45, 50, 53, 57, 66–69, 73–75, 78, 79, 93, 94, 96, 101, 102, 104, 105, 111, 117, 120, 127, 128, 131–134, 136–138, 142–148, 151, 154–156, 158, 159, 161, 162, 164, 169, 173, 174, 181–183, 187, 194, 200, 207–209, 213, 216, 217, 219, 222–226, 228
outputs, 3, 19, 145, 154

P
Participatory approaches, 209, 221
Participatory evaluation, 71, 179, 221
Partnerships, 2, 9–11, 49, 55, 59, 84, 90, 101, 105–108, 111, 114, 115, 117, 118, 145, 146, 152, 157, 164, 169, 171, 174, 181, 224, 227
Peripheral stakeholders, 121, 122, 127
Policy diffusion, 88, 167
Policy networks, 32, 33, 50–52, 79–85, 89, 91, 112, 167
Policy network theory, 49, 51, 52
Policy silos. *See* Components (network)
Population health, 9, 17, 48
Positional variables, 75, 76
Power analysis, 220
Power concentration/distribution
power dynamics, 1, 8, 22, 118, 128, 159, 192, 193, 202, 213, 215, 226, 228
power relations, 14, 16, 25, 52, 73, 133, 148, 149, 151, 154, 211
Process evaluation, 94, 208
Program accountability, 207
Program effects, 133, 145, 146, 158, 215
Program implementation, 3, 19, 20, 57, 104, 126, 127, 142, 143, 146, 149, 153, 154, 162, 200, 228
Program plan, 78, 132, 133, 214, 222. *See also* Action plan
Program scope, 133–137, 139, 158
Program theory, 19, 65, 72, 74, 75, 94–96, 105, 112, 119, 120, 122, 123, 131–140, 142–144, 146, 147, 149, 154–156, 158, 159, 162, 164, 172–174, 180, 182–184, 186, 197, 200, 201, 219, 227, 228
Public health interventions, 3, 6, 9
Public health outcomes, 1, 3, 7

Q
Qualitative network inquiry, 163
Quantitative network data, 181, 185, 209

R
Reachability, 77, 79–81, 88, 92
Readiness assessment, 19, 39, 87, 103, 104, 113, 117, 127, 128, 185, 214, 218, 228
Realist evaluation, 22, 24, 148, 215–217
Reciprocity (networks), 46, 48, 54–56, 75, 83, 84, 90, 98, 135–137, 145, 147, 151, 157, 182
Reflexivity, 4, 6, 8, 25, 196, 200, 201, 220
Relational data, 66, 71, 103, 107, 108, 113, 114, 117, 118, 122, 140, 162, 163, 165, 171, 174–176, 180, 186, 193
Relational dynamics, 3, 4, 6, 8, 18, 20, 23, 25, 41, 45, 50, 69, 73, 93, 94, 101, 104, 105, 109, 117, 118, 120, 122, 123, 126, 127, 129, 135, 158, 159, 162, 172, 201, 208, 209, 226
Relational mechanisms, 9, 10, 22–24, 45, 78, 96, 104, 105, 111, 132, 145, 157–159, 164, 172–174, 180–182, 218, 219, 226–228
Relational variables, 75, 76, 164
Reporting, 70, 106, 113, 125, 163, 184–189, 191, 193, 194, 196–198, 200, 202
Resource allocation, 22, 31, 34, 68, 94, 102, 121, 141, 153, 168, 209
Resource flows, 2, 8, 17, 18, 21, 25, 34, 101, 133, 150, 152, 158, 164, 208, 224
Resource networks, 150, 152
Responsiveness, 7, 24, 52, 53, 55–57, 66, 68, 71–73, 80, 96, 97, 125, 126, 142, 162, 174, 186, 193, 221
Robustness (network), 51, 69, 86, 147, 197, 209

S
Self-organization, 34, 40
Sensemaking, 13, 67, 185–188, 190, 192, 214, 221
Small-world properties, 86, 92
Social capital

bonding, 46
bridging, 46, 48
Social determinants of health (SDOH), 10, 11, 15, 17, 18, 20, 25, 31–33, 36, 59, 60
Social inquiry, 207, 208
Social network analysis (SNA)
network analysis, 16, 17, 32, 35, 37, 41–47, 50–52, 74, 76, 92, 109, 111, 117, 118, 135, 136, 140, 146, 151, 155, 156, 158, 167, 168, 176, 179, 181, 183, 184, 193, 199, 217, 219–221, 224, 228
ego-network analysis, 35, 37, 38, 54, 162
policy network analysis, 51, 52
whole-network analysis, 41, 43, 162, 181
Stakeholder
analysis, 95, 102, 104, 106, 113, 114, 119–123, 127, 213
engagement, 21, 25, 71, 72, 81, 87, 94, 95, 102, 103, 113, 127, 141, 148, 153, 162, 172, 175, 186, 191, 193, 201, 209, 214, 217, 221
identification, 52, 87, 93, 107, 113, 119–121, 123–126, 136, 222
input, 132, 201, 214
mapping, 107, 113, 126, 127, 214
Structural barriers, 2, 15, 23, 25, 47, 59, 68, 79, 80, 85, 128, 228
Structural control
dependency concentration, 81, 89, 152
gatekeeping, 89
Structural differentiation
inequality, 48, 85
segmentation, 85, 91, 181
Structural holes, 10, 11, 16, 17, 31, 35, 46, 48, 51, 52, 135–137, 139, 140, 143, 208
Structural position. *See* Centrality
Structural properties. *See* Network properties
Structural span. *See* Diameter (network)
Summative evaluation, 188, 208
Sustainability, 66, 72, 73, 78, 87, 115, 139, 140, 144, 150, 152, 164, 221, 222, 224
System mapping, 104
System readiness, 123, 173
Systems perspective, 57
Systems thinking, 5, 7, 23, 70, 131, 214–217, 221, 228
System transformation, 5

T

Theory-driven evaluation, 22, 23, 68, 131, 132, 134, 145, 149, 154, 155, 164
Tie strength, 54, 73, 75, 76, 83, 84, 90, 151, 153, 174
Trust, 5, 7, 13, 31, 34, 36, 41, 45, 48, 49, 53, 54, 56–59, 66, 69, 70, 76, 84, 90, 97, 98, 103, 105, 113, 122, 129, 136, 137, 139, 140, 144, 148, 151, 157, 183, 200, 203, 208, 220, 224, 228

U

Utilization-focused evaluation, 22, 23, 69, 104, 111, 112, 120, 126, 209

V

Value-based evaluation, 117, 209, 213
Value-free, 4
Values, 2, 4, 5, 82, 92, 161, 209, 213

W

Whole-network analysis, 162, 172

The manufacturer's authorised representative in the EU is Springer Nature Customer Service Centre GmbH, Europaplatz 3, 69115 Heidelberg, Germany. If you have any concerns regarding our products, please contact ProductSafety@springernature.com

Printed and bound by CPI Group (UK) Ltd, Croydon, CR0 4YY
07/10/2026
02229357-0006